Personal and Vocational Relationships in Practical Nursing

Personal and Vocational Relationships in Practical Nursing

Fifth Edition

Carmen F. Ross, R.N., Ed.D.

Professor of Nursing, University of Miami School of Nursing;
Formerly President, Florida State Board of Nursing; Director,
School of Practical Nursing, and Director of Nursing and Nursing
Education, Mount Sinai Hospital of Greater Miami, Florida

J. B. Lippincott Company Philadelphia · London
Mexico City · New York · St. Louis · São Paulo · Sydney

Library of Congress Cataloging in Publication Data

Ross, Carmen F
 Personal and vocational relationships in practical
nursing.

 Includes index.
 1. Practical nursing. 2. Practical nursing —
Vocational guidance. I. Title. [DNLM: 1. Ethics,
Nursing. 2. Nurse–patient relations.
3. Nursing, Practical. WY 16 R823p]
RT62.R6 1981 610.73'0693 80-25066
ISBN 0-397-54281-X

Printed in the United States of America

This book is affectionately dedicated to my mother, Johanna Frank, and to my husband, Joe Ross, whose understanding ways have helped a dream to become a reality.

This book is also dedicated to the nurses whose humanistic care makes the difference in the quality of life our patients/clients lead along life's way.

> The light of life is a finite flame. Like a candle, life is kindled: it burns, it glows, it is radiant with warmth and beauty. But soon it fades, its substance is consumed, and it is no more.

> In light we see, in light we are seen. The flames dance and our lives are full. But as night follows day, the candle of our life burns down and gutters. There is an end to the flames. We see no more and are no more seen. Yet we do not despair, for we are more than a memory slowly fading into the darkness. With our lives we give life. Something of us can never die. We move in the eternal cycle of darkness and death, of light and life.*

*Reproduced with permission from the Central Conference of American Rabbis: Gates of Repentance, p 73. New York, 1978.

Contents

Appendices   257

Index   277

Preface

It is 20 years since the first edition of Personal and Vocational Relationships in Practical Nursing was published. Nursing has changed and, so too, has the content of this text. The fifth edition, like the first four, is designed as a primary text in the course covering personal and vocational relationships in practical nursing or as a supplementary text when the subject is integrated with other nursing courses. It will also serve as a valuable reference for the licensed practical or vocational nurse, whose increasingly important role on the health team necessitates awareness of new trends and constant refreshing of basic knowledge.

This edition has been updated and revised to reflect today's role of the licensed practical/vocational nurse in delivering humanistic nursing care. Each chapter is prefaced with reader-oriented objectives to enhance learning. Of particular mention are the following additions to the text:

1. Chapter 2, "Nursing History and Trends," includes the "Competencies of Graduates of Educational Programs in Practical Nursing" as approved by the National League for Nursing Council of Practical Nursing Programs in 1979, a section on the status of women, and a discussion of the future for the practical/vocational nurse.

2. Chapter 3, "The Nursing Team," contains information on the nurse practitioner, primary nursing, computers, and the National Federation of Licensed Practical Nurses, Inc.'s newly adopted "Nursing Practice Standards for the Licensed Practical/Vocational Nurse."

3. Chapter 4, "Personal Considerations," has been enriched with sections on Erikson's psychosocial theory, assertiveness, and human sexuality and with new material on marijuana, diet, and sexually transmitted diseases.

4. Chapter 5, "Health Care Facilities and You," includes new information on health system agencies, hospices, acupuncture, pharmacies, comprehensive health services, and community mental health centers.

5. Chapter 6, "Your Patient," has been rewritten to include such topics as economics of health care, transcultural nursing, problem-oriented record, quality assurance programs, the gay patient, vegetarians, and Muslims.

6. Chapter 7, "Ethical and Legal Responsibilities," encompasses an interpretation of the 1979 N.F.L.P.N. "Code of Ethics," civil and criminal laws, informed consent, and duty of care.

7. Chapter 8, "Organizations," covers the reorganization of the former Department of Health, Education and Welfare, the national vocational organization for students (H.O.S.A.), and the National Consumer's League.

8. Chapter 9, "Career Opportunities and Responsibilities," contains material on the resume, collective bargaining, and rape/sexual assault.

9. N.A.P.N.E.S.' "Declaration of Functions of the L.P./V.N." has been added to the Appendix.

To assist the student, questions with the correct answers continue to appear at the end of each chapter. Additionally the comprehensive review test and its answers have been retained in the students' self-evaluation. The Directory of State Boards of Nursing or Nurse Examiners has been updated and, along with a job description for the LPN charge nurse, is found in the Appendix.

A major task of education is to motivate the learner to study not only for today but also for the future. It is the author's hope that this book will assist students, instructors, and others to become more humanistic and realistic in their personal and patient care activities.

Carmen F. Ross, R.N., Ed.D.

Acknowledgments

The author wishes to express her gratitude to the many people who have helped with this edition. Recognition must be given to Sister Mary J. Walsh, Director of NLN's Division of Practical Nursing Programs; Elizabeth Cannata, Program Consultant, Division of Vocational Education, Florida State Department of Education; Gloria Hogue, Chairman of Practical Nursing, Miami-Dade Community College; and the practical nurse educators at Broward County Practical Nursing Programs, Lindsey Hopkins Technical Education Center, and South Technical Education Center, Boynton Beach for their valuable suggestions.

Sincere appreciation is extended to Rabbi Solomon Schiff, Director of Chaplaincy, Greater Miami Jewish Federation and Executive Vice President, Rabbinical Association of Greater Miami; and to these University of Miami Chaplains: Ms. Polly Cook, Director, Wesley Foundation; Dr. Francis J. Lechiara, St. Augustine Catholic Church and Student Center; and Dr. Henry N. F. Minich, Episcopal Church Center for their contributions and suggestions in the section, "The Patient's Religion." Finally, the author wishes to thank Barton H. Lippincott, David T. Miller, Paul R. Hill, and Eleanor Faven of J. B. Lippincott Company for their encouragement, support, and editorial help.

1

Orientation

Student Council ● *Learning* ● *Intelligence* ●
Problem Solving ● *Studying* ● *Tests and Exam-*
inations ● *Assignments* ● *Reference Reading* ●
Questions and Answers

Objectives

On completion of this chapter you should be able to
1. understand the importance of adjusting in a practical nursing education program
2. discuss the functions of the Student Council
3. understand the learning process and the role of intelligence
4. name and apply the steps in the problem-solving process
5. identify needed study habits
6. function effectively as a test taker and student in carrying out required assignments.

Entering an educational program in practical nursing means for many of you a new career in the offing and a fresh start in life. It will also mean some new problems. However, at the time of enrollment it will help you to realize that (1) the program will consist of new, required information that is sometimes difficult to learn and understand, (2) the hours may be long and tiring, (3) you will constantly be meeting people, and (4) you will have to accustom yourself to ways of thinking and acting that are probably completely unfamiliar. You will then be prepared to meet the hurdles of the first few months of your nursing career with greater ease and confidence.

Although some students will live at home and have family and other responsibilities while attending school, others may be separated from their families for the first time with the attendant problem of adjusting to a new way of life. Furthermore, all students must accept (regardless of age) certain regulations governing group behavior as established by the school. On and off duty, in the classroom, in the hospital, and in the residence, they will be expected to conform to these rules, even if it is necessary to reorganize their habits. If you are in a career ladder program, working and studying part time, be sure to retain your identity as a nursing assistant at work and as a student in school. Of course, the disciplined person will adjust at a more rapid rate than the undisciplined one.

1

Most schools of practicl nursing plan an orientation program to help students adjust to their new environment. During this period the student becomes familiar with the physical facilities of the school, and if entering a vocational program, may be taken to visit the affiliated hospitals. In addition, various faculty members will discuss school regulations, the health service, class and hospital conduct, residence rules, student government activities, and course content. The student who accepts these regulations as a necessary part of the educational program and realizes that every well-organized school must have them has begun a satisfactory adjustment.

The process of becoming accustomed to any new situation requires thought, effort, and understanding on the part of the individual. When you realize this and understand that you must work at making adjustments, you will be better able to analyze some of your own feelings. It is not always easy to judge what you see. Perhaps you will find that you cannot make friends quickly, or are homesick, or cannot make a satisfactory adjustment because you are not readily accepted as a member of the student group. The reasons for such things are often difficult to understand. In these instances be sure to turn to a faculty member for guidance in dealing with your problems.

Each student should receive whatever guidance is necessary for scholastic as well as social adjustment. As you learn to discuss your difficulties with faculty members or the assigned guidance counselor, you will become more and more secure in your understanding of the program. Until you have learned to meet your own daily student problems and are able to solve them, you will certainly find it difficult to learn the complicated process of taking care of others.

STUDENT COUNCIL

During your high school days you may have participated in student government or board-council activities. In schools of practical nursing the student body is smaller, and unless the honor system, student residence regulations, and hospital problems demand a complex structure, the bylaws can be very simple. A member of the faculty elected by the students and an appointed alumnae representative may serve as advisers to the Council, which is composed of elected class officers. (See Chapter 8 for alumnae associations and parliamentary procedure.)

The Council should be responsible for recommending rules governing the student body, planning social, recreational, and other extracurricular activities, and represent the students' interests. Through council activities you will prepare yourself for your future role in nursing organizations, promote a harmonious relationship among students, faculty, and hospital personnel, and set standards of behavior that are acceptable in the educational and social activities of your school program.

The primary responsibility of the Council is to recommend disciplinary action for all infractions of school regulations. These infractions may be brought to the Council by any student, Council member, or member of the faculty, and they must be presented in writing. Any action or recommendation handed down by the Council must also be submitted in writing to the faculty adviser for approval.

Approved copies are then sent to those concerned and to the Director of the school. Copies of the minutes of meetings, recommendations made, and action handed down by the Council should be submitted to the faculty adviser at the earliest possible time.

LEARNING

Thinking, reasoning, solving problems, becoming proficient in new skills, and acquiring ideas are all phases of the learning process. Learning is development through experience, practice, and insight. This active process is self-initiated and self-motivated. An instructor can only guide or assist the learner to find the pertinent information and experiences. This situation is similar to that of the farmer who can lead the horses to water, but cannot make them drink. As a student, you must be motivated—you must *want* to reach certain goals.

Your enthusiasm for nursing should certainly motivate you to learn the subject matter. Practice and repetition are essential in order for learning to take place and also so that errors can be detected and corrected immediately. As you demonstrate adeptness at nursing procedures and skills, whether it be making an empty bed or doing a catheterization, the mastery of these skills will depend a great deal on your interest and your ability to grasp the subject matter (background material), your motor control, and the amount of practice you have had under your instructor's guidance.

Memory is related closely to the learning process. Material that has immediate meaning to you usually is memorized and retained easily. Only when you learn thoroughly will you be able to keep from forgetting; material only half-learned is forgotten more rapidly than that which is really studied. Repetition will help to fix the desired information in your mind so that it will not be forgotten quickly.

INTELLIGENCE

Intelligence is the capacity to adjust to new and unforeseen situations. It includes all those abilities that you have acquired and retained. Your memory, imagination, past learning, and judgment will all be used. Individual differences in intelligence are great and are measured by standardized tests, which show the intellectual development in terms of the ability of average individuals of a given age. Intelligence is dependent on heredity and environment (that is, what you have inherited and what you have been exposed to), and both play an important role in determining capabilities. However, inherited potentialities reach their fruition only through the environment. Intelligence is associated closely with general scholastic success, especially in subjects that demand linguistic ability and the understanding of abstract ideas.

Psychological surveys have shown that there is a direct relationship between the level of a person's intelligence and success in a particular occupation. These studies show that persons may not succeed if they are either too low or too high in intelligence. Individuals with intelligence too low for their jobs soon become helpless and frustrated, whereas the highly intelligent individual becomes bored and uninterested. Success in practical nursing depends not only on intelligence but also on good health, the ability to work with people, interest, personality, and the ability to solve everyday problems.

PROBLEM SOLVING

Whenever you are faced with a situation that is perplexing or difficult, and the course of action appears to be uncertain, you are confronted with a problem. A mature person will resist the temptation to act impulsively and will devote time and mental energy to the systematic exploration of a problem before attempting to solve it. The first step in solving any problem is to state the problem in words — define it as accurately as you can. It is amazing how far this one step will take you toward the solution. It not only banishes most irrelevant considerations, but also helps to eliminate the mental paralysis caused by the emotional impact of the dilemma. Gather all the facts that may have created the problem. Examine the cause or causes before you try to do anything at all about it.

Once you have gathered all the facts and have evaluated them, think of the solution or several possible solutions, then review each by considering the purpose of your actions. Consider how you can best accomplish your goal without upsetting anyone. Make sure that you take into account every pertinent fact; make a genuine effort to suppress emotional coloring as you try to reach the truth of the matter. Try to see the situation as a whole instead of acting on only a part of it. Be certain that you are dealing directly with facts and not with distortions of them acquired secondhand or thirdhand. Then take your time and weigh every pertinent sign and symptom before making your diagnosis. When you have decided on the best possible solution, ask yourself, "Am I going to handle this personally? Do I need the help of my charge nurse, instructor, or family? Should I refer this to a higher echelon? Will this be against any established policies or regulations?" After you have answered one or more of these questions to the best of your ability, proceed with your solution.

The best aid to problem solving is creative thinking. This is achieved by using past experiences to understand present situations and by directing your thinking toward the clarification and solution of your immediate problem. Remember, you may not know every aspect; therefore, you must avoid "set" thinking. It is remarkable how radically a situation may change if we force ourselves to look at a difficult problem from the other person's point of view. If you must question authority, do so tactfully and intelligently, realizing that you may be aware of only one side of the problem. Thinking becomes truly creative if imagination is applied along with logic. After all, many a problem is insolvable by the use of reason alone.

Competence in problem solving increases gradually with experience. Knowledge and linguistic development also influence this ability. However, even young children—preschoolers, in fact—have demonstrated that they can reason. Research has shown that the ability to reason develops continually. The ability to search for, evaluate, and organize factual information, and also to find the best answer to any question, is probably the most important habit that you can ever develop.

In summary, solving a problem involves:

1. Defining the problem. Is it clear? Do not confuse the symptoms with the cause.
2. Establishing your objectives. What do you want to accomplish? Be realistic and use common sense.
3. Gathering the facts. Do you have the whole story?
4. Weighing and deciding. Take your time, do not jump to conclusions—be flexible and make adjustments.
5. Taking action. Don't "pass the buck." Get beyond fault-finding and seek advice if needed. Then make up your mind.
6. Evaluating action. Did you reach your objectives? If not, try another approach and repeat steps 3 through 6 of the process.

STUDYING

During the first part of the practical nursing program you probably will find that your most difficult problem will be meeting the scholastic requirements. Keen competition exists among students of various educational backgrounds and ages. The schedule of classes is planned to meet modern curriculum requirements and is therefore more extensive and comprehensive than the usual high school program. It is not uncommon for students to have an average of six to eight hours of classwork daily during the early months of the program. Thus, it is necessary to keep up with this heavy volume of work in order to maintain passing grades. To learn at this rate is not difficult, provided that you have some system or method for studying. Another reason for adopting a method of study is that many of you have probably been away from high school long enough to be out of practice in this respect. Therefore, make some rules for yourself and abide by them.

Good study habits will enable you to take more pertinent notes in class, distinguish the important meaning of your reading assignments, enjoy your classes, and, above all, enable you to maintain a passing grade. Of prime importance in establishing a system of study is incentive. You must want to do it, realizing that only through study will you be able to understand the relationship between the classroom and your hospital experience. By performing the tasks assigned and by carrying out your faculty's instructions, you will be able to acquire the knowledge and the skills so necessary for success in your nursing career. It is important for you to realize that many failures in these educational programs are due to ineffectual study methods and lack of application, rather than to an inability to learn subject matter. Students who are well prepared will enjoy their classes far more, and they will feel much more at ease if there should be a quiz, or if they are asked a question by the instructor. Actually, you will probably discover that, although you will have to devote much more intensive effort to your nursing subjects than you ever did to your high school courses, learning will be a correspondingly greater pleasure. You will find a real purpose in applying yourself, and you will also have the satisfaction of putting your new knowledge to use for the benefit of your patients.

Privacy and quiet are important. Your study materials should be at hand; a good light, proper ventilation, and a table or a desk with a comfortable chair are other essentials. Plan your time so that you will not be interrupted. Try to have a definite place and time for your studies—on a daily basis. Do not spend time talking and worrying about when and how to study, but *get right down to it*. The power of concentration is most important for successful studying, as most of us have a strictly limited attention span. Therefore, shorter periods of concentrated study are more beneficial than longer periods, which usually include interruptions, day-dreaming, and other distractions. As a rule, students are able to study much more effectively in the library than in their rooms, because others are studying there at the same time, reference books are at hand, and the atmosphere of the library usually stimulates one to study. For students who must study at home, it is often the bedroom that provides the best atmosphere.

Your thoughts should be free of personal problems, and it is most important that you turn to what you *must* think about rather than what you may *want* to think about. Get the telephone calls out of the way, make the trips to the snack bar and the bathroom, and eliminate all possible distractions. Get your mind into harness, and keep it from straying; once you have started to study, you will find that your interest will develop, and you will forget everything else. Be honest with yourself and do not overrate yourself when judging your study habits. Discover your weaknesses and discuss them with faculty members so that they can help you to overcome them. Here are some suggestions for improving your studying:

1. Review the notes of the previous class before studying the assigned lesson and keep separate notes for each course. If you use a tape recorder to record the speaker(s), be sure you obtain permission. Tape recorders can be very helpful in reviewing lecture content later.

2. Ask questions in class if you do not understand the lecture content. Join in class discussions.

3. Study with adequate light and without radio or television turned on.

4. Get adequate sleep and rise early enough to allow time for a healthy breakfast each day.

5. Follow a daily plan and budget your time to include study, recreation, and personal affairs.

6. Use the recommended or standard-size looseleaf notebook (8½ × 11), and recopy your class notes into this notebook so that they will be neat and easy to read.

7. Study for an examination from these notes, with the emphasis on learning and remembering rather than on just passing the test.

8. Go over the mistakes that you made on a test and find the right answer. If you received a failing grade, discuss this further with the instructor.

9. Decide that you will enjoy attending classes. Be attentive and turn in your written assignments when due.

10. As you read, pay close attention to charts, photographs, diagrams, and other illustrations. Very often "one picture can tell more than a thousand words."

11. Take brief but useful notes while studying, so that you can tie into your actual nursing practice the theory that you have learned from your reading.

12. Words or phrases should beunderlined only in your own books or magazines. Write in the margins, so that you may pay special attention to important passages.

13. Use the library not only for a place to study but also as a "friend" to help you locate reference books, magazines, and other necessary literature. One of the great pleasures of the library is to browse and discover books that you never imagined existed. Once in a while do this merely for the fun of it. You will be amazed how much useful information you can pick up without really trying. This practice also keeps your curiosity nicely stimulated.

14. Study and practice your nursing skills with a friend. Teaching another person is an excellent way to learn.

TESTS AND EXAMINATIONS

As a student you will be tested many times. Even though the grade does not necessarily reveal all you know or do not know about the subject, it is one of the important yardsticks by which the faculty evaluates your progress. You, too, can use grades for setting your standards, realizing what you must improve on, knowing what you should review, and finding what you must "learn all over again" to prepare yourself for the State Board examination.

Your success in passing examinations depends a great deal on your ability to retain classroom material and to complete your daily assignments. If you have established good study habits and study regularly, if you review previously learned material and do not procrastinate in "getting ready for that test," you should be able to evaluate and answer each question carefully and maintain a passing grade.

Multiple choice, true or false, statement completion, matching, and other types of questions requiring careful evaluation, judgment, and factual knowledge are methods of testing that are preferred by most instructors. Essay questions will test not only your knowledge of facts but also your spelling and your ability to use English correctly. Samples of different questions will appear throughout this book. At the end of each chapter you will have an opportunity to test your acquired knowledge.

Prepare systematically for your examinations by beginning the day after a test to study for the next one. Arrange your schedule for continued review of lecture notes and textbook assignments, setting aside a definite study time throughout the week. Cramming on the night before an examination, as a concentrated review, is ineffective unless you are familiar with the material. Try to ascertain the type of test that will be given, the precise material to be covered, and the questions your instructors might include. Keep all previous tests for review and analyze them to determine your weak areas.

Since the State Board examination is objective, most instructors prefer using this type of test. Read the directions twice and be sure you understand them before beginning to read the questions. Careful reading is most essential. Answer the questions as you read them, putting aside all debatable ones (consider these later). If it is a "timed test," do not spend too much time on any one question; if you cannot recall the answer, come back to it later. Other questions may give you clues to this one. As you read the questions, be on the lookout for such words as *always, usually, never,* and so on, and read the question very carefully. Restate it, if necessary, to clarify it. When you have finished the test questions, reread them all and check for carelessness. Rely on your first answer when in doubt. If there is no penalty for a wrong answer, you lose nothing by guessing.

Cheating on examinations is a temptation to some people. Nurses must be honest, dependable, and reliable; therefore, there is no excuse for letting anyone "get away with it." If a fellow student cheats, gets away with it, and passes the course, what kind of nurse will he or she be? If you were aware of this cheating and did not report it, would you feel safe with the nursing care this person would give? What will this do to your school standards? What will happen during State Board examinations, when cheating is impossible? Do not cheat or condone the cheating of others.

ASSIGNMENTS

Often, your teachers may assign specific field trips, group projects, audio visual materials, including tapes and films, term papers, programmed instructions, independent study, patient care studies, and other supplementary materials for your use. These are carefully selected, planned, and evaluated by your instructors to augment classroom instruction and thereby help you retain more knowledge. Be sure to follow your instructors' directions and complete the assignment by the due date. Punctuality, ability to follow directions, and accepting the responsibility for one's own actions are *MUSTS* for nurses.

Reading Assignments

One of the most effective ways of studying reading assignments is by the PQRST method. The five letters stand for Preview, Question, Read, State, and Test.

By *previewing* the assignment you will get a general idea of what the author is trying to convey. Read headings, topic sentences, italicized words, and summaries. This will enable you to understand the "why" of the material. As you are previewing, make up *questions* or be familiar with those usually found at the end of the chapter. There are only a limited number of good questions possible, and as you become familiar with the type of questions your instructors ask, you will be able to make up similar ones as you preview.

The third step is *reading,* which is discussed more fully in Chapter 4. You must react as you read. Don't let your mind relax; read ideas and react effectively. The next step is *stating* in your own words what you have read. You may wish to do this by making an outline or listing new words as you come across them. You should not only write this material down but also be able to state it orally. As you think about the topic and put it in your own words you are problem solving and thinking the assignment through. You are also improving your memory.

The final step is *testing.* Review what you have read by testing yourself on the content of the material you have stated. This fifth step is very important and should not be done hurriedly. You will discover the hazy areas in which you need to reread and review before your examination.

The PQRST method has been used very effectively by many students. It takes time to develop, but as your skill improves you should note a marked improvement in your grades. Another name for this effective method, as developed at Ohio State University, is SQ3R—Survey, Question, Read, Recite, and Review. The letters may be different but the important points are similar.

REFERENCE READING

In your classroom sessions the instructors cannot possibly provide you with all the information necessary about any given topic; therefore, the interested student will seek further knowledge by reading about the subject. Magazines, pamphlets, and books—such as nursing texts, dictionaries, encyclopedias, and other source materials—should be referred to frequently. It is surprising how much you can learn about a subject by reading more than one version of it. For example, if you read in your basic text about the action of the kidney, it may or may not mean anything to you. But go to the library, pick up a slightly more advanced text and read about the kidney once again. The chances are that suddenly a great deal will become clearer to you. Many instructors distribute various pamphlets during their class sessions and assign readings. Reference reading is done easily if you know how to use a library, in particular the card catalogue, which assists you in locating books, journals, and pamphlets. If your school does not have a library or a librarian, you should use the public library in your community. Usually, librarians will be most helpful in assisting you.

Most hospitals have up-to-date medical libraries, and in addition, "floor libraries" may be established in each clinical unit. These libraries usually will provide current information, reference books and tapes, audiovisual aids, and other material for the use of the entire hospital staff, but maintained primarily for the convenience of medical and nursing personnel.

Once you have had a little practice in using references and have become familiar with their typical plan of organization, you will be able to find information very quickly. In the back of most books is the index, arranged alphabetically, which will help you to locate specific items by indicating the page(s) on which the subject is discussed. The table of contents appears in the front of the book and serves as a guide to the chapters and to the divisions of a chapter. Although the table of contents will give clues as to the section of the book the topic you are looking for may be, the use of the index will save you valuable time.

When you are using the facilities of the library and wish to borrow tapes, audiovisual aids, and books, become acquainted with the proper methods of caring for them and "signing them out." Do not mutilate library material by tearing out pages or handling it carelessly. Library regulations are usually simple and reasonable; they include common courtesies, such as not disturbing others by unnecessary talking or noise, returning borrowed books when due, and not losing the books.

Nurses are encouraged to build their own reference libraries at home by purchasing books that they feel will be of most use to them, by writing for the many free pamphlets available to them, and by subscribing to the magazines that will keep them currently informed about their career responsibilities.

Following are suggested lists of references that you may find especially useful.

Pamphlets

Write to the voluntary and official health and welfare organizations outlined in Chapter 8 for their many free or very inexpensive educational materials and publications lists. Usually, your local or state health department will have a compilation of various pamphlets pertaining to health subjects, and you can obtain these by noting the topic of interest. In addition, pharmaceutical companies have free drug information leaflets available, from which you can build an accurate and current reference file.

Pamphlets are excellent teaching tools for patients, but need to be evaluated for content, advertising, and suitability. Many will come in bilingual editions, whereas others may only be available in translation. Feel free to write for these materials; file them alphabetically for easier use.

Journals

Helpful and informative articles are published in the official magazines of various nursing organizations and in those journals sponsored by reliable associations. By reading magazine articles and browsing through the various monthly publications in the library or in your home, you will be able to keep yourself currently informed on nursing. Although it would be advantageous to subscribe to these magazines, financially you might not be able to; however, group subscriptions are available to you at a reduced rate. Very often for the nurse who "has everything" these periodicals make excellent gifts. Here are only a few listed for your information:

The American Journal of Nursing American Journal of Nursing Co.
Nursing Outlook 555 W. 57th St.
New York, N.Y. 10019

The Journal of Practical Nursing	The National Association of Practical Nurse Education and Service, Inc. 122 E. 42nd St. New York, N.Y. 10017
The Journal of Nursing Care	The National Federation of Licensed Practical Nurses, Inc. 888 7th Ave. New York, N.Y. 10019
RN	P.O. Box 374 Oradell, N.J. 07649
Nursing and Health Care	Technomonic Publishing Co., Inc. 265 Post Rd. Westport, Conn. 06880
Nursing Homes	222 Wisconsin Ave. Lake Forest, Ill. 60045
Nursing '81, '82, and so forth	Intermed Communications, Inc. 132 Welsh Rd. Horsham, Pa. 19044

Books

The reference books you keep should cover your field as thoroughly as possible. Books are nice to have, but make sure that they are useful as well. Progress in nursing is rapid, and books are being revised constantly. See to it that yours are up to date. Do not buy books indiscriminately; evaluate them carefully with respect to their overall value to you.

Questions

A. True or False. Write *T* or *F* in answer space.

_____ 1. Memory is related to the learning process.
_____ 2. A person's intelligence influences success or failure in a particular occupation.
_____ 3. The first step in solving a problem is to define it.
_____ 4. The power of concentration is not important for successful study.
_____ 5. When reading, you should skip pictures and charts.
_____ 6. Cramming is an effective study technic.
_____ 7. When in doubt, rely on your first answer when taking a test.
_____ 8. The PQRST method should be used when reading assignments.
_____ 9. The PQRST method should be used in problem solving.
_____ 10. Beginning the day after a test to study for the next one is a good plan.

B. Select the correct answer and circle the number that answers the question best.

1. The Student Council is usually responsible for (A) planning extracurricular activities, (B) promoting harmonious relationships between faculty and students, (C) recommending disciplinary action for infraction of school regulations, (D) setting standards of behavior for students.

    1. All except A
    2. All except C
    3. All except D
    4. All of these

2. Intelligence is primarily dependent upon (A) heredity, (B) environment, (C) religion, (D) nationality.

   1. All of these
   2. All except B
   3. All except D
   4. A, B

3. The learning process includes (A) acquiring new ideas, (B) problem solving, (C) reasoning ability, (D) thinking.

   1. All of these
   2. All except B
   3. All except D
   4. A, C

4. When taking a test, you should (A) read the directions at least twice and be sure you understand them before beginning to answer, (B) answer the questions as you read them, omit debatable ones and come back to them, (C) watch carefully for words such as *always, usually, never,* and so forth, (D) prepare by predicting the type of questions the instructor might ask.

   1. All of these
   2. All except A
   3. All except B
   4. All except D

5. Problem solving includes (A) defining the problem, (B) establishing objectives, (C) gathering facts, (D) taking action.

   1. All except A
   2. All except D
   3. All of these
   4. B, C

6. In establishing objectives within problem solving, one must (A) jump to conclusions, (B) go beyond fault-finding, (C) be realistic, (D) use common sense.

   1. All except A
   2. All except B
   3. C, D
   4. All of these

7. Previewing an assignment includes (A) reading headings, (B) making up questions, (C) skipping summaries, (D) skipping questions.

   1. All except C
   2. All except D
   3. A
   4. A, B

8. Improvement in your study habits may result from (A) reviewing notes before starting to study, (B) following a daily personal plan, (C) budgeting time for social needs, (D) joining in class discussions.

   1. All except B
   2. All except C
   3. All except D
   4. All of these

Answers

A. True or False (2 points each)

   1. T
   2. T
   3. T
   4. F
   5. F
   6. F
   7. T
   8. T
   9. F
   10. T

B. Multiple Choice (10 points each)

   1. 4
   2. 4
   3. 1
   4. 1
   5. 3
   6. 1
   7. 4
   8. 4

2

Nursing History and Trends

Nursing in Ancient Civilizations • Nursing in Early Christian Times • The Dark Ages (400–1000) • The Medieval Period (1000–1450) • The Decline of Nursing—The Renaissance to the 19th Century • The Beginning of Modern Nursing • To the Present Time • Status of Women • The Future • Questions and Answers

Objectives

Upon completion of this chapter you should be able to
1. describe the development of nursing from ancient times to modern day
2. trace the development of practical nursing
3. cite, by name and accomplishment, the contributions of those who influenced nursing and practical nursing
4. identify important studies in nursing
5. understand your future role in promoting practical nursing.

Not the least of the satisfactions found in nursing is pride in the ancient tradition of selfless service. As a career, nursing is comparatively recent, but as an instinctive act it dates back to the time when the first woman nursed her child or served as a midwife. In most primitive societies the ministrations of the men and women of the tribe supplemented the efforts of the witch doctor in tending to the sick and the wounded. The communal spirit of nursing dates from the very earliest times. It is difficult for today's student, accustomed to equal rights for all, to imagine what nursing, medicine, and society were like in the past. Nursing is interwoven with general history, and the political and social forces that influence society also affect nursing.

NURSING IN ANCIENT CIVILIZATIONS

For thousands of years before Christ an advanced and stable civilization flourished along the river Nile in Egypt. Medicine of a kind was practiced widely (Egyptian physicians were adept at treating fractures), and medical specialties were known to have existed. Although there is no direct evidence of a segment of the population devoted to nursing the sick, there are written records of procedures followed in ancient Egypt that could be classified only as nursing. Probably, nursing was actively carried on, since the physicians could hardly have undertaken these duties themselves.

Elements of professional nursing were also part of the culture of the ancient Hebrews. The civilization of the Hebrew people, part of whose writings became the Old Testament, had a tradition of hospitality and healing: "Thou shalt love thy neighbor as thyself." The Hebrews erected sick-houses and homes for the aged; to them the sick and homeless stranger was welcome. The Hebrew people initiated many principles of personal hygiene and public sanitation as well, and a number of present-day Jewish dietary laws stem from these ancient health measures.

Among the greatest civilizations of all time was that of the Greeks, who attained the height of their power and influence about 450 B.C. A trio of Greek philosophers—Socrates, Plato, and Aristotle—gave to Western civilization their characteristic system of logical thought. If you think that nobody before Columbus believed the earth was round, consider this: not only did learned Greeks take that for granted, but one of them actually measured the earth's circumference within a few hundred miles—an incredible feat of human intelligence characteristic of the Greeks.

In the late fifth century B.C., a Greek named Hippocrates (the "Father of Medicine") introduced a system whereby observations of symptoms and the application of other carefully reasoned scientific principles replaced the superstitions and the illogical concepts of primitive medicine. The Hippocratic ethical code is still the basis of modern medical practice.

The method of healing devised by Hippocrates was to assist nature in doing the work—a clear implication of the need for systematic nursing care. By all rights the Greeks ought to have invented the trained nurse, but strangely enough, they did not. One reason is that in Greece, women were forced to occupy a subordinate position in society and were not considered worthy of being trained in medicine or nursing. What nurses there were usually occupied household positions as retainers or domestics and frequently were slaves. They tended to the children and other family members, whereas the Hippocratic nursing procedures for the sick were carried out by the physician or his pupils.

In time Greece declined (though Greek innovations were never forgotten), whereas the Roman Empire grew to become the mightiest political power the Western world had ever known. Rome was primarily a military state and established military hospitals, but organized nursing care was not widespread until the advent of Christianity.

The Caduceus, the physician's emblem (adapted as the insignia of the Medical

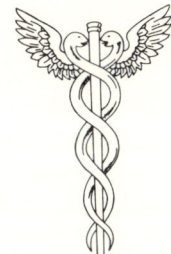

FIGURE 2-1. *The Caduceus.*

Corps of the United States Army) originated in Greek and Roman mythology (Figure 2–1). In legend, Apollo gave Mercury a magic wand (formed by two entwined, winged snakes) that had the power to turn things to gold, to control life and death, and to conduct the souls of the dead to the lower world.

In the Orient at about the same time, Emperor Shen Nung, "father of Chinese medicine" was developing the technic of acupuncture, which began to be practiced about 170 A.D.

NURSING IN EARLY CHRISTIAN TIMES

Roman power reached its peak at about the time of Christ's birth. Christianity was outlawed at first, but as the centuries passed, it became tolerated, then respectable, and finally it was the offical religion of Rome (about 325 A.D.). In the process, Rome itself declined. With the growth of Christianity, organized nursing developed as an expression of the Christian ideal of charity. Christian nursing included men as well as women, each concerned with the care of those of his or her own sex. About 30 years after the Crucifixion, St. Paul introduced into Rome a woman named Phoebe of Cenchreae, an ordained *diakonos* (minister or servant) of the church, among whose duties was ministering to the sick. The word "diakonos" has become "deaconess"; Phoebe is known as the first Deaconess and also the first visiting nurse. In addition to the Deaconesses, other orders of Christian women converts who were dedicated to serving the poor and the infirm were founded. One, a lay group, was the Order of Widows; another was called the Order of Virgins—nuns enrolled in the service of the church, who lived humbly and piously and spent their lives doing charitable deeds.

St. Jerome (345–420 A.D.), who translated the Bible into Latin, had a wealthy protégée named Fabiola. In atonement for her earlier sins, Fabiola founded a hospital in Rome and with her own hands rendered personal nursing care to the maimed and the hopelessly diseased.

THE DARK AGES (400–1000)

In the year 476, the Roman Empire, which had been besieged for centuries by Germanic and other barbarian peoples, finally yielded to its invaders and came to an end. For the next 500 years or so all Europe fell into that long night of chaos and violence known as the Dark Ages. Rival chieftains fought each other back and forth over the land, dynasties rose and fell, and all the while Europe was slowly being divided into a multiplicity of great and small kingdoms.

In this dangerous era the adherents of the Christian Church retreated behind the walls of convents and monasteries, which became small islands of peace, order, and intellectual endeavor in that sea of anarchy. Within these monastic orders learning was kept alive, and the spiritual and worldly power of the Church quietly gathered momentum. In time the church had the strength to assume a role as the controlling force of the Middle Ages. During the Dark Ages several great hospitals were founded by the Church: Hôtel Dieu (Lyons) in 542, Hôtel Dieu (Paris) in 650, and Santo Spirito (Rome) in 717. Several religious orders included in their duties care of the sick as well as conversion of the heathen.

THE MEDIEVAL PERIOD (1000–1450)

In the Medieval period (also called the Middle Ages) Europe emerged from the Dark Ages completely transformed; now, instead of a monolithic Empire, a collection of small states existed, with the Church as supreme head of them all. Never before or since has the Christian religion so completely dominated the Western world in every respect—philosophy, politics, art, even the everyday thoughts and deeds of ordinary people. During the Middle Ages the great cathedrals were built, and outstanding universities were founded, such as those of Oxford and Paris. Commerce was begun, first between cities and then between European nations, and finally, the Crusades started the flow of commerce and culture between Europe and the Orient. With commerce, a middle class emerged, which eventually was to change the whole fabric of society. It was the time of knights, troubadours, feudal barons with their serfs, Crusaders, theologians, and saints. The period was one of extraordinary piety, enterprise, vitality, and color.

Both men and women were involved in nursing now, since monks and nuns continued to share most of the burden of nursing care during the Middle Ages. Many more monastic orders were founded, among them military orders known as Knights Hospitalers, who were trained to fight the enemy as well as to tend the sick in their fortified hospitals. Nursing brotherhoods included the Brothers of Mercy, the Franciscans, the Alexians, and the Brothers of St. John of God.

A great medieval mystic, St. Francis of Assisi, founded the Franciscan order, which was committed to wandering, poverty, preaching, and nursing of the sick and the destitute. A disciple of Francis was Clara of Assisi, who founded the Franciscan order of nuns known as Poor Clares. This group also tended the sick, particularly lepers.

The history of nursing during this period is characterized by stories of highborn ladies who renounced their heritage for the sake of the poor and the infirm— among them Clara herself, Agnes of Bohemia, and St. Elizabeth of Hungary. For instance, St. Catherine of Siena, a remarkable combination of mystic and practical organizer, could have lived only in the Middle Ages. She had unearthly visions, she was granted the bodily marks of stigmata (wounds of Christ), she brought the Papacy back to Rome after its long Avignon exile, and she was a first-rate hospital nurse, specializing in cases that nobody else would undertake.

As the Middle Ages wore on, the Church's power began to wane. Most young people no longer found monastic life attractive. Several secular orders were founded at this period of decline by people who still wanted to serve humanity but were unwilling to place themselves under Church authority. The Beguines of Flanders are a notable example of such a group.

THE DECLINE OF NURSING— THE RENAISSANCE TO THE 19TH CENTURY

At the end of the Middle Ages, Europe seemed to be old and worn out. Society was disrupted, great plagues and wars swept over the land, and millions died. Religious fervor was replaced to a great extent by cynicism and despair. Yet, simultaneous with the dissolution of medieval society came the emergence of a new Europe of large and powerful monarchies and the development of what is now recognized as the modern mind. The word "Renaissance" means "rebirth," and it marks the period of about 1450–1650, when the ancient learning of the Greek and the Roman worlds was brought to light and put to use again, the effect of which was to discipline and thereby set free the mind of the common man. The Greeks were scientifically oriented; that is, they inquired into the nature of things and formed their conclusions only after careful observation and reasoning, an example of this was the method employed by Hippocrates some 2,000 years before. Now it was rediscovered, and as Church authority declined, people adopted the scientific method to reassess the world in their own way. There began the great age of science, exploration, and discovery that has continued without a break to this very day.

It is a peculiar historical fact that the progress of medicine seems at variance with that of nursing; only in our own time did they finally become interrelated services. In Greece, as you will recall, Hippocratic medicine developed, but there was no real nursing. In the period of monasticism nursing orders proliferated, but there was no medicine (Hippocrates had been forgotten). Now, in the Renaissance the disciplines of anatomy, physiology, and scientific healing were founded, but nursing suddenly declined and was almost forgotten until the 19th century. There are two main reasons for this. During the Renaissance came that period of religious upheaval known as the Reformation, in which the Church split into Catholic and Protestant factions. In Protestant countries, such as England and Germany, monasticism nearly came to an end and with it nursing, most of which had been carried on by the religious orders. Also, since the comparatively modern concept of social service was not yet common, secular nursing practically disappeared.

Even though the common man achieved greater personal freedom during and after the Renaissance, and an extension of individualism, the tradition of unselfish service to humanity was neglected almost to the point of extinction. It was a cruel age, callous to the plight of the poor, the homeless, and the diseased. The communal spirit of charity was desperately lacking—it remained for one man, St. Vincent de Paul, to found organized charity almost singlehandedly. A French priest of the 17th century, Vincent dedicated his life to righting the wrongs of his time. He attracted many disciples from the aristocracy and succeeded in making charity fashionable. With a follower, Louise de Marillac, Vincent founded the Sisters of Charity, an order that to this day has devoted its efforts exclusively to caring for the poor and the sick.

With the 18th century came widespread industrialization, resulting in a disruption of the old agricultural society. The population shot up, and cities sprawled far beyond their ancient boundaries. In the provinces widespread unemployment and misery abounded; in the cities slums grew, full of poverty, crime, and disease. The end of the 18th century saw the appearance of a most modern and desperately needed figure—the social reformer. The most influential of these reformers was John Howard, who traveled from England to Russia, visiting jails, almshouses, asylums, penthouses, hospitals, and infirmaries. Howard's voluminous reports of the horrors that he saw served to awaken the conscience of the society of his time, preparing the way for the sweeping social reforms that were first launched in the 19th century and continue to the present day.

THE BEGINNING OF MODERN NURSING

By the end of the 18th century nursing in secular institutions had become practically nonexistent, particularly in Protestant countries, where the services of the Sisters of Charity were not generally available. Typical of the hospital nurse at that time was the ignorant, gin-soaked slattern personified by Sairey Gamp and Betsy Prig in Charles Dickens' *Martin Chuzzlewit*. It was clear that an entirely new type of nurse was needed, one who was not only intelligent and dedicated but who was also technically trained. It is true that various attempts had been made in the past to train nurses. The Sisters of Charity had their own program, and in certain American hospitals (for instance, Pennsylvania Hospital, founded in 1751, and New York Hospital, founded in 1771) limited courses of instruction were instituted. However, it was not until 1836 that the first real school of nursing was founded.

In that year a German pastor, Theodor Fliedner, established a hospital in his parish at Kaiserswerth. An experienced nurse, Gertrude Reichardt, was engaged, and to Pastor Fliedner's parish came a group of women who were the nucleus of a modern order of deaconesses, whose duties were nursing the sick and performing other charitable acts. At the hospital they received formal instruction in nursing principles. Many of the graduates of the Kaiserswerth Deaconess Institution settled in other parts of the world to found similar training programs.

For a time Kaiserswerth had a famous pupil, the person from whom all modern nursing dates; she stands in relation to nursing as Hippocrates did to medicine—Florence Nightingale.

Florence Nightingale (1820–1910)

The history of nursing may be divided into two epochs: before Nightingale and after Nightingale. Florence Nightingale was the founder of modern nursing; it was she who made nursing the highly respected career that it is today. She was born May 12, 1820 in Florence, Italy to a wealthy English family, and when she was one year old the family, including an older sister, returned to England, where Florence Nightingale was reared and educated. She received a remarkably thorough education and was well schooled in subjects such as French, German, Latin, Greek, Hebrew, history, mathematics, and philosophy, and by family tradition she was taught the social graces and manners befitting a girl of her rank. Despite these advantages, however, Miss Nightingale's ambition was unfulfilled for many years. She was possessed by a need to serve humanity, and specifically to nurse the sick. However, for a woman of her station to be a nurse was unthinkable. Only "Gamps" and "Prigs" did public nursing in those days.

In 1844, when she announced that she wished to be a nurse, her family was violently opposed to this venture, but with the encouragement of Elizabeth Blackwell, America's first woman physician, she entered the Deaconess School at Kaiserswerth. In addition, she studied the work of the Sisters of Charity in Paris and investigated various hospitals and religious houses. Finally, she obtained the position of superintendent of a small institution in London, where she was able to gain valuable experience in hospital administration as well as in nursing. In 1854, when the Crimean War erupted, with England, France, and Turkey allied against Russia, the inefficiency of the English Army medical authorities was soon evident to the people back home. The wounded of France were cared for by the Sisters of Charity, the Russian casualties by the Sisters of Mercy, but the wounded of England were almost completely neglected. A loud public outcry ensued. Eventually, with the aid of Sidney Herbert, the Secretary of War, Florence Nightingale and 38 nurses were allowed to sail from England to the Crimea to attend the wounded.

At Marseilles she outfitted herself with a large stock of supplies despite the Army's declaration that it was in need of nothing. The conditions that she found in the military hospitals of the Crimea were appalling. The hospitals were overcrowded and without soap, linen, chairs, tables, or lamps. The wounded lay on the floors in their battle uniforms, in indescribable filth. Miss Nightingale's stock of supplies was decisive in persuading the authorities to allow her to help, and in spite of the reluctance of the Army, mountains of red tape, and unclear channels of authority, she set to work, taking things into her own hands. She personally raised funds to purchase supplies that doctors could not obtain for the Army. She hired people to clean up the hospitals and established laundries to wash linens and uniforms. Her early training in organization and administration came into use in this crisis, and her calm manner helped to maintain a rigid discipline over her nurses and other helpers. Her endless rounds, comforting the wounded, created the picture in the public mind that made her famous. The men adored her, and to them she was their "Lady with the Lamp." Six months after her arrival the fruits of her labor were apparent. The death rate among the wounded dropped from 420 per 1000 to only 22 per 1000. There was order and cleanliness; well-prepared meals and an efficient distribution of supplies had replaced the former chaos. Miss Nightingale was seemingly tireless, and stayed on until the war ended and the last soldier had left. Finally, she herself became ill with Crimean fever and could no longer walk.

In 1856, she returned to England amid wide acclaim as the heroine of the Crimean War. She modestly avoided all public demonstrations, and sick and exhausted, she disappeared from public view. Many supposed her dead, but she actually lived for 54 years after her return, working to improve conditions at home as she had in the Crimea. She initiated reforms in both military and civilian hospitals. The public showed its appreciation by establishing a training school for nurses called the Nightingale School, the first institution of its kind and the model of the modern school of nursing. Miss Nightingale wrote many books on nursing; of these the most widely read is *Notes on Nursing*. She emphasized the importance of high moral character in addition to the nurse's technical skill, and her philosophy included the principle of absolute obedience. She believed that nurses should work only in hospitals, not in private duty; to her, nursing was a sacred calling and not a business. Despite the evidence that licensure was necessary in order to distinguish qualified nurses from the unqualified, Miss Nightingale was against it. To her, obtaining a license was too much like joining a union—a nurse was above such practices.

Miss Nightingale died in 1910 at the age of 90 years, three years after receiving the Order of Merit from King Edward VII, the highest British honor ever bestowed on a woman.

Late 19th and 20th Centuries

The greatest strides in the development of modern nursing took place during and after the Nightingale era. The reforms of this period spread throughout the world. In 1863, J. H. Dunant, who was Swiss, founded the Red Cross with the object of creating an international health organization to serve as a neutral body in time of war and to be available for assistance in peacetime in the event of disaster. In 1882 Clara Barton organized the American Red Cross along the same lines. After the Civil War, American women assumed a new interest in public affairs and were instrumental in reforming Bellevue Hospital according to the Nightingale tradition. A new training school was founded there in 1873, patterned after the original Nightingale School in England. In 1888, the Mills Training School for Male Nurses was established at Bellevue. Thereafter, one new school after another was founded. The first official nursing textbooks and uniforms for secular nurses appeared. The public lavished great adoration and praise on the early pioneers of trained nursing, appreciating the long hours of labor they devoted to the welfare of patients.

Meanwhile, medicine and nursing were both making revolutionary progress. An era of medicine based on bacteriology had been ushered in by Louis Pasteur and Robert Koch. Joseph Lister was the "father of modern aseptic surgery," and the work of Semmelweis practically banished the dreaded child-bed fever (puerperal sepsis) from the hospitals of Vienna and ultimately from all the hospitals of the civilized world. Nursing followed the example of medicine, and a number of outstanding women arose to give direction and scope to the new profession. Dorothea Dix was an ''American John Howard,'' conducting a lone and relentless campaign to improve the barbarous treatment of the insane. During the Civil War she served as Superintendent of U. S. Army nursing. Linda Richards, the first trained nurse in America, organized the school of nursing at Massachusetts General Hospital. Isabel Hampton Robb launched and brilliantly managed the school of nursing at Johns Hopkins Hospital.

America's first black graduate nurse, Mary E. Mahoney, pressed for integration and better working conditions and health care facilities in the Boston area. Mary Breckenridge started the Frontier Nursing Service of Kentucky, which offers maternal-child care services in the remote Cumberland Mountains.

The famous Henry Street Settlement in New York, which began the community movement of visiting nursing, was founded by Lillian Wald. The role of the nurse in society broadened considerably with the establishment of various social agencies: Red Cross Societies, YMCA, YWCA, settlement houses, and others.

When America entered World War I in 1917, the American Red Cross Nursing Services, through the efforts of Jane Delano, enrolled many nurses for service with the Army and Navy Nurse Corps. In 1918 the Army School of Nursing was opened with Annie W. Goodrich as director. After the war, the emphasis in American medicine shifted to improving health education; nursing instruction kept pace to meet the challenge of the times. Medical men as well as hospital officials came forward with measures for promoting a higher level of medical practice. Nurses were expected to be able to meet the additional demands placed on them. Surveys were made, which concluded that in addition to hospital training, nursing education should include college-level courses leading to licensure, and should offer postgraduate courses as preparation for administrative and teaching positions. In 1907, M. Adelaide Nutting (who with Lavinia Dock wrote the monumental *History of Nursing*) established the first college-level nursing program at Teachers College, Columbia University. There was a fresh, critical examination of nursing schools; new standards were set that placed the emphasis on education rather than on service or training through service.

The need for nurses kept increasing, and during 1943 in the midst of World War II, the United States Cadet Nurse Corps was established through the efforts of Mrs. Frances Payne Bolton and an emergency measure of Congress. Thousands of young women desirous of becoming professional nurses were extended financial aid and thereby encouraged to enter schools of nursing. At the conclusion of World War II the shortage of nurses became even more critical. Many nurses who had become active during the war years retired or entered advanced education programs, others went into doctors' offices or accepted nursing positions in industry. At the same time, many of the married or retired nurses who had given their valuable assistance and service left the profession again when the emergency was over.

In 1951, Mildred L. Montag's doctoral thesis, ''Education of Nursing Technicians'' proposed that a new position, nurse technician, above the level of the practical nurse and below the level of the professional nurse be established. Under Dr. Montag's leadership these programs have been instituted in junior and community colleges. At this time there are almost 700 Associate Degree of Nursing (ADN) programs throughout the United States.

In 1979 there were 1,389 nursing programs educating students to be registered nurses. About 50% of these programs are ADN, 24% are diploma (or hospital) schools, and 26% are baccalaureate programs in college or universities.

Practical Nursing

To cope with the shortage of nurses, or perhaps with the problem of better use of nursing personnel, the practical nurse attained an important permanent place on the health team. The need for better education of practical nurses was recognized early, and in 1893 the Ballard School, the first practical nursing school in America, opened in New York with a three-month program. In 1907, the Thompson School was founded in Brattleboro, Vermont, and in 1918 the Household Nursing Association School of Attendant Nursing was begun in Boston with the purpose of training practical nurses to work in the home. These pioneer institutions were the forerunners of the practical nursing schools of today. The last two are still going strong, although the Boston school was later renamed the Shepard-Gill School of Practical Nursing. Training of the practical nurse has recently extended into hospitals, junior and community colleges, and vocational/technical institutes.

It was not until the 1940s that those in practical nursing education felt the need to form an association that would be concerned with practical nursing. In 1941, 28 people met in Chicago and founded the Association of Practical Nurse Schools. Hilda M. Torrop, Director of the Ballard School; Etta Creech, Director of the Family Health Association in Cleveland; and Katherine Shepard, Executive Director of the Household Nursing Association in Boston were founders and officers of the Association. Later, Hilda Torrop became its first executive director. The next year (1942) membership was opened to practical nurses, and the name of the Association was changed to the National Association of Practical Nurse Education (NAPNE). In 1945, NAPNE established an accrediting service for schools of practical nursing; in 1950 it began conducting a summer school and workshops for directors and instructors; and in 1951 it initiated the first practical nursing magazine (now titled *The Journal of Practical Nursing*). By 1953, it was sponsoring summer courses at colleges and universities for practical nurses. As time went on, the continuing education and welfare of practical nurses received more and more emphasis. In 1959, a Department of Service to State Practical Nursing Associations, as well as a Department of Education, were established, and the title of the Association was changed to the National Association for Practical Nurse Education and Service (NAPNES).

The National Federation of Licensed Practical Nurses was organized as the official membership organization for LP/VNs in 1949 by Lillian Kuster, who also became the Executive Director. Through the efforts of NAPNES and NFLPN the public became aware of practical nursing, its educational programs, and the licensure of practical nurses.

The issuance of the "Statement of Functions of the Licensed Practical Nurse" in 1957, as approved by the Board of Directors of both the American Nurses Association and the NFLPN, provided the impetus for an all out public awareness program. The Council on Practical Nursing was established in 1957 under the auspices of the National League for Nursing (NLN) and in 1961 became a department within the Division of Nursing Education. The NFLPN in 1962 founded the National Licensed Practical Nurses Educational Foundation for the purposes of research, awarding of scholarships, and development of continuing education programs for LP/VNs. In the late 1970s, the National League for Nursing Councils (see Chapter 8) developed, adopted, and published competency statements for graduates of various nursing education programs. The competencies of graduates of educational programs in practical nursing were finalized in 1979* and state that

Practical nursing students are prepared in educational programs that stress clinical experiences primarily in structured care settings such as hospitals and nursing homes. Clinical practice is correlated with basic therapeutic knowledge and introductory content from the biological and behavioral sciences. Planned and supervised experiences are directed toward teaching students to perform nursing measures with precision, safety, and efficiency consistent with current nursing concepts and practices. Communication skills and mental health concepts are integrated into the total curriculum. Qualified nurse educators guide students in the nursing process and care planning.

Assessing

- Contributes to the identification of basic physical, emotional, and cultural needs of the health care client.
- Identifies basic communication techniques in a structured care setting.
- Interviews health care clients to obtain specified information.
- Identifies overt learning needs of the health care client.
- Observes the health care client and communicates significant findings to the health care team.
- Identifies appropriate resources in some other agencies within the health care delivery system.

Planning

- Contributes to the development of basic nursing care plans in an institutional setting.

- Contributes, with assistance, to the development of health plans for health care clients and/or families.

* Division of Practical Nursing Programs, *Competencies of Graduates of Educational Programs in Practical Nursing* (New York: National League for Nursing, 1979).

Implementing

- Safely performs basic therapeutic and preventive nursing procedures, incorporating fundamental biological and psychological principles in giving individualized care.

- Shows respect for the dignity of individuals.
- Applies basic communication techniques in a structured care setting.
- Demonstrates the ability to do incidental teaching during routine care.
- Shares assigned responsibility for health care delivery in structured situations.

Evaluating

- Seeks guidance as needed in evaluating the care given and making necessary adjustments.
- Identifies own strengths and weaknesses and seeks assistance for improvement of performance.

Role As A Member
Within The Profession
Of Nursing

- Recognizes own role as an LPN/LVN in the health care delivery system.

- Seeks out and takes advantage of learning situations and opportunities for own continuing education.

The National League for Nursing competencies are the minimal expectations of the new graduate. Additionally, the Nurse Practice Act of each state specifies the role and functions of the LPN/LVN within the framework of nursing. Licensed practical or vocational nurses are prepared to work under the guidance of a registered nurse or licensed physician as responsible members of the health care team. They are concerned with basic therapeutic, rehabilitative, and preventive care for people of all ages and cultures in various stages of dependencies.

TO THE PRESENT TIME

Along with the increased tempo of life, politics, and sweeping social change of the 1960s and 1970s, nursing and nursing education began to experience enormous change and progress. As a result, nursing has begun to put forward a new image. No longer are nurses limited to being the "doctor's helper." In many areas of the country independent nurse practitioners are now engaged in private nursing practice or work as members of medical teams. In some areas nurse-midwives are delivering babies in hospital settings. Many nurses are now giving physical examinations and making initial patient assessments and diagnoses.

At the same time, practical nurses are facing added responsibilities every day.

With increased hospital costs and limited numbers of hospital personnel, the practical nurse has had to assume more duties than ever before. Often, the practical nurse will be making crucial decisions in moments of crisis. This is the nature of the age in which we live—we are in a time of "future shock," and change, as we know it, will continue to become increasingly rapid as it pertains to every aspect of our lives.

In the past few years research and numerous studies have been carried out to improve patient care and nursing education. Grants from official and voluntary agencies have supported various programs dealing with the changing roles of the practical and the registered nurse, problems involved in nursing care patterns, and the proper preparation and use of all nursing personnel.

In 1963, the Surgeon General's Consultant Group on Nursing determined the needs and goals of nursing. These were released in the publication, *Toward Quality in Nursing,* and still serve as an excellent reference. The Group's recommendations included (1) a study of the present system of nursing education in relation to the responsibility and the skill levels required for high-quality patient care, (2) an expansion of efforts to give financial and other assistance for recruitment in nursing and other health programs, and (3) the availability of federal funds to provide scholarships to attract and prepare more nurses in basic and advanced programs, to help offset the costs of construction and expansion for educational facilities, to promote in-service education, on-the-job training, and continuing education for nursing service personnel, and to increase research programs that improve the quality and the quantity of patient care.

Although the Congress of the United States had done much in the area of recommendations, the second and third, it was not until 1967 that an independent National Commission was appointed to do a major comprehensive study of nursing and nursing education in the United States. The National Commission for the Study of Nursing and Nursing Education (NCSNNE) published its report *An Abstract for Action** in 1970. This report was based on a two-and-one-half-year study by the Commission and its staff under the leadership of Jerome P. Lysaught, Ed.D., Director.

He concluded that nursing is of vital concern to the future of health care in America, and he summed up the paradoxes and frustrations of the nursing profession as follows:

> Yet nursing has been and is a troubled occupation. It is an occupation that fails in every characteristic to achieve the status of a full profession, despite the fact that its best practitioners are professional in every sense of that word. It is an occupation that has never controlled its own destiny, but has suffered severe consequences when it has failed to meet the demands imposed by our society. It is an occupation fraught with paradox and promise—and it holds within itself the key to whether or not the vast majority of our people will receive quality health care ... Nursing cannot continue to be the stepchild of the health professions ... Nursing must take the opportunity afforded by these recommendations, capitalize on them, and emerge as a full profession, dedicated and capable.

* Jerome Lysaught, *An Abstract for Action* (New York: McGraw-Hill, 1970), pp. 155–164.

Any less achievement will represent less than optimum health care for all Americans, in all likelihood, for generations to come. Reveille sounds not for nursing alone, but for all those who want American society to enjoy the promise of the best health care, sensitively and humanely dispensed.

In 1979, the American Nurses' Association released a "Study of Credentialing in Nursing." The report advocates the establishment of a central agency to coordinate all credentialing activities related to nursing practice and education. The objectives of this national nursing credentialing center would be to study, develop, coordinate, and provide services in the areas of accreditation, certification, registration, and licensing. This report has received much criticism, and early feedback indicates that the recommendations are very debatable.

STATUS OF WOMEN

Women in general have held a demeaning and powerless status in American society. Although not all women assumed the culturally prescribed subservient role, nurses were notorious for accepting this role and image. In 1963, the Commission on the Status of Women found that many states used laws to discriminate against women. Although the Constitution covers all persons in the due process clauses of both the fifth and 14th amendments, women were not generally included as "persons." The National Organization of Women (NOW) and other women's rights organizations were instrumental during the 1970s in creating new anti-discrimination laws. Civil rights movement groups monitored court decisions supporting the feminist position and assisted in promotion of new legislation affecting women's status. Backlash from these activities is probably the reason that the Equal Rights Amendment (ERA), passed by Congress in 1972, has not been ratified by 38 states.

Nurses must become visible in the political arena. The feminist movement is trying to raise consciousness levels and provide equal rights for all persons. This means elimination of sex discrimination practices in employment and media stereotyping of roles. It also includes working for the passage of the ERA, promoting equal job training and educational opportunities, implementing laws that would allow for child and home care expenses for working women, and providing better child care centers.

Changes must be brought about in our cultural orientation. You as a nurse must assume a leadership role both in the elimination of sexism in the delivery of health care and in the education of health care personnel. The status of women and of nurses will then be recognized.

THE FUTURE

The National Advisory Council on Vocational Education (NACVE) was established by Congress to study vocational education and advise the President, the Congress, and the U.S. Commission of Education regarding the status and needs of such programs. In March, 1979 this group unanimously adopted the following resolution:

> Whereas: The American Nurses' Association has taken position that minimum preparation for beginning professional nursing practice should be baccalaureate degree education in nursing and that all associate degree nurses should serve as professional nurses' assistants; and
>
> Whereas: There is no conclusive evidence that this proposal will result in improved health care services; and
>
> Whereas: Implementation of the position would eliminate the diploma nurse and the licensed practical nurse; and
>
> Whereas: Diploma nurse training programs, licensed practical nurse training programs and associate degree programs currently offer viable options to persons desiring a career as a nurse;
>
> Whereas: All four types of nurse training programs produce valuable members of the health care delivery system; and
>
> Whereas: Implementation of the American Nurses' Association's position would increase the cost of health care services;
>
> THEREFORE, BE IT RESOLVED: That the National Advisory Council on Vocational Education oppose the position of the American Nurses' Association and support the continuance of all four routes to a career in nursing: baccalaureate degree, associate degree, diploma, and licensure of practical nurses.

Additionally, they also moved that:

> NACVE communicate the position that it has taken, together with its background findings, to all interested parties, including the State Advisory Councils on Vocational Education, professional associations, members of Congress, state legislatures, state attorney generals and others.

It is felt that this is the type of action that is needed and it must be communicated to health care consumers and state and national legislators. Many feel that the opposition to the ANA 1985 proposal should be voiced and demonstrated. Furthermore, the public must be educated so that the impact of the proposal is understood. This is the challenge in the early 1980s to licensed practical and vocational nurses. You are a vital part of the total health care team. The American Association of Community and Junior Colleges, American Health Care Association, American Vocational Association, National Association for Practical Nurse Education and Services, National League for Nurses, and others are opposed to ANA's position and will support you.

You are advised to unite your organizations, increase your membership, support lobbyists on state and federal levels, and prove that your patient care contributions do *make the difference* in the delivery of health care. Demonstrate that LPNs are caring nurses who give quality care with only one year of basic educational preparation and, therefore, are cost-effective and valuable contributors in meeting the health care needs of our country.

Some of you may wish to enroll in career ladder transition programs and become registered nurses (see Chapter 9). Many of the graduate practical nurses I taught at Mt. Sinai Medical Center, Miami Beach continued their education and became registered nurses. Some of them earned baccalaureate, master, and doctorate degrees. However, the great majority of practical nurses should remain at the patient's side giving quality care. That is where the need is greatest and where most LPNs gain personal satisfaction. It is important that you are happy in your chosen career—be a happy and contended LPN, not a frustrated RN.

Your destiny as a practical or vocational nurse is in your hands. Become an advocate not only for quality patient care but also for yourself. Be involved in your organization and community. Know the political climate and get to know the politicians on an individual basis. Your destiny will then become secure.

Questions

A. Complete the following statements.
   1. The "Father of Medicine" was _____
   2. Florence Nightingale was born on (date) _____
   3. The American Red Cross was organized by _____
   4. The first trained nurse in the United States was _____
   5. Dorothea Dix improved the treatment for _____
   6. Lillian Wald founded the _____
   7. The Ballard School was established in (year) _____
   8. A founder and Executive Director of NAPNES was _____
   9. Lillian Kuster founded the _____
  10. The "Lady with the Lamp" was _____

B. Select the *one* correct expression that will complete the sentence, and place the letter in the answer space.
   1. The first visiting nurse was (A) St. Francis, (B) Fabiola, (C) Phoebe, (D) St. Catherine.   ____
   2. Church hospitals were founded during (A) the Early Christian Era, (B) the Dark Ages, (C) the Medieval period, (D) the Renaissance   ____
   3. The "Father of Modern Aseptic Surgery" was (A) Dunant, (B) Blackwell, (C) Fliedner, (D) Lister.   ____
   4. Florence Nightingale studied nursing (A) at Kaiserswerth, (B) in England, (C) in Italy, (D) at Hôtel Dieu (Lyons).   ____
   5. One of the first Practical Nursing Schools in the United States was (A) Bolton, (B) Henry Street, (C) Thompson, (D) Torrop.   ____
   6. The National Commission for the Study of Nursing and Nursing Education was directed by (A) Mildred Montag, (B) Lillian Kuster, (C) Jerome Lysaught, (D) John Howard.   ____
   7. "An Abstract for Action" is the report of the (A) NCSNNE, (B) NAPNES, (C) NFLPN, (D) NLN.   ____
   8. The official membership organization for licensed practical nurses is (A) NAPNES, (B) NFLPN, (C) NLN, (D) NLPVNO.   ____
   9. The "Technical Nurse" Program was founded by (A) Lillian Wald, (B) Hilda Torrop, (C) Mildred Montag, (D) Lillian Kuster.   ____

10. The newest, up-to-date report on nursing is (A) ''Toward Quality in Nursing,'' (B) ''Surgeon General's Report,'' (C) ''An Abstract for Action,'' (D) ''Study of Credentialing in Nursing''.   ____

Answers (5 points each)

A. Completion
1. Hippocrates
2. May 12, 1820
3. Clara Barton
4. Linda Richards
5. the insane
6. Henry Street Settlement
7. 1893
8. Hilda Torrop
9. National Federation of Licensed Practical Nurses
10. Florence Nightingale

B. Multiple Choice
1. C
2. B
3. D
4. A
5. C
6. C
7. A
8. B
9. C
10. D

3

The Nursing Team

Nursing Defined • The Team Members • Other Nursing Personnel • Nursing Care Patterns • Questions and Answers

Objectives

On the completion of this chapter you should be able to

1. define nursing
2. identify and compare the various types of nursing education programs
3. describe the role and functions of the members of the nursing team
4. summarize NFLPN's "Nursing Practice Standards for Licensed Practical Nurse"
5. interpret the different nursing care patterns

NURSING DEFINED

The meaning of nursing is simple. To define the *scope* of nursing is more difficult. Many nursing educators have attempted to do so, and perhaps the simple dictionary phrases, "to care, cherish, support, nourish, foster, bring up," and so forth are as definitive as the more formal ones. Nursing implies helping people who cannot help themselves. Although you may think of nursing only in connection with the care of the sick and the disabled, modern nursing also includes the prevention of illness in the hospital and the community, health education, rehabilitation, and many other areas in which patient needs are met.

In *Guides for Developing Curricula for the Education of Practical Nurses*, published by the Office of Education, Department of Health, Education, and Welfare, nursing is discussed as follows:

> Nursing is practiced in its primitive form whenever one person helps another to meet daily needs for personal care when the person assisted can no longer care for himself because of some physical or mental incapacity. The initial and continuing development of nursing and the continued spread of nursing practice rests on the inabilities of people to care for themselves at times when they need assistance because of their state of personal health. Assistance as used here means assistance in the activities of daily living which is special, and not in the common pattern of

the life of the individual. For example, many adults have their meals prepared for them by other persons, but only when there is personal incapacity does an adult need to be fed by another.

Nursing is perhaps best described as the giving of direct assistance to a person, as required, because of the person's specific inabilities in self-care resulting from a situation of personal health. Care as required may be continuous or periodic. Self-care means the care which all persons require each day. It is the personal care which adults give to themselves, including attention to ordinary health requirements, and the following of the medical directives of their physicians. Nursing may be required by persons in any age group, but it is the situation of health and not the dependencies arising from age which initiates requirements for nursing. Requirements for nursing are modified and eventually eliminated when there is progressive favorable change in the state of health of the individual, or when he learns to be self-directing in daily self-care. . . .

The most common description of nursing is "an art and a science." It is not a pure science—the pursuit of knowledge for its own sake—in the sense that physiology, chemistry, or physics is, but rather it draws from these sciences' facts and laws and applies them for immediately practical reasons. In the application is the art. Art is the knack of drawing on principles and technics from many sources to create something that by general agreement has excellence. Sculptors draw on their knowledge of materials as well as on the science of anatomy. Painters use these and, in addition, their scientific knowledge of color. What artists do with this knowledge is their art. The same principle applies to nurses. They study social science, for instance, because it will help them to develop the supreme art of creating a constructive, helpful human relationship with patients.

Nursing is a delicate combination of many fields, achieved by blending the physical, biological, social, psychological, and medical sciences with "nursing arts," so that the technics of the nurse are exercised in the best manner possible to render patient care. In addition to technics, the art of getting along and working with people—patients, coworkers, fellow students, and others—will be given equal importance.

Because of scientific advances and discoveries, today's nurse must continually learn new procedures that will be used as technical tools in the practice of nursing. However, the mechanical aspects of these methods should never interfere with the establishment of harmonious relationships with patients. Professional nursing emphasizes the importance of good human relations on the premise that nursing care is a service to mankind; therefore, it is the *spirit* in which the nurse renders patient care that really counts.

Good nursing, as it applies in almost any setting, is a personal service to a patient, tailored to the individual personality, specific illness, and general physical condition. In meeting these nursing needs there are three main principles to consider. The first deals with recognizing the patient as an individual with a unique personality pattern and personal problems. The second pertains to maintaining body functions, and the third stresses the importance of protection against illness or accident. Therefore, nursing implies not only the care of the sick but also the prevention of illness and the promotion of health.

The nursing needs of patients may require anything from simple nursing measures to a high degree of diversified scientific knowledge. Usually, they include

1. Establishing good rapport (harmonious relationships) with the patient, family, and friends, and with the members of the health team who are concerned with giving care.

2. Observing, recording, and reporting facts of the patient's physical and emotional state that would have significance in the diagnosis and treatment of the illness.

3. Assisting the patient in meeting normal physical needs, such as eating, personal hygiene, and so forth (activities of daily living).

4. Preparing the equipment required for treatment, and assisting the physician with all necessary treatments and tests.

5. Giving all nursing treatments and medications as prescribed by the physician and observing the patient for reactions to them.

6. Protecting the patient from infections, accidents, and other health hazards.

7. Assisting in providing a pleasant and clean environment to help the patient feel secure and comfortable.

8. Teaching the patient health maintenance and independence, as much as is possible.

9. Helping the patient adjust to any limitations that may be the result of illness, by personal assistance or referral to community agencies.

10. Meeting any unforeseen circumstances or emergency situations promptly, calmly, and intelligently.

From the foregoing list you can readily see that although a short definition of nursing is easily stated, the implications of the term are almost endless. There are many occupational divisions within nursing; it is a career with room for individuals who have very different educational preparation, interests, and abilities. Yet all who choose it feel that they can contribute in some fashion to improving the health of the nation. Also, they know they will have the satisfaction of being vitally needed.

THE TEAM MEMBERS

In the last decade the education, functions, and composition of nursing personnel in hospitals and other health and welfare agencies have undergone profound changes in order to keep pace with many new demands. Scientific and medical advances, changes in medical practices, increases in the number of hospital admissions, greater patient expectations, shorter hospital stays, and the complexity of nursing care performed are all contributing factors. Although the supply of nurses is steadily growing, a shortage still exists, and the use of nonprofessional personnel is becoming more widespread.

The ratio of nurses to population varies widely throughout the United States, with the New England states having the highest ratio of both registered and practical nurses. It is estimated that about one half of all registered nurses (RNs) and three quarters of all recent graduate practical nurses are employed in general hospitals. At the present time there are more than 961,000 RNs, 489,000 practical nurses, and one million aides and orderlies employed. Even though the number of hospital nursing employees is increasing constantly, the need for professional nurses will continue to grow. Therefore, the proper use of the practical nurse is of great concern today.

Today nursing service includes both professional and nonprofessional nursing personnel—registered and practical nurses, aides and orderlies, receptionists and nursing clerks, and sometimes even floor (unit) managers who render direct and indirect patient care. Through various educational programs, particularly those for the practical nurse, the supply of better-prepared nonprofessional nursing personnel is increasing constantly.

The following appears in *Opportunities for Education in Nursing, a Statement on Nursing Education,* distributed by the National League for Nursing, Inc.:

> Nursing as an educational subject can be developed on different levels with proportionate foundations. The range of levels extends all the way from that adapted to short inservice training of auxiliary personnel to that appropriate for graduate professional education leading to a doctoral degree, based upon and including breadth and depth of scientific knowledge and humanistic understanding.
>
> Various types of educational programs are needed to attract diverse groups and prepare them for usefulness and satisfaction in nursing roles suited to each. . . .
>
> The educational programs now available in the field offer a variety and range of opportunities adapted to: this diversity of interests and needs among potential nursing students; this wide range of needed functions, educational possibilities, and career opportunities in nursing; and this extensive need of society for nursing services.
>
> The opportunities for education in nursing are therefore now similar to those provided by the general system of American education which has evolved over the years to meet similar needs of students, occupations, and society. They include:
>
> 1. Basic programs that prepare new candidates for beginning practice as licensed practical nurses or registered nurses
>
> 2. Programs that provide the means for registered nurses previously graduated from diploma or associate degree programs to obtain senior college or university preparation for the field
>
> 3. Programs in nursing on the graduate level that prepare for advanced functions

Since this statement was issued, career ladder programs have been introduced at both the community college and university levels. In these programs the nurse aide, practical nurse, or ADN/diploma graduate may enroll at present experience level in a program that will lead to a higher degree. Thus, a graduate nurse can enter a career ladder program and, if qualified, can graduate from an ADN program within one year or more. The ADN/diploma graduate may enroll in a baccalaureate program and graduate with a BSN degree (Fig. 3-1).

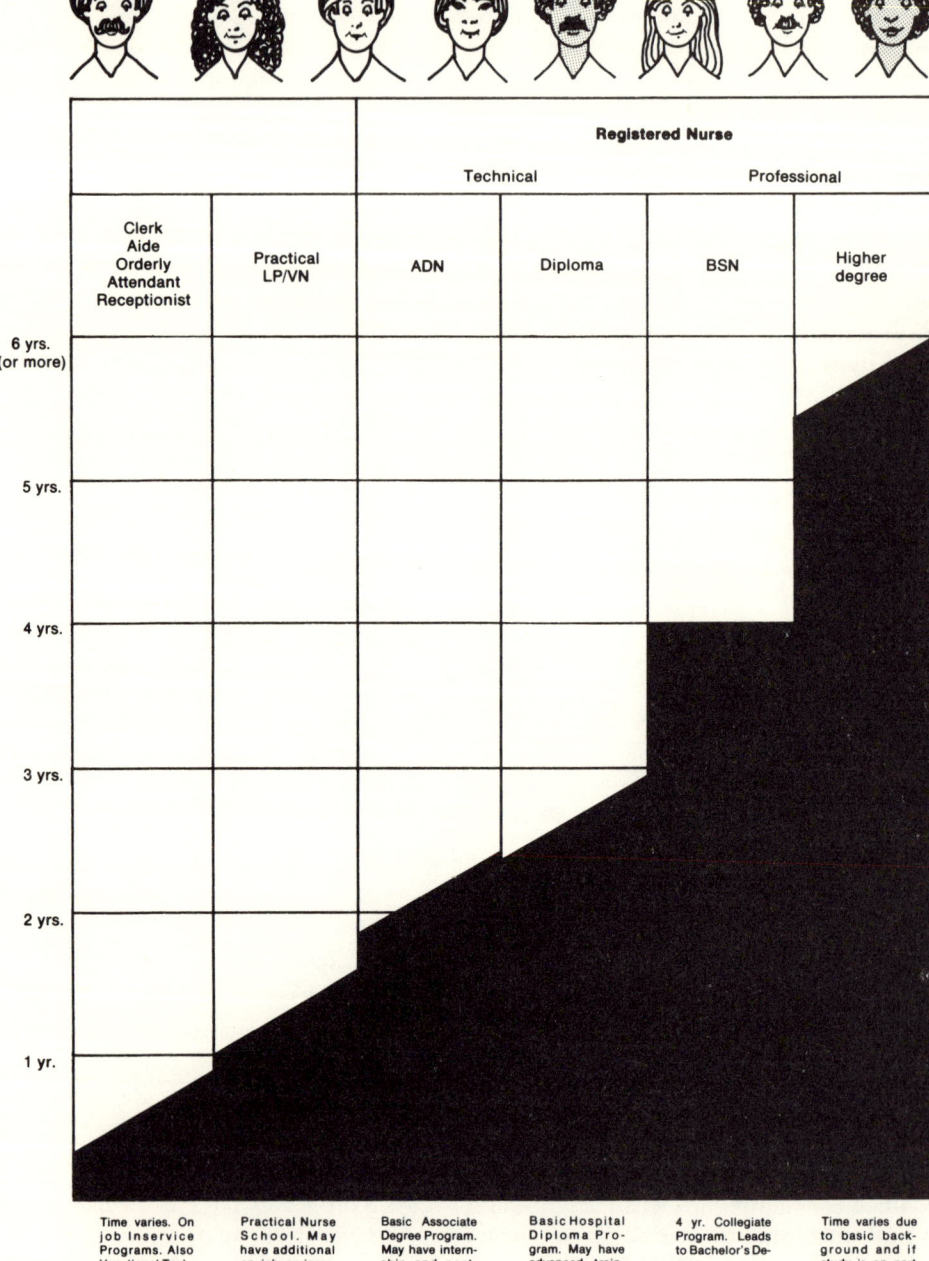

		Registered Nurse			
		Technical		Professional	
Clerk Aide Orderly Attendant Receptionist	Practical LP/VN	ADN	Diploma	BSN	Higher degree
Time varies. On job Inservice Programs. Also Vocational Technical courses and programs.	Practical Nurse School. May have additional on job or inservice, extension, and postgraduate education.	Basic Associate Degree Program. May have internship and postgraduate education.	Basic Hospital Diploma Program. May have advanced training and postgraduate education.	4 yr. Collegiate Program. Leads to Bachelor's Degree.	Time varies due to basic background and if study is on part of full time basis. Leads to Master's and Doctorate degree.

y-axis labels: 6 yrs. (or more), 5 yrs., 4 yrs., 3 yrs., 2 yrs., 1 yr.

FIGURE 3-1. *Nursing Personnel Educational Preparation.*

Nursing Enrollments

Nursing education statistics are shown in Tables 3-1 and 3-2. Baccalaureate and associate degree programs are growing in number, whereas diploma and practical nurse programs are declining, reflecting a gradual movement of nursing education into institutions of higher learning.

To be eligible to take a licensure examination, the applicant must be a graduate of a state-approved school of nursing. Additionally, many schools of nursing are accredited by the National League for Nursing, with new programs being accredited annually. The League is recognized as the national accrediting agency for masters, baccalaureate, and associate degree nursing programs by the National Commission on Accrediting and is additionally certified as an accrediting source for masters, baccalaureate, associate degree, diploma, and practical nursing programs by the U.S. Office of Education.

Men in Nursing

In 1978, 6,383 men were admitted to basic programs preparing RNs; this is about 6.3% of all admissions to these programs. During this time, 2,365 men were admitted to practical or vocational programs, representing 4.5% of all admissions. It was also reported that 3,902 men graduated from the RN basic programs, whereas 1,395 men graduated from the practical nursing programs. Various position papers by nursing organizations such as the National League for Nursing emphasize the importance of recruiting members of minorities, and specifically men, into the nursing programs.

The Registered Nurse

The more you know about registered nursing, the better able you will be to understand your own field of practical nursing and to compare them in terms of similarities as well as differences.

The American Nurses' Association defines an RN as "one who has met all legal requirements for registration in a state, and who may practice nursing by virtue of her technical knowledge and practical ability." The RN may have had anywhere from two to four years or more of education, as will be discussed later.

The following definition of a technical nurse was approved in 1967 by the NLN Division of Member Agencies, Council of Associate Degree Programs:

> A registered nurse with an associate degree in nursing licensed for the practice of nursing who carries out nursing and other therapeutic measures with a high degree of skill, using principles from an ever-expanding body of science. The technical nurse performs nursing functions with patients who are under the supervision of a physician and/or a professsional nurse and assists in planning the day-to-day care of patients: evaluating the patient's physical and emotional reactions to therapy, taking measures to alleviate distress, using treatment modalities with knowledge and precision, and supervising other workers in the technical aspects of care.

TABLE 3–1. NURSING EDUCATION STATISTICS—1979

Type of Program	Number of Programs	Admissions*	Graduation*
Practical	1,318	57,953	45,066
Associate degree	688	54,131	36,763
Diploma	333	18,499	15,820
Baccalaureate	368	36,087	25,349
Total Basic RN Programs	1,389	108,717	77,932

*Academic year 1978–1979.

TABLE 3–2. NUMBERS OF REGISTERED NURSING AND PRACTICAL OR VOCATIONAL NURSING PROGRAMS, 1968–1979

Academic Year	Associate Degree	Diploma	Baccalaureate Degree	Total Basic RN Programs	Practical or Vocational	Grand Total
1968	330	728	235	1,293	1,191	2,484
1970	444	641	270	1,355	1,253	2,608
1972	541	543	293	1,377	1,310	2,687
1974	598	461	313	1,372	1,315	2,687
1976	642	390	341	1,373	1,339	2,712
1978	677	344	353	1,374	1,329	2,703
1979	688	333	368	1,389	1,318	2,707

You will note that the term RN indicates the passing of the same licensure examination as professional nurses. However, under the American Nurses' Association's newer concepts, the RN—a graduate of an associate degree or diploma program—would, therefore, not be considered professional. However, until State Boards of Nursing have separate licensure examinations or credentials for graduates of different RN programs (associate, diploma, baccalaureate), the terms "professional" and "registered" nurse will be used by most people as meaning a graduate of any one of the three programs who has passed the licensure examination and is, therefore, *registered* to practice professional and/or technical nursing.

The ANA, State and Territorial Boards of Nursing, and other groups are deliberating the implications of licensure, titles, and credentialing, not only of nurses but also of other health-related personnel.

RN Education

In 1873, nursing schools, patterned after the Nightingale School in London, began to be established in the United States. The early schools offered approximately one year of training, but with scientific progress the programs increased in scope and length, so that by the early part of the 20th century the three-year course was the generally accepted one. Today there are 1,389 state-approved schools of registered nursing in the United States, admitting 108,717 students yearly into three distinct programs, from which there are 77,932 graduates yearly. Regardless of the type of program, the graduate nurse must take the State Board or licensure examination, and upon passing it, will obtain a license and will then have the legal title of RN.

Basic Programs.   Basic education programs for the registered nurse are found in junior or community colleges, in which a two-year program usually leads to an associate degree; in the hospital or diploma program, which is two to three years in length; and in the senior college or university program, which leads to a baccalaureate degree after four years of study and experience. Although each program has its distinctive purposes and features, they all prepare the student for the licensure examination.

The *associate degree program* (the newest program in nursing education) prepares graduates to give patient care in various nursing positions. Graduate ADNs have a scientific background; they have gained an understanding of human behavior and have been given selected, well-supervised hospital patient-care experiences. Some go on to finish their college work while working either full-time or part-time, and others in ADN baccalaureate ladder programs finish while still in school. The junior college programs are becoming more and more popular. There are 688 of these programs in existence.

The *diploma program* is conducted in and controlled by a hospital. This program serves the interests and the needs of qualified high school graduates who desire an educational experience that is centered in a hospital and, therefore, will give them an early and continuing opportunity to be with patients. Instruction and experience are available in all areas of hospital nursing and usually include liberal experience with medical and surgical patients, obstetrics and pediatrics, certain communicable diseases, psychiatric nursing, and other specialties.

There are approximately 330 of these programs in the United States. The hospital-based diploma programs are declining in number. This has been attributed to the rapid development of the associate degree programs and the ANA's *Position Paper on Education for Nursing*. The American Hospital Association and the National League for Nursing have officially gone on record as supporting the diploma hospital schools. Many of these programs have adjusted their curriculum to include junior college courses and have reduced the traditional three-year program to 30 months or less.

Graduates of these programs usually are skillful in planning and rendering patient care, with the knowledge and the ability to become primary nurses or team leaders. They advance quickly in the hospital setting; many of them later attend colleges and universities, either part-time or full-time, in order to obtain their degrees.

College or *university programs* offering bachelor of science in nursing degrees give an opportunity to those nursing students who prefer a collegiate atmosphere, since the student nurse becomes an integral part of the student body. The program is organized into four years or more of college, and the courses in nursing are usually offered after the sciences, the humanities, and other subjects are mastered, most often after one or two years. The completion of the college program prepares the graduate to give skillful nursing care in various hospital or community settings.

In view of the educational background required, the BSN graduate should be able to interpret and to understand patients' needs better than graduate nurses of shorter programs. Therefore, besides being eligible for the usual first-level positions available, the baccalaureate graduate can also enter the field of community health nursing. Many of these graduates go on to advanced study leading to a master's degree for teaching, supervision, and administration, on either a part-time or a full-time basis. Over 365 colleges and universities conduct baccalaureate programs.

Graduate or Advanced Education. Postgraduate education for RNs who have graduated from basic programs (other than a baccalaureate program) and want to add a college degree to their RN, is available in many colleges and universities. Qualifications for this degree will depend on the school. The content and the quality of the individual's preparation will be compared with the educational background required. Courses leading to the baccalaureate degree are drawn from the sciences, the humanities, the arts, and other contributing fields, so that the nurse with a degree will be well versed in a number of areas.

Once the baccalaureate degree (usually a BSN) is earned, graduates continue in nursing education, first on the master's level (MSN, MA, MS) and later on the doctoral degree level (PhD, EdD, DNSc). This advanced study permits the nurse to engage in systematic study concentrating on some field of interest in nursing, such as obstetric and pediatric nursing, medical and surgical nursing, teaching, supervision, administration, or others, either separately or in combination. Solid foundations are built in the selected area, both in theory and practice, before the degree is awarded. Graduates of these programs usually function as clinical specialists, instructors, administrators, and independent nurse practitioners.

The Nurse Practitioner (NP)

Although the term "nurse practitioner" was first used in a demonstration project at the University of Colorado in 1965, there still is no uniformity in the educational preparation of this nurse. Various states have adopted rules and regulations defining the scope and practice of the nurse practitioner and some have used terms such as advanced registered nurse practitioner (ARNP) and registered nurse practitioner (RNP). It is recommended, to ensure competence and quality care, that NPs hold a master's degree in nursing. This is advocated primarily because the NP role is highly autonomous, whether inside or outside of institutions. This autonomy requires a great deal of independent decision making and accountability. NPs should be able to give comprehensive health care, in some instances through collaboration with physicians, and in other instances independently.

NPs and other nurses may be reimbursed for their services through certified rural health clinics under the Rural Health Clinics Act of 1977.

The Practical Nurse

Various sources have placed the number of employed licensed practical nurses (LPNs) in the nation around 500,000. The majority of practical nurses are employed in hospitals, and more and more licensed, graduate practical nurses are entering the fields of industrial, public health, office, and institutional nursing. In the past 15 years there has been expansion and improvement in practical nursing programs, as well as a better use of the practical nurse.

The role of the practical nurse has been defined and redefined and is constantly being revised, so that today opinions vary widely as to the types of duties to be performed. Perhaps the best way to assess the qualifications of the practical nurse is to consider the great differences in background still permissible. There are trained as well as untrained practical nurses. There are those who have had sound experience and received their licenses by waiver (the state allows experience to substitute for the usual education for licensure; it "waives" these formal requirements) but have had no training or supervised experience except possibly on a very limited home-nursing basis. Then, too, there are some LPNs who have had good extension courses, in-service or on-the-job education, and nursing care supervision. To summarize the practical nursing picture, one might say that both the quality and the quantity of educational background and experience vary with the individual. If you are a student or a recent graduate from an approved practical nursing school, you will realize that educational programs differ widely, and even your job responsibilities after graduation will vary from one institution to another. However, do not be disturbed by this, because it is a part of the dynamic growth and change that characterizes the vocation; and in the not-too-distant future no doubt there will be more uniformity in the educational requirements of practical nurses, with universal recognition of their abilities.

Practical Nurse Standards

An important step that helped to clarify the duties of the LPN was the *Statement of Functions of the Licensed Practical Nurse,* which was prepared by the Executive Board of the National Federation of Licensed Practical Nurses in June, 1970, and revised in April, 1972. However, in October, 1979, the NFLPN House of Delegates adopted the following landmark statement on the practice of practical nursing.*

Preface

The Standards replace the "Statement of Functions and Qualifications" as approved by the Executive Board of the National Federation of Licensed Practical Nurses in June 1970 and revised in April 1972 and were developed and adopted by the NFLPN to provide a basic model whereby the quality of health service and nursing care given by LP/VNs may be measured and evaluated.

These nursing practice standards are applicable in any practice setting. The degree to which individual standards are applied will vary according to the individual needs of the patient, the type of health care agency or services and the community resources.

The scope of practice of licensed practical nursing has extended into specialized nursing services. Therefore, specialized fields of nursing are included in this document.

* National Federation of Licensed Practical Nurses (NFLPN), *The Journal of Nursing Care* (Westport, Conn.: Technomic Publications, Inc., 1979).

INTRODUCTORY STATEMENT

Practical/vocational nursing means the performance for compensation of authorized acts of nursing which utilize specialized knowledge and skills and which meet the health needs of people in a variety of settings under the direction of qualified health professionals.

Scope

Practical/vocational nursing comprises the common core of nursing and therefore is a valid entry into the nursing profession.

Opportunities exist for practicing in a milieu where different professions unite their particular skills in a team effort for one common objective—to preserve or improve an individual patient's functioning.

Opportunities also exist for upward mobility within the nursing profession through formal education and lateral expansion of knowledge and expertise through both formal and informal education.

STANDARDS

Licensed Practical/Vocational Nurses
should adhere to the following Standards

Education

1. Shall complete a formal education program in practical nursing approved by the appropriate nursing authority in a state.
2. Shall participate in initial orientation within the employing institution.

Legal/Ethical Status

1. Shall hold a current license to practice nursing as an LP/VN in accordance with the law of the state wherein employed.
2. Shall know the scope of nursing practice authorized by the Nurse Practice Act in the state wherein employed.
3. Shall have a personal commitment to fulfill the legal responsibilities inherent in good nursing practice.
4. Shall take responsible actions in situations wherein there is unprofessional conduct by a health care provider.
5. Shall recognize and have a commitment to meet the ethical and moral obligations of the practice of nursing.

Practice

1. Shall accept assigned responsibilities as an accountable member of the health care team.
2. Shall function within the limits of educational preparation and experience as related to the assigned duties.
3. Shall function with other members of the health care team in promoting and maintaining health, preventing disease and disability, caring for and rehabilitating individuals who are experiencing altered health state.
4. Shall know and utilize the nursing process in planning, implementing, and evaluating health services and nursing care to the individual patient or group.
   a. Planning: The planning of nursing includes:
      - assessment of health status of the individual patient, the family and community groups

- an analysis of the information gained from assessment
- the identification of health goals

b. Implementation: The plan for nursing care is implemented to achieve the stated goals:

  - observing, recording and reporting significant changes which require intervention or different goals
  - applying of nursing knowledge and skills to promote and maintain health, to prevent disease and disability and to optimize functional capabilities of an individual patient
  - assisting the patient and family with activities of daily living and encouraging self-care as appropriate
  - carrying out therapeutic regimens prescribed by a physician or other authorized health care providers

c. Evaluation: The plan for nursing care and its implementation are evaluated to measure the progress toward the stated goals and will include appropriate persons and/or groups to determine:

  - the relevancy of current goals in relation to the progress of the individual patient, the family and community
  - the involvement of the recipients of care in the evaluation process
  - the quality of the nursing action in the implementation of the plan
  - a re-ordering of priorities or new goal setting in the care plan

5. Shall participate in peer review and other evaluative processes.
6. Shall participate in the development of policies concerning the health and nursing needs of society and in the roles and functions of the LP/VN.

Continuing Education

1. Shall be responsible for maintaining the highest possible level of professional competence at all times.
2. Shall periodically reassess career goals and select continuing education activities which will help to achieve these goals.
3. Shall take advantage of continuing education opportunities which will lead to personal growth and professional development including: reading new publications and periodicals; self-study programs; membership in their professional organization; seminars and community health activities.
4. Shall seek and participate in formal continuing education activities which are measurable such as the nationally accepted and recognized CEU.

Specialized Nursing Practice

1. Shall have had at least one year's experience in general nursing at the staff level.
2. Shall present personal qualifications that are indicative of potential abilities for practice in the chosen specialized nursing area.
3. Shall present evidence of completion of a program or course that is approved by an appropriate agency to provide the knowledge and skills necessary for effective nursing services in the specialized field.
4. Shall meet all of the standards of practice as set forth in this document.

Glossary

Authorized (Acts of Nursing)—Legalized through State Nurse Practice Acts

CEU*—One continuing education unit is defined as: "Ten contact hours of participation in an organized continuing education experience under responsible sponsorship, capable direction and qualified instruction and which is of sufficient merit to be documented in permanent form on the record of the individual participant."**

Continuing Education—The updating and upgrading of knowledge and skills following graduation from a basic education program

Health Care Professionals—Persons with specialized education and experience who perform a variety of functions related to total health care

Lateral Expansion of Knowledge—Extension of the basic core of information learned in the school of practical nursing

Peer Review—Evaluation of performance on the job by other LP/VNs

Specialized Nursing Practice—A restricted field of nursing in which a person is particularly skilled and has specific knowledge

Therapeutic Regimens—Regulated plans designed to bring about effective treatment of disease

Upward Mobility—Change of career goal, e.g. Licensed Practical/Vocational Nurse to Registered Nurse

LP/VN—The LPN is the same as the LVN in California and Texas

Milieu—Environment and surroundings

The *Nursing Practice Standards* can be interpreted very broadly; therefore, we have listed some of the skills that may be part of your responsibilities. See which procedures you would need more experience in, and ask your charge nurse or a faculty member to help you to perfect those that your hospital considers to be your responsibility. Remember that this list is only an approximate one. There is a tendency for functions to change, and, therefore, so will this list. Remember also that the institution controls the functions of its staff in relation to the degree of illness of the patient. Under certain circumstances only a doctor will change a dressing; under others, a practical nurse may change the dressing.

Admission and discharge of patient	Catheterization
Aerosol inhalation	Charting
Apical-radial pulse	Colonic irrigation
Bandaging	Colostomy care and irrigation
Baths—bed, tub, sitz, medicated, and so forth	Comfort measures
	Crutch gaits
Bedpan—giving and removing	Dental and denture care
Binders—all types	Doctors' orders—processing
Bladder instillation	Drainage collection
Bladder irrigation	Dressings—all types
Blood pressure	Ear instillation
Blood transfusion—assist	Ear irrigation—assist

* Quoted from "The Continuing Education Unit—Criteria and Guidelines" prepared by the National Council on the Continuing Education Unit.

** NFLPN keeps records for LP/VNs in a computerized data bank.

Electric pad and cradle
Enemas—all types
Eye instillation
Eye irrigations—assist
Feeding patients
Fetal heart beat
Gastric gavage
Gastric lavage
Hair care, shampoo, pediculosis treatment
Heat lamp
Hot-water-bag application
Hypodermoclysis—assist
Icecap and collar application
Intake and output—recording and measuring
Intravenous infusion—assist
Lumbar puncture—assist
Medications—all except intravenous therapy
Mouth care
Moving patient
Nose instillation
Nose irrigation—assist
Nursing care plan
Ordering supplies
Orthopedic care and appliances
Oxygen therapy
Paracentesis—assist
Perineal care

Physical examination—assist
Positioning patient
Postmortem care
Postoperative care
Precaution (isolation) technic
Preoperative care—complete
Preps—surgical, obstetrical
Pulse rate
Respiration rate
Restraints
Rotating tourniquet
Side rails
Slings
Soaks
Specimen collections—all types
Sponge bath
Steam inhalations
Sugar and acetone (ketone) urine test
Suture removal—assist
Temperature rate
Terminal care of unit
Thoracentesis—assist
Throat irrigation
Tracheostomy care
Transfer of patient
Urinal—giving and removing
Vaginal douche
Vaginal instillation
Weighing of patient

Over the years the roles of the RN and practical nurse have been changing. The rapid advances in scientific knowledge and technology, increased consumer demands, greater availability of health personnel, and innovations in the care of patients have magnified the need for change in nursing practice. Legally, you as a practical nurse, are responsible for what you do or do not do in the care of your patients. However, under certain circumstances you may be asked to perform duties beyond your normal ones. Ask yourself—is this safe for and in the best interest of the patient? Have I been adequately taught this function and judged to be competent in performing this skill? Will I be supported by the RNs and physicians if I perform this function? Do I have their consultation readily available? If you answer "yes" to all these questions, let your conscience be your guide! (See Chapter 7, Negligence and Malpractice.)

Practical Nurse Education

Practical nurse programs grew rapidly from their beginning in the 1890s, not only in numbers but also in quality and scope. In the 1940s there were about 50 approved programs. With the organization of the practical nursing associations, the efforts of the National Association for Practical Nurse Education and Services, Inc., as well as the interest of the U.S. Office of Education, standardization began to appear in the practical nurse curriculum. The tremendous need for these schools, as well as the availability of governmental and private funds to establish them, helped to increase their number, so that by 1955 there were almost 400 approved programs. About 15,000 students entered these programs annually, and about 10,000 of these graduated a year later.

In 1956, Public Law 911, passed by Congress and signed by President Eisenhower, was directed toward the improvement and the expansion of practical nurse training, and a sum of several million dollars was appropriated for this purpose. Under the supervision of the Assistant Commissioner for Vocational Education of the Office of Education, this sum was allocated to local Boards of Education. Vocational schools of practical nursing were enlarged, new ones were started, and in addition, a practical nurse education service was established in the Office of Education by the Department of Health, Education, and Welfare. Professional staff members made field visits and conducted and participated in workshops, conferences, and consultations, and new programs were developed, with the cooperation and the interest of the state.

The rate of training practical nurses increased rapidly in subsequent years under the impetus of federal assistance. About five million dollars a year was authorized under the George-Barden Act on a dollar-to-dollar state matching grant. Additional aid became available under the Manpower Development and Training Act (MDTA) of 1962, which established a program of training unemployed and underemployed men and women to meet present and future manpower shortages. Practical nursing programs have demonstrated their cost effectiveness and are continuing to improve the quality of the graduates they prepare. They reached an all-time high of 1,337 programs in 1976.

Basic Program.   Today there are more than 1,315 state-approved programs. In 1978–1979, 57,953 students were admitted in the one-year basic program that combines classroom work with supervised hospital experience. These programs are conducted in public schools, in which they are part of the vocational school or adult education programs; in private schools, under the auspices of hospitals or other community agencies; or in junior or community colleges and universities.

The programs usually include courses in or exposure to body structure and function, general psychology, microbiology, basic nursing, medical/surgical nursing of adults and children, maternity nursing, personal and vocational relationships, nutrition, pharmacology, mental health nursing, and geriatrics. The supervised experience includes patient care in medical/surgical, pediatric, and maternity nursing and may include specialties such as labor and delivery, nursery, operating and recovery rooms, as well as other areas—emergency, "cast" and minor surgery rooms, central service, the outpatient department, and occasionally, psychiatric nursing. The program content and experience may vary with each school and the facilities available; however, owing to state and national accreditation agencies, uniformity in the basic program is being achieved.

The entire program usually lasts one calendar year and is divided into two phases. The foundation period, often called the preclinical area, covers the first four months, more or less, of basic teaching and is conducted primarily in the classroom setting. The clinical phase, referred to as the experience period, covers the remainder of the 12 months and consists mostly of closely supervised hospital experience, with some classroom work. There are also vacations, holidays and, an ill-time allowance—as permitted by the state-approving agencies. All programs must meet the approval of the State Boards of Nursing, so that the graduate becomes eligible to take the licensure examination, which, when passed successfully, enables one to be called an LP/VN. In addition, many programs are approved at the national level by the National Association for Practical Nurse Education and Service, Inc., and the National League for Nursing.

Extension Programs.   The LP/VN who has not graduated from an accredited program but became licensed on the basis of experience has an excellent opportunity to be brought up to date on trends of nursing care by attending extension courses sponsored by vocational schools, community colleges, LPN organizations (NFLPN), or through the National Association for Practical Nurse Education and Service.

Continuing Education.   LP/VNs may continue their education by investigating courses in topics, leadership, medications, communications, psychology, and the many other courses, or programs sponsored by NAPNES, NFLPN, junior colleges, and vocational/technical schools. Courses taken under junior college auspices often offer college credit, and you are urged to investigate the opportunities for you to continue your education and perhaps become an RN. Many qualified and interested practical nurses have enrolled in these career ladder or transition programs and have become RNs. The NLN Board of Directors in support of these programs issued the following statement in 1970:

> An open curriculum in nursing education is a system which takes into account the different purposes of the various types of programs but recognizes common areas of achievement. Such a system permits student mobility in the light of ability, changing career goals, and changing aspirations. It also requires clear delineation of the achievement expectations of nursing programs, from practical nursing through graduate education. It recognizes the possibility of mobility from other health related fields. It is an interrelated system of achievement in nursing education with open doors rather than quantitive serial steps.

> The National League for Nursing believes that:

>> Individuals who wish to change career goals should have the opportunity to do so.

>> Educational opportunities should be provided for those who are interested in upward mobility without lowering standards.

>> In any type of nursing program opportunity should be provided to validate previous education and experience.

Sound educational plans must be developed to avoid unsound projects and programs.

More effective guidance is urgently needed at all stages of student development.

If projects and endeavors in this area are to be successful, nursing must accept the above concept of the open curriculum.

There are various ways to receive some credit for your past knowledge, education, and skill. See Chapter 9, Continuing Your Education, for further information.

Legal Title

A currently licensed practical nurse may use the letters LPN after his or her name. In Texas and California the term licensed vocational nurse is used, and the initials LVN are legally accepted. In many schools the student practical nurses will be asked to use SPN after their names to indicate their status. Until you graduate and take a licensure examination, you may be called graduate nurse; however, since graduates of registered nursing programs also use this term, it is recommended that the title, graduate practical nurse, be used to avoid confusion. All practical nursing graduates must take the State Board examination the first time it is offered after graduation.

There is no difference between the license obtained by the graduate practical nurse and that granted to the waiver nurse. The licenses are identical and entail the same legal obligations. Graduate practical nurses should wear their school emblems proudly and be prepared to discuss logically the differences between the graduate and the nongraduate, yet still recognize the valuable services given by practical nurses for many years when no schools for them existed. (See Chapter 7, Legal Aspects.)

OTHER NURSING PERSONNEL

Besides registered and practical nurses, there are many other people who render direct and indirect patient care. These include orderlies and aides, sometimes called attendants, who give direct patient care under the supervision of RNs. To relieve RNs—especially those in administrative, teaching, and supervisory roles—of many nonprofessional nursing duties, clerical personnel have been added to the nursing staff. These include floor clerks, receptionists, and secretaries who primarily render indirect patient care and therefore play a valuable part in the nursing service administration. The clerical personnel are usually under the direct supervision of an RN. In some institutions in which floor managers are employed, the clerical personnel may be under their jurisdiction.

In the 1976–1977 Health Resources Statistics Report, Department of Health, Education, and Welfare, Public Health Service, it was pointed out that hospitals employ far more nonprofessional nursing personnel than RNs. In community hospitals the number of professional and nonprofessional nursing personnel is almost equal, but in other types of hospitals and specially in nursing homes there is a higher percentage of nonprofessional workers. In 1976 more than 2,450,000 nursing personnel were employed. The newer concepts of floor secretary, receptionist, or even floor manager were not included. In many of the larger hospitals today we find the floor receptionist or clerk, who is a valuable assistant to the supervisor or head nurse.

Aides, Orderlies, or Attendants

Although more registered and practical nurses are employed in community hospitals every year, there is still an apparent shortage of these nurses. In order to help them spend more time with their patients, nursing aides and orderlies have been employed to assist in patient care. In some institutions they are called attendants, since they ''attend'' patients; these employees are also called ''subsidiary or auxiliary personnel'' and are prepared through in-service and on-the-job training. Some aides may have had the Red Cross course or some other volunteer training program, whereas others may have graduated from private and vocational school programs or those offered by junior and community colleges.

Under the supervision of the RN and/or LP/VN they are permitted to give simple and limited nursing care to patients. Their work is semiskilled in nature and usually involves simple patient care and cleansing procedures. They must have an adequate knowledge of personal hygiene, including the maintenance of normal body functions and the prevention of disease. In addition, they must be able to understand patients as individuals and establish good relationships with them and hospital personnel.

They work under close supervision at all times and should never be placed in positions in which they will need to exceed their designated duties. It must be impressed upon them that they are employed to provide simple care measures for the patient, and that if a patient's request requires the attention of a more skilled person, they must report this immediately to the nurse in charge. The condition of the patient usually determines whether the nursing care can be given by an orderly or a nursing aide. This decision rests with the charge nurse.

The duties of these attendants include assisting registered and practical nurses with the admission and the discharge of patients, caring for hospital equipment and the patients' surroundings, collecting simple specimens, and offering and removing bedpans and urinals. Although some institutions may assign them other duties, such as changing sterile dressings, giving colostomy care and irrigations, taking blood pressure, giving enemas and douches, and doing ''preps,'' these duties usually do not fall into the list of nursing aides' and orderlies' duties acceptable to some State Boards of Nursing in their interpretation of the Nurse Practice Acts.

Clerical and Secretarial Personnel

The clerical nursing personnel are usually receptionists, floor clerks, and, sometimes, secretaries. Clerical employees, beside having many administrative and clerical duties to perform, such as all the paper and desk work, may also double as host and public relations contacts. The coordination of communications for all professional and nonprofessional personnel may be their responsibility in addition to overseeing the general appearance of the nursing station area and its contents. This would include preparing the requisitions for all supplies and necessary patient care equipment, answering telephones and signal lights, taking and relaying messages, and freeing the nurse of other time consuming paper work.

In some hospitals floor secretaries are employed, whose duties include charting, taking and processing doctors' orders, and recording dictation, as well as other vital information, on patients' charts. These employees probably have had secretarial experience before they receive additional on-the-job training.

Clerical and secretarial personnel are usually responsible to the charge nurse, but in those institutions that employ floor managers they may be under their supervision.

Floor (Unit) Managers

Some institutions have experimented very successfully with floor managers, who are administrative employees responsible for the management of an entire nursing floor or unit. They may come under a supervisor or a hospital administrator. The floor manager is assigned to assist and support the nursing staff. The function of the manager is to serve the needs of the head nurse or supervisor by coordinating, supervising, and participating in the indirect patient care activities performed in a nursing unit.

Their duties usually are planned so that nursing personnel do not need to spend time away from the patient. The floor managers contact various departments, such as housekeeping, engineering, dietary, and the pharmacy, for supplies, cleaning, repairs, and so forth; they keep various reports, maintain the file, the floor library, and the bulletin boards; they check patients' charts; and they transcribe doctors' orders.

Some of these managers have background experience in business, management, or hospital administration, or a combination of these fields. Sometimes nursing personnel who are physically limited or are not interested in direct patient contact are oriented to these duties through in-service education. A few colleges offer special programs to train floor managers.

NURSING CARE PATTERNS

Every hospital is interested in rendering good nursing care while still achieving efficiency and economy. There are many different nursing care patterns, and how efficiently and economically nursing care may be performed will depend on the selection and the use of the personnel previously discussed. The method used in one hospital is not necessarily effective in another. In 1978 there were more than 37.2 million hospital admissions, with a daily average of 1,042,000 patients expecting good nursing care. The nursing care that these patients received was not necessarily always to their liking, but probably it was the best that the hospial could provide within the limitations of its existing staff and facilities. Perhaps the public would be more tolerant if it were better informed of the ways in which hospitals use personnel for the maximum benefit to everyone.

Nursing care is considered, first of all, as either direct or indirect. *Indirect care* is that which is performed away from patients but on their behalf, whereas *direct care* means bedside nursing.

The Functional Method

The oldest acceptable method in providing patient care is known as the functional method. It is called functional because each nursing employee is assigned specific duties (functions) that are carried out on all patients in a given unit. The RN may check orders, the LPN may give treatments and medications, whereas the aides and the orderlies may make beds, give baths, and distribute meals.

Team Nursing

Team nursing has become perhaps one of the most practical methods of rendering patient care, since under this plan nursing personnel are used to the maximum of their ability. The nursing team is under the supervision of an RN who acts as leader. The team leader knows and understands the patients' conditions and is able to plan the care of each by assigning the team members—practical nurses, aides, and orderlies—to tasks best suited to their individual capabilities and personalities.

Guidelines for team nursing include well-planned patient care assignments, daily patient care team conferences, use of nursing care plans and nursing histories, use of problem-oriented records, and frequent communication between team leaders and team members. Although the RN is usually the team leader in the hospital, qualified LP/VNs have assumed these responsibilities in nursing homes, extended care facilities, and on selected hospital units.

Total Patient Care—Comprehensive Nursing—Primary Nursing

Total patient care is another method, perhaps the most satisfactory one for the patient. In this type of care the nurse, whether registered or practical, is responsible for all the patient's needs, and this includes all phases of bedside nursing. One advantage of this system is that the nurse has an opportunity to get to know the patients more readily.

Comprehensive nursing is a term that is sometimes used interchangeably with total patient care (TPC) or patient-centered care. The simple dictionary definition for comprehensive is "including much," and that describes its meaning best of all. In the fourth edition of Fuerst and Wolff's *Fundamentals of Nursing,* the following three nursing care guides are given for total patient care.

> **MAINTAINING THE INDIVIDUALITY OF MAN:**
> *Each person is an individual member of society and has rights, privileges and immunities which should be respected, regardless of race, creed, social or economic status, and has personal fears and needs which usually are exaggerated when there is a threat to his well-being.*

MAINTAINING PHYSIOLOGIC FUNCTIONS IN MAN:
The human body requires that certain physiologic activities be maintained if the body is to function effectively.

PROTECTING MAN AGAINST EXTERNAL CAUSES OF ILLNESS:
Appropriate precautionary measures will help to reduce or eliminate physical, chemical or biologic factors in the environment which cause illness or injury to man.

Each of these guides is a composite of many factors, and in most patient care situations, all three are applicable. Therefore, these are the foundations of comprehensive or total patient care nursing.

This type of care evolves through the *nursing process,* which is usually expedited by the RN. This process has four major components: assessment, planning, implementation, and evaluation. First, the needs of the patient are estimated; next, a plan of care is instituted, using the nursing history and nursing care plan. This plan is then carried out by means of the proper use of personnel and resources, and an accurate interpretation of physician and nursing orders. Finally the evaluation is made, based on audit and conferring with the patient and personnel involved to ascertain the extent to which the plan of care has been effective. The nursing process is sometimes called the problem-solving method for quality care. The nursing care plan, problem-oriented record, and quality assurance, part of comprehensive nursing, are discussed in Chapter 6.

Primary nursing is considered the best method for delivering individualized comprehensive nursing. In primary nursing, one nurse is assigned the total care of the patient and the "primary nurse," usually a professional nurse, is responsible for the patient 24 hours a day. The primary nurse is assisted by "associate nurses," usually technical and practical nurses, who are held accountable for the continuity of patient care on the other tours of duty and when the primary nurse is off duty. Primary nursing should not be confused with primary care, the usual entry point of patients into the health care system.

Whatever the type of patient care, it should be designed to suit the particular institution by using nursing employees to the maximum of their ability in the existing physical conditions, centering on individual patient needs.

Sometimes there may be a combination of the three methods discussed. As one director of nursing put it, "We use the functional team method in rendering comprehensive patient care!" Regardless of the method used, the object of each is good nursing care and satisfied patients.

Progressive Patient Care (PPC)

This concept is an attempt to furnish better care in many hospitals. In this method the patients are grouped according to degree of illness and need for care. Nurses are assigned according to their capabilities and interests. There are four or five divisions or units in this plan, depending on the type of hospital, and each one is designed to meet the medical and the nursing needs of the patient.

For instance, in the *intensive care unit,* the critically or seriously ill patients are segregated. These patients are under the constant observation of expert nurses who have all the necessary life-saving emergency equipment, drugs, and requisite knowledge.

In the *intermediate care unit,* the patients who require a moderate amount of nursing are taken care of. This includes those who may be ambulatory for short periods of time, the terminally ill, and those who need a great deal of health teaching and rehabilitative care.

Self-sufficient patients requiring only certain of the hospital's services are admitted to the *self-care unit.* Here, in a homelike atmosphere, they may wear street clothers, eat in a community dining room, and avail themselves of the recreational and other facilities offered. These patients are directed to the clinical and the diagnostic units for their specific tests and therapy, and they return to the self-care unit unless more care is necessary, in which case they are transferred to the intermediate or the long-term unit.

The *long-term unit* accommodates those patients who require extensive and lengthy care, particularly rehabilitation as well as physical and occupational therapy.

The *home-care unit* is an extended hospital service that reaches into the patient's home. Physicians, nurses, and other personnel—as well as equipment—are provided by the hospital or the community health and welfare agencies. Members of the family are trained to care for the patient at home, and much emphasis is placed on rehabilitation, health education, and prevention. The benefits of progressive patient care programs are being evaluated constantly, and it appears that the patient, the physician, the nurse, the hospital, and the community do gain, because maximum use is made of the existing services, staff, and facilities.

Specialized Care

In order to improve nursing care and to offer an opportunity for *specialized care,* many hospitals assign the patients to certain units according to their diagnoses (or age group), so that there may be separate units for psychiatric, communicable disease, maternity, pediatric, adolescent, orthopedic, and other patients. Included also would be a surgical unit with divisions for urology, gynecology, ophthalmology, renal dialysis, and others. In addition to the operating rooms, the recovery room, or the postanesthesia room, there may be a minor surgery area, which would perhaps include a room for "contaminated cases," another room for the application and the removal of casts, and other specialized areas—depending on the patient census figures. In the medical unit there may be a division for cardiovascular disease, and this division, in turn, may include an intensive care unit (ICU) or coronary care unit (CCU).

Private Duty and Group Nursing

Private duty nursing is taking care of a patient privately and on an individual basis. This type of nursing care is discussed more fully in Chapter 9.

Group nursing is a "share-the-nurse" service, whereby three or four patients usually share the extra cost and the nursing care rendered by professional and/or practical nurses, if the services of private duty nurses are not available or desirable. Patients receive more individualized care from these nurses, and nurses may receive more personal satisfaction because they are able to render complete care to a few patients.

Computers

With the rising cost of health care, many of the nation's hospitals have become involved in computer-based information systems. Computers definitely are an asset in the delivery of care. The following can be processed by computer: nurses' notes, admissions records, laboratory reports, work schedules, unit reports, dietary orders, x-ray requests, patient scheduling, billing, issuing of drugs, and the cardiac monitoring system. Another positive factor of the computer system is the elimination of illegible handwriting.

It is anticipated that the computer will eventually eliminate the traditional nursing Kardex system, preparation of medicine tickets, and traditional patient charting. The nursing care plan, generated at the time of admission, will be tailored to meet the individual patient's needs and will be kept up to date by calling out information and rekeyboarding data. Medications ordered by the physician will be processed by computer, and the tickets will arrive in the nursing station when the medications are delivered. Hopefully, with this type of automation, nurses will be able to spend more time in teaching patients care and health maintenance.

The computer is an important tool in modern health care delivery. It is important that the nurse become familiar with the computer system.

Questions

A. Select the correct answer and circle the number that answers the question best.

1. Accredited Practical Nurse programs are conducted in (A) junior and community colleges, (B) hospitals, (C) correspondence schools (D) vocational/technical schools.
   1. All of these
   2. All except B
   3. All except C
   4. All except A

2. The state sets the title that the practical nurse may use in its licensing laws. Some of the titles used are (A) LPN, (B) RN, (C) PN, (D) LA, (E) LVN.
   1. All except B
   2. All except D
   3. A, B, D
   4. A, C, E

3. *Registered nurses* may have graduated from the following nursing programs (A) vocational, (B) diploma, (C) associate degree, (D) correspondence, (E) baccalaureate degree.
   1. All of these
   2. All except D
   3. B, C, E
   4. A, B, C

4. Progressive patient care usually includes the following units: (A) intensive care, (B) functional care, (C) intermediate care, (D) self-care, (E) group care.
   1. All of these
   2. All except B
   3. A, C, D
   4. A, C, E

5. The *Statement of Functions of the Licensed Practical Nurse* was approved by the (A) National Association for Practical Nurses, (B) American Nurses Association (C) National Federation of Licensed Practical Nurses, (D) National League for Nursing, (E) Department of Health, Education, and Welfare.

1. A, B
2. C
3. C, D
4. C, E

6. "Nursing team" members giving direct patient care include (A) registered nurses, (B) practical nurses, (C) aides, (D) clerks, (E) floor (unit) managers, (F) orderlies.

1. All except D
2. All except E and F
3. All except C and E
4. All except D and E

7. The nursing process includes (A) assessment, (B) planning, (C) implementation, (D) evaluation.

1. All of these
2. B, C, E
3. A, C, D
4. B, C

8. NLN is the recognized national accrediting body for the following nursing education programs (A) practical, (B) diploma, (C) technical, (D) baccalaureate.

1. All of these
2. A, C, B
3. A, C, D
4. A and D

9. The concept of team nursing is based on (A) functional assignment, (B) daily patient care conferences, (C) use of nursing care plans, (D) use of nursing histories.

1. All of these
2. A, C
3. B, C
4. B, C, D

10. Comprehensive nursing is based on the following guides—the patient (A) should be protected against external causes of illness, (B) must have physiological functions maintained, (C) is an individual member of society, (D) should be respected regardless of race, creed, social, or economic status.

1. All of these
2. B, C, D
3. A, B, C
4. D

B. Match the best associated expression from column *B* with column *A* and insert the letter in the space provided.

A	*B*
____ 1. associate degree	A. two years
____ 2. bathing patient	B. LVN
____ 3. progressive patient care	C. ICU
____ 4. LPN	D. ANA
____ 5. diploma program	E. direct care
____ 6. vocational program	F. Board of Nursing
____ 7. state accreditation	G. three years
____ 8. *Toward Quality in Nursing*	H. NFLPN
____ 9. processing orders	I. indirect care
____ 10. *Statement of Functions*	J. special care
	K. State Board of Education
	L. four years
	M. NAPNES
	N. Surgeon General

C. True or False. Write *T* or *F* in answer space.

_____   1. There are more professional than nonprofessional nursing personnel in hospitals today.

_____   2. Junior colleges conduct associate degree programs.

_____   3. LPN and LVN are legally the same.

_____   4. NLN and NFLPN approved the Nursing Practice Standards.

_____   5. There are more vocational than hospital schools of practical nursing.

_____   6. Intermediate Care and Long-Term units usually are part of PPC.

_____   7. Comprehensive and total patient care are used interchangeably.

_____   8. Unit managers give direct patient care.

_____   9. Eliminating physical, chemical, or biological factors in the environment that cause illness or injury to man is a guide to action in nursing practice.

_____   10. Primary nursing is an example of comprehensive nursing.

Answers (3⅓ points each)

A. Multiple Choice	B. Matching	C. True or False
1. 3	1. A	1. F
2. 4	2. E	2. T
3. 3	3. C	3. T
4. 3	4. B	4. F
5. 2	5. G	5. T
6. 4	6. K	6. T
7. 1	7. F	7. T
8. 1	8. N	8. F
9. 4	9. I	9. T
10. 1	10. H	10. T

4

Personal Considerations

Understanding Yourself • Mental Health • Culture • Communications • Appearance and Grooming • Your Health • Questions and Answers

Objectives

Upon completion of this chapter you should be able to

1. describe personality development
2. explain Freud's personality theory
3. summarize the three characteristics of people with good mental health
4. identify seven defense or protective mechanisms
5. arrange Maslow's hierarchy of human needs according to priorities
6. list Erikson's eight critical stages of development
7. discuss self-awareness groups and transactional analysis
8. illustrate appropriate assertive behavior at home, school, or work
9. review cultural and ethnic differences in people
10. explain how prejudice develops and how it can be corrected
11. discuss the importance of appearance, grooming, and good health for nurses
12. list the "do's and don'ts" when wearing the uniform.

UNDERSTANDING YOURSELF

In order to be able to understand others (one of the most desirable attributes of a nurse), you must first of all understand yourself. Your attitudes and actions influence others, but how do they affect you? To what extent do you really know yourself? Are you willing to face the truth about yourself? Self-awareness or insight into our own personal qualities is most complex, but it starts with an understanding of personality.

Although you may have excelled scholastically and perform at the highest level of technical competence, the patients, co-workers, supervisors, faculty members, and others with whom you work may still feel that you are not the type of nurse you should be. One of your classmates may have scored highest on the State Board licensure examination, whereas another may have only barely passed; yet it is not necessarily the nurse with the higher marks who is most liked by the patients. Perhaps the personality of the high scorer does not inspire confidence or a rapport with others. You cannot be a success in nursing or in any other kind of service of an intensely personal nature unless your personality affects patients and co-workers positively.

Personality

Your personality is you—everything that you are, were, and are to become. The building blocks of your personality were established by heredity; they were influenced by your environment and family life during your earlier years, and later they were affected by cultural conditioning and the accumulation of experiences. Your talents, strengths, weaknesses, innermost likes and dislikes, emotional response to events and experiences in general are all random bits and pieces of your personality; you can probably name many more. To have a personality is as inescapable as having organs within your body. Your personality is unique—no two are alike. Since nurses meet patients of all ages and cultural backgrounds, displaying a wide variety of personality traits, the nurse's own personality is a critical factor in the achievement of success—more so than in many other fields of employment. A stenographer, for example, usually is able to hide those aspects of personality that may impede the smooth running of an office. But because the nurse's duties are by their nature intimate, and patients in their helplessness come to depend so heavily upon the nurse's understanding, one's innermost resources are constantly required. The conduct you display toward others will reflect the type of person you are, and the type of person you are is the foundation upon which you will build your nursing career.

Personality development is dynamic. It is constantly changing. You can modify your personality by conscious acts of will. In this respect your personality is not a fixed part of you, like the color of your eyes, the size of your feet, or the shape of your nose. However, you do not become an entirely new person in a moment or even in a year. The development is a continuous process—one of improvement, hopefully, as no doubt you will be eager to show the best of yourself in your chosen career. To acquire some of those difficult-to-define traits of personality that will differentiate you as a superior nurse rather than one who is merely competent will take time, sincere effort, patience, and sometimes guidance from your faculty and supervisors. The person with the adequate personality is able to adjust satisfactorily to life and its demands. Do not imitate blindly someone who your judgment has told you is outstanding; rather, try to define those characteristics that give that person particular distinction and make them your own.

Freud's Personality Theory

Although many theories have evolved regarding the development of personality and how it functions, the theory of Sigmund Freud the Viennese psychiatrist (1856–1939), is one of the most widely modified and accepted. Freud felt that there were three "levels of the mind"—the conscious (which contains all that we are immediately aware of), the subconscious (which contains memories that are easy to recall), and the unconscious (which stores memories that are much more difficult to recall).

He described the forces that determine our behavior or actions as the *id,* the *ego,* and the *superego.* The *id* follows the pleasure-seeking principle, is primitive and entirely unconscious; it does what it wants to when it wants to! The newborn baby is an excellent example of "all *id*." The *ego*, partly conscious and partly unconscious, is responsible for behavior of "the self"—the "me, myself, and I" aspect, which encounters reality and modifies behavior in accordance with the influence of social forces. The *ego* activity is greatly influenced by our parents, teachers, friends, or other "hero" models. The *superego* is our conscience, telling us "what we have to do," and restraining the activity of the *ego* and *id*. To illustrate this more clearly—it would be the *superego* that reminds the *ego* that it is time for our annual physical check-up. We then call to make an appointment with the family physician. The appointed day comes and passes. Suddenly we realize that we missed this important appointment; unconsciously we avoided going to the physician. The *id* was at work.

This type of behavior involves the unconscious use of what some authorities call defense or protective mechanisms, and which are referred to by others as mental adjustment mechanisms. I am sure that you or some of your friends have used one or more of these reactions unconsciously to maintain your ego equilibrium when a conflict arose involving social conscience or cultural conditioning. A few of the common ones follow:

1. *Compensation*—to obtain gratification from a second choice, e.g., the unpopular student who becomes an outstanding scholar.

2. *Conversion*—to change emotional difficulties into physical symptoms, e.g., the "convenient headache" that prevents you from studying.

3. *Fantasy* (daydreaming)—to imagine past, present, or future experiences, e.g., the adolescent who enjoys daydreams about love and future mate.

4. *Identification*—to assume the attributes of another person, e.g., the student who admires a team leader and imitates that behavior.

5. *Rationalization*—to justify behavior by reasoning, e.g., the excuse for not studying that "studying will not help me, since the teacher never tests me on what I do study."

6. *Sublimation*—to replace a frustrated basic drive with socially acceptable behavior, e.g., the married woman who is frustrated by housekeeping duties and volunteers her services in the pediatric unit of a hospital.

7. *Regression*—to retreat to a less mature level of adjustment, e.g., the adult's "temper tantrum" that has worked so effectively in childhood.

Since the well-adjusted person accepts a certain amount of anxiety in everyday living and adjusts accordingly, it is important that you recognize the use of these and other defense mechanisms in yourself and that you do not resort to their excessive use.

MENTAL HEALTH

In the instance of the scholarly and technically capable nurse who nevertheless does not seem to have what it takes, it may be that personality development has been hampered by poor mental health. What exactly is meant by this term?

The National Association for Mental Health in a little pamphlet reproduced here in part (see Figure 4-1) tells us that mental health is something that all of us want for ourselves, whether we know it by name or not. Mental health does not mean the absence of mental illness but rather the presence of something positive: the happiness, the peace of mind, the enjoyment, and the satisfaction that we derive from living. Mental health is associated with everybody's everyday life. It means the overall way that people get along in their families, at school or work, at play, and in their communities. It concerns the way that each person comes to terms with desires, ambitions, ideals, feelings, and conscience, in order to meet the demands of life and face them realistically.

There is no line that neatly divides the mentally healthy from those who are not, and there are many different degrees of mental health. No single characteristic by itself can be taken as evidence of good mental health, nor can the lack of one be evidence of mental illness. Whether it is a neurosis or a more serious psychosis, mental illness is a true illness. A "ruptured psyche" is often as painful and as crippling in its way as a ruptured appendix, and the afflicted person is equally in need of professional medical help. It has been estimated that at least one out of every 10 Americans, at some time, will need help for a personality disorder.

Good mental health is an absolute "must" for nurses. The "1-2-3 table" in Figure 4-1 is a handy index for judging your own status in this respect. Be as honest as you can with yourself, and try to determine where there can be room for self-improvement. Remember that this table is not merely a convenient check list; it is more than that. In the aggregate, the items represent an overall attitude toward life, an ideal to which you may aspire not only for your own sake but also for that of your patients.

A person with good mental health is usually considered "mature." What is maturity? A simple definition is "full development" or being "grown up." Consider a baby, for example—the most selfish and demanding creature imaginable. This is certainly excusable, because we expect this behavior from a virtually helpless infant. However, as a person grows to physical maturity, we expect growth in independence and understanding and less preoccupation with one's self—that is, to grow to emotional maturity. A mature nurse accepts responsibilities as a team member and must be able to follow orders and ask for further directions if so indicated, and in addition, the nurse must be willing and able to

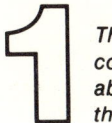 *They feel comfortable about themselves.*

They are not bowled over by their own emotions—by their fears, anger, love, jealousy, guilt or worries.

They can take life's disappointments in their stride.

They have a tolerant, easy-going attitude towards themselves as well as others; they can laugh at themselves.

They neither under-estimate nor over-estimate their abilities.

They can accept their own shortcomings.

They have self-respect.

They feel able to deal with most situations that come their way.

They get satisfaction from the simple, every-day pleasures.

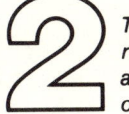 *They feel right about other people.*

They are able to give love and to consider the interests of others.

They have personal relationships that are satisfying and lasting.

They expect to like and trust others, and take it for granted that others will like and trust them.

They respect the many differences they find in people.

They do not push people around, nor do they allow themselves to be pushed around.

They can feel they are part of a group.

They feel a sense of responsibility to their neighbors and fellow men.

 *They are able to meet the demands of life.*

They do something about their problems as they arise.

They accept their responsibilities.

They shape their environment whenever possible; they adjust to it whenever necessary.

They plan ahead but do not fear the future.

They welcome new experiences and new ideas.

They make use of their natural capacities.

They set realistic goals for themselves.

They are able to think for themselves and make their own decisions.

They put their best effort into what they do, and get satisfaction out of doing it.

FIGURE4-1. *Characteristics of people with good mental health. (National Association for Mental Health)*

take on other duties and responsibilities when necessary. Rather than being governed by wishful thinking, you, the mature nurse, will face problems as they really are. You must not be afraid to consult your superiors when in doubt, making it a rule never to carry out any measures that have not been taught or have never been performed under supervision. You should derive great satisfaction from giving good care to patients and not be rigid either in ideas or in feelings. Perhaps, above all, the mature nurse recognizes both intellectually and emotionally that patients are human beings who will respond favorably if shown genuine interest.

Habits

The word "habit" has been used to mean any type of repetitive behavior—good or bad. Habits usually are related to interests, attitudes, and personality. The capacity to acquire habits is inborn in human beings and animals, and this innate quality plays a vital role in their development. All through life we adopt new habits, modify old ones, and discard those that are undesirable. We have a strong natural tendency to repeat any pattern of behavior that we establish. For example, once a baby takes a certain toy to bed, this choice is likely to be repeated. Despite the fact that some habits are bad for us, we form them because we gain satisfaction from them. For example, we may not enjoy being fat, but most of us enjoy good food and are not in the habit of counting calories.

It may be comforting to know that when you really want to break a habit, and are willing to work at beaking it, it can be done. However, you must have a real desire. Habits are personal and uniquely individual, and as long as they do not harm anyone else, it is up to you to decide whether or not you want to continue them. Smoking is an example. You may decide that you cannot or do not want to give it up, or you may have followed the Surgeon General's warning and have given it up because of the fear of eventual illness. Alternatively, you may have learned to get around it by substituting another habit, such as eating candy. When it comes to habits, you are the only master. Nevertheless, it often is difficult to change habits that are emotional in nature, even though we are aware that they may be unreasonable.

How do you break an undersirable habit, even one that has been with you for a lifetime? Here are some simple suggestions. First of all, analyze the habit. List the good features as well as the bad features. This will help you to decide if you really want to give it up. Then set "D" or Discard Day. Tell your friends of your intentions. Invite them to participate by offering five dollars to anyone who witnesses your breaking it. Burn your bridges behind you, and get temptations out of the way. Permit no exceptions. Stick to your convictions, and when you feel it necessary, say to yourself, "I know this is wrong; therefore I will not do it." This is effective with conscious habits as well as those that are almost unconscious. If you have a new habit substitute, make it work for you, and stay on guard until you are completely sure the old habit is gone. Test yourself, "Can you resist it?" You will never know until you try.

Coping With Tensions

Within the last few years we have heard much about the relationship of mind and body; we are told that they are closely linked. This relationship may be considered and accepted as the "whole person" holistic concept and is the basis for psychosomatic medicine (*psycho*—mind; *soma*—body). In your everyday experiences you may find that some emotions may affect your body functions. You may blush when you are embarrassed, or you may have a tight feeling in your chest or feel that your stomach is "tied into a pretzel" just before an examination or while waiting outside your supervisor's office. Also, you may perspire more freely, or your heart may pound more rapidly when you are excited or afraid. These are normal reactions of your body to emotional tensions and usually will disappear quickly once the cause has been removed. Tensions are natural and are often useful in our complex lives, provided that you know what should be done about them.

Here are some helpful suggestions. When something bothers you, talk about it. Confide your problem or worry to someone you can trust—a relative, a friend, a supervisor, a faculty member, or a coworker. Exchanging views on your problem will help to relieve your stress and will enable you to see things in a clearer light, and it often may help you to see the solution, too. If the "someone" you would like to confide in is not available, write yourself a letter. Put down exactly how you feel. "Get it off your chest" while writing about it. Tell about the sense of injustice or injury you have, and how you have been mistreated. Go into detail, elaborating on and illustrating the situation. When you have finished, tear it up. It has served its purpose and has given you a useful outlet. Sometimes this works even better if the letter is addressed to the one against whom you have the grievance—a nagging supervisor, an unfair head nurse, or an aggressive fellow student. At times you may have to rewrite the letter, and at other times just starting it may be sufficient.

Work anger or hostility out of your system. You will find that by doing something constructive—whether it be working at your hobby, cleaning out the utility room, or attacking some other worthwhile project—you will "cool off" and be better prepared to understand and handle your anger. Do not talk back when someone has provoked or upset you, and do not raise your voice or become impatient, but rather do something constructive until you can handle the situation calmly and with dignity.

Hierarchy of Needs

Dr. Abraham H. Maslow, a recognized authority on human needs, arranges them according to priorities. He classifies needs into five categories: physical needs, safety, belonging, recognition, and fulfillment. (An adaptation of these is given in Figure 4–2.)

The physical needs are the most basic and the first to be met. These physiological needs include food, water, shelter, rest, oxygen, and so forth. They form the base of the hierarchy and satisfy the instinct for survival. Most of us have come to understand these basic needs and realize what happens if we skip breakfast and lunch or stay up until 2 or 3 o'clock AM, even though we have an early morning class. The second category includes the need for safety or protection against danger or deprivation. These safety needs are also known as "security" and may have emotional, economic, and physical aspects. To illustrate, you may feel insecure about a coming examination or the possible hazards to cope with during your first day in the hospital. Third in the hierarchy is the need to belong. Included in this category is the need to be liked as a person, friendship and affection, fellowship, the feeling of being part of a group, and the need to love and be loved.

Once the survival, safety, and social needs are met, one tries to satisfy the need for recognition or self-esteem. This includes the desire for self-confidence, respect, and competence. These desires are rarely fully satisfied but are very important to the individual. You may recall many an incident when your needs for status and recognition by your family, classmates, hospital personnel, and instructors may have been thwarted; however, when your patient says, "you are the best nurse ever," you will experience an almost unbelievable degree of emotional satisfaction. You will need to develop a real understanding of yourself when it comes to this need, since many people (including patients) are often too busy or careless to offer this kind of recognition. However, your own self-respect may compensate for the need of respect and recognition from others.

The last or highest need of the hierarchy is that of self-actualization or fulfillment. This need is the most difficult to achieve, and most people do not attain it,

FIGURE 4-2. *Common human needs based on Maslow's hierarchical motivation theory. (Adapted from Maslow In Keller MJ, May WT: Occupational Health Content in Baccalaureate Nursing Education. Cincinnati, U.S. Department of Health, Education, and Welfare, 1970)*

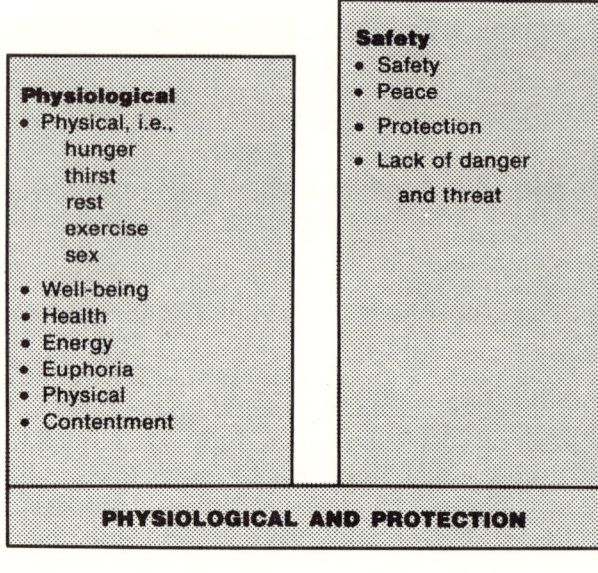

as realization of one's potential is difficult. This challenge motivates us to achieve more and more by satisfying our curiosity about ourselves and the potential in each of us. "Being fully oneself" involves increased acceptance of self, others, and the world around us. Fulfillment is something the nursing profession can lead to, because in sharing and lessening the hardships of people who cannot help themselves, the nurse reaches toward the highest levels of human achievement.

Your application of the hierarchy of needs to yourself and your patients will strengthen your interpersonal relations. You will become much more tolerant and understanding of the needs of others and realize that when the needs of a patient, or a coworker, or your own needs are not met, you will be settling for a lesser degree of satisfaction.

Erikson's Psychosocial Theory

Erik Erikson's theory of personality development builds on Freud's analytical concept. Erikson emphasizes the continuous role of the ego throughout the life cycle. The theory stresses that developing individuals attempt to strike a balance between two priorities during eight critical stages of development. These begin

Love and Belonging	Esteem	Self-actualization

Self-actualization
- Self-actualization
- Self-fulfillment
- Realization of one's
  potentials (thru
  complete development,
  fruition of resources,
  growth)
- Fitness
- Suitability
- Learning
  satisfied
  curiosity
  learning and knowing
  large amounts

Esteem
- Self-reliance
  -respect
  -esteem
  -confidence
  -trust
- Reputation
  ability
  achievement
  competence
  success
  ego strength
  respectworthiness
  prestige (status)
  leadership
  autonomy
  independence

Love and Belonging
- Belongingness
  being one of a group
  identification with
  group goals and
  triumph
- Acceptance
- Having a place
- Giving and receiving
  of friendship and love
  being loved
  being loveworthy
  love identification

SOCIAL   **EGO**

with the concept of trust versus mistrust (birth to about one year) followed by autonomy versus shame and doubt (between two and four years), initiative versus guilt (about four to five years), industry versus inferiority (approximately six to 11 years), identity and repudiation versus identity diffusion (approximately 12 to 18 years), intimacy versus isolation (young adulthood), generativity versus self-absorption or stagnation (middle years), and conclude with integrity versus despair (old age).

Sensitivity, Encounter, and (T)Training Groups

These self-awareness groups involve small numbers of people intent on exploring their own interpersonal feelings and attitudes with the help of a qualified group leader competent in dealing with group data and intergroup relationships. Through open communication, sharing of emotions and feelings, and sometimes body handling and touching, group members learn about themselves and others. Feedback plays an important role, and through it the participants learn to understand themselves and others. It must be pointed out that much of this feedback and much of the communication is in the form of feelings and emotions rather than facts. An outcome of this kind of self-examination is often an expansion of openness and awareness. Group participants often gain an increased tendency to be free of inhibitions and to say what they think and feel without embarrassment or fear.

There exist, however, mixed feelings about the use of sensitivity and encounter group methods in understanding and learning situations. When used effectively, all these technics encourage openness of individual and group feelings and sensitivity, so that attitudes towards self and others become more responsive and manageable. You may wish to check with your instructor before becoming involved in a group.

Group therapy has come to be regarded as a valuable therapeutic technique. "T" or training groups use a multidisciplinary approach that may include nurses, psychiatric residents, social workers, psychologists, and others drawn from the mental health discipline to prepare trainers for group therapy sessions. Many nurses involved have found that the group training program affects their nursing practice for the better. They report increased awareness of their own feelings, improved communication skills with patients, family, and coworkers, and greater confidence in dealing with others.

Transactional Analysis

Dr. Eric Berne is the originator of transactional analysis, a method of analyzing interactions between two (or more) people, which was developed from several schools of thought. He based his concept on the premise that a person is responsible for what happens in the future, no matter what has happened in the past. He theorized that each person has three basic elements in his personality: the parent, the adult, and the child (P-A-C). The parent relates to the earliest years of development when the "do's and don'ts" are implanted. The child represents the "seeing and hearing and feeling and understanding" body of data that is reflected in emotions. The adult is a data-processing computer, which grinds out decisions after logically evaluating the facts. By describing our feelings and interactions, we can often analyze whether it is the parent or the adult operating in us.

Dr. Thomas Harris, in his book *I'm OK, You're OK: A Practical Guide to Transactional Analysis,* explains the application of P-A-C to problem solving in our every day situations. He also outlines four positions that underlie people's behavior. They are: "I'm Not OK, You're OK" (anxious dependency of the immature); "I'm not OK, you are not OK" (despair); "I'm OK, you are not OK" (criminal); and "I'm OK—You're OK" (mature adult). If it is relevant, apply transactional analysis to your classroom and clinical situations. It will help you understand your own behavior and that of others.

Assertiveness

Assertive behavior will help you overcome personal frustrations and tensions encountered in daily life. Assertion is self-respect; it involves standing up for your personal rights and expressing your thoughts, feelings, and beliefs in an honest and appropriate manner without infringing on the rights of others. Assertive behavior is based on the premise that self-respect exists only when the rights of others also are respected. Openness to different points of view reduces tension levels and promotes self-confidence. Assertive behavior maintains a balance between aggression and nonassertive behavior. It means being able to say "no" when refusing a request. The assertive nurse is able to discuss both sides of an issue and compromises when necessary.

Some illustrations of assertive behavior include statements such as:

> (1) "I feel that I need your help. Practical nursing education is very demanding and I just can't continue unless I can depend on you to prepare dinner the nights I have clinical experience." (2) "I know how difficult it must be for you to be on this diet. Let's find out what foods you like and dislike so that I can help you plan appropriately." (3) "When you don't answer my questions, I feel very angry and put out. Please answer them." (4) "I enjoy giving quality nursing care and you are a pleasant person to care for." (5) "No, I'd rather not. I have had Mrs. Jones as my patient three times already, while some other L.P.N.s have not had her at all. I think someone who hasn't had her should take her before I take her again. I understood that we would rotate very difficult patients." (6) "I understand that you would like to smoke in bed, however, smoking in bed is against hospital regulations because it presents a fire hazard and disturbs your roommate. Smoking is permitted in the visitors' lounge. Let's check with your doctor and see if he would write an order for you to be able to walk to the visitors' lounge."

CULTURE

The recognition of cultural differences is most important in giving us an understanding of the behavior of both ourselves and others. Culture in its broadest sense refers to all distinctively human activities that are passed from one generation to the next. More narrowly, it applies to the collective ways of life in a group of people. It includes such basics as mating and family bonds, language, government, wars, religious observances, food preferences, clothing, shelter, and daily maintenance of life. Although most people have similar fundamental needs, no two cultures are exactly alike. Social scientists who specialize in studying present-day culture patterns believe that there may be "cultures within cultural settings."

All cultures have certain common denominators and certain differences. These are dependent upon the natural conditions in which we live (climate, available food, and other natural resources) and are influenced by existing factors such as technological changes, institutions, languages, arts, and systems of values and beliefs. *"Technology"* generally refers to the basic tools for everyday living; this may include labor-saving machines to obtain food, clothing, and shelter. *"Institution"* refers to a group of people who either live together or meet regularly for common purposes. The family is one of the basic and the simplest institutions found everywhere. Others include the political, economic, religious, and other private or voluntary organizations formed because of some common interest among a group. *Language* provides a system of communication. The *desire for beauty,* and thus, the creation of art, exists in all cultures and includes various forms of expression: dance, song, sculpture, painting, instrumental music, or myths, tales, and legends.

We are born into a society that teaches us a system of values and beliefs that are necessary to the functioning of a group with interdependent members. Every culture has rules of behavior and ethics and offers general patterns involving what, how, and when to eat, what to wear, how to get along and communicate with others, and how to care for oneself. Most members learn to be consistent with the patterns accepted by the group. Some examples of cultural groups are those that are familial, racial, national, economic, and social.

The following is an example of a simple cultural difference: you have to eat to live, but whether you prefer steaks to eel is determined by your culture. What may be a delicacy in one culture may be repulsive in another. Also, you need to wear clothes, but your personal appearance—the type and style of your garments—will vary; you need to communicate with others, but which language and accent you use is part of learned behavior, or culture. Although intracultural education has helped people to understand similarities and differences, many barriers still exist. For example, in only a few nations is the same official language spoken (in Russia between 150 and 200 separate languages and dialects are used).

The food tastes and customs of many lands can be seen in the diets of most Americans today. Bread, for example, varies with the national heritage of the baker and consumer. Dark pumpernickel has long been associated with the Germans, white loaves in different shapes with the Italians, the slim, long shape with the French, and the flat breads with the Norwegians and Armenians.

French and Creole cookery is still prevalent in New Orleans; in the Southwest the hot, spiced foods of Mexican origin are dominant. The culinary arts of the Chinese and Japanese have left a visible influence along the West Coast. Hot breads, cornbread, hominy grits, and black-eyed peas with salt pork are favorites of many southerners in the United States.

The Mexicans' use of corn and other whole-grain products, the Puerto Ricans' preference for rice and legumes, and the Italians' dependency on pasta or macaroni products all illustrate national food customs and traditions.

Some cultural differences are so slight that we tend to disregard them in our everyday life. However, in nursing we should take them seriously, since little things become magnified to a sick person. People who are accustomed to highly seasoned food may seem to be unduly critical of the bland diet ordered by the doctor; the lady who "never takes a bath during her menstrual period" may be difficult during routine morning bath care; the patient who complains about a window being opened during the night may have been taught that this caused "lung congestion"; the quiet little girl in the children's unit, who is embarrassed when some other children question her "giving thanks" before meals, was probably raised in a devout family. These are situations requiring tact, patience, and ingenuity.

You will note that patients react differently to pain, often according to cultural influences. Some people will "grin and bear" pain, whereas others may groan, moan, and even cry. Although stereotyping of nationality groups is misleading, social behaviorists report that Orientals accept pain without displaying their emotions, whereas Italians, French, and other southern European groups are generally more demonstrative. Therefore, to become familiar with your patients' cultural standards helps you toward a better understanding of them as individuals.

Ethnic Differences

"Ethnic" is derived from the Greek word *"ethnos,"* originally referring to a group of people living together; later, to a tribe, a group of people, or a nation. In the United States, the major ethnic groups are differentiated by the concept of minority groups of a given society, based on the following factors: race, religion, nationality, politics, and language. (Differences in the major religious faiths will be discussed in another chapter.)

Scientists generally agree that all human beings are descended from the same ancestral stock, which came into existence between 600,000 to a million years ago, probably in Africa. Far too much misunderstanding and ill-feeling have grown out of ignorance in the matter of race. Because racial prejudice is largely acquired, and a great deal of pseudoscientific nonsense has been propagated by the hatemongers of our own day, we should have a brief look at the real meaning of race.

There is no generally accepted classification of races. Although some scholars still feel that humankind is divided into Negroid, Caucasoid, and Mongoloid races, there are disagreements even among them. For example, the Australian aborigines are dark skinned (from which some would classify them as Negroid), but they also have wavy hair, which is sometimes brown and even blond (from which some would assign them to the Caucasoid race). The reason that race is so difficult to classify is that the world's populations have always been transient. Humans have always conquered or been conquered. For example, as early as 5,000 years ago Europe was invaded by tribal groups who spoke related languages (the ancestors of Greek, Latin, and present-day European languages). Many scholars believe that the invaders came from the border region between Europe and Asia. About 1,500 years ago the Huns and other warlike tribes left northern and central Asia to invade Europe. Shortly thereafter, southern Europe was conquered by Goths and Vandals from northern Europe. A few hundred years later Muslims from North Africa invaded Spain and Portugal. The story goes on and on and is as valid for Africa and Asia as for Europe. What is clear is that there is no such thing as a pure race in Europe, Africa, or Asia. All people are the product of intermingled cultures. Wherever there has been a migration of people, there has been intermarriage and intermixing of cultures.

Even though there is no generally accepted classification of race, there are at least acceptable guidelines for distinguishing what is not a race. There is no such thing as the "American race" or "Irish race" or "Jewish race." Race cannot be classified by nationality or religion. Recent history has in fact proved that false or erroneous classification can lead to disaster. An example of this is Germany's treatment of the "Jewish race" before and during World War II. This will be discussed in more detail in the section on prejudice.

Despite what seems to remain a controversy among a small group of scientists, the vast majority of scientific researchers have concluded that given similar social, economic, and environmental backgrounds, with equal educational opportunities, the members of any given race will do about as well as those of any other; no race is more inherently intelligent than any other.

The races are distinguished from one another in only one respect: slight physical differences, such as skin color, shape of the head, and average size. Probably these distinctive characteristics came about through the natural process of evolution, that is, adaptation of the individual to different environmental conditions. However, beyond these physical characteristics no differences exist. There is no such thing as a "superior" or an "inferior" category of human beings.

In order to grow and develop as a healthy human being, one needs an environment to reach the highest potential. In a healthy society, there is no room for racial, national, or religious prejudice. The principle of equal rights and opportunities for full development applies to all human beings. (See the section on transcultural nursing, Chapter 6.)

Prejudices

What is prejudice? The word means "prejudgment," and in the sense in which we ordinarily use it, it implies that we have already formed an opinion, usually unfavorable, about a person or a thing for insufficient reasons—that is, we have not bothered to make an intelligent inquiry or examine the available evidence. In Figure 4-1 you read that a well-adjusted person is relatively free from prejudices against other people. It should also be noted that almost every person is prejudiced in some way against some person or thing. Lack of prejudice in nursing is not just desirable, it is essential. No one is completely free from some degree of prejudice, but if you are affected seriously by a person's religious belief or racial origin, your attitude will be reflected in your work, despite your efforts to hide it. The remedy is not concealment, it is a reappraisal that must originate within you.

All prejudices are acquired from others. You are not born prejudiced. However, slowly and surely, just as your other emotions and attitudes were developed during your childhood, so, too, were your prejudices. When you heard your parents and other adults speak unfavorably about certain things and (more important) about certain people, you learned from them. By the time you were able to think and make your own decisions, the seeds of prejudice were deeply rooted. Prejudices usually are based not on realistic judgments but on preconceived ideas and emotionally labeled stereotypes.

Prejudice usually is not caused by conscious ill-will but rather is the result of emotional reactions stemming from ignorance, fear, insecurity, and inferiority. Most of us are prejudiced in one way or another, and we must make every attempt to overcome this handicap. First of all, we must examine ourselves honestly and appraise our attitudes toward those of other races, religions, or nationalities. Then let us study the teachings of our own faiths about brotherhood and the equality of human beings, and take into account the scientific facts. We must recognize and assume the responsibility for overcoming our own prejudices and be able to discuss this with others, to help them overcome theirs.

ARE YOU PREJUDICED?

Do you	No	Yes
• Choose your friends only from among your "own" racial and religious group?		
• Believe that God created different races so that some might be "inferior" to others?		
• Believe that certain jobs should be denied to people because of race or religion regardless of their qualifications?		
• Feel that people should be treated, spoken to, or thought of as being "different" because of their race or religion?		
• Think that a family, because of its color or religion should be deprived of the right to buy or live in any home it can afford?		
Total		

Do you	No	Yes
• Believe that houses of worship should be divided into racially segregated congregations?		
• *Habitually* speak of other racial and religious groups as "they" and your own as "we"?		
• Believe that any racial or religious group can be characterized by such terms as happy, rhythmic, lazy, shrewd, dirty, clean, or prejudiced?		
• Feel it necessary to praise members of other racial groups whenever you speak of them, and frequently refer to your own freedom from prejudice?		
• Get more irritated (or less irritated) by an offense from a member of another race or religion than by one from a member of your own group?		
Total		

FIGURE 4-3. *(Anti-Defamation League of B'nai B'rith.)*

Prejudice is sometimes used as a political instrument to exploit people. An example of this is what happened in World War II, when Adolf Hitler was responsible for the slaughter of six million Jews and other minorities. His concept of the supremacy of the noble race ("Aryan race") and the inferiority of the "Jewish race" led to one of history's most tragic events. It should be noted that Hitler's hatred of Jews was influenced greatly by the writings of a Frenchman named Gobineau and an Englishman named Chamberlain, each of whom was greatly prejudiced against Jews. It could be claimed that Gobineau's prejudice in the mid-1800s was partially responsible for the murder of six million people one century later.

Social scientists are hard pressed when they are asked to describe and analyze human attitudes. In the past 15 years, attitudinal changes have occurred whereby stereotyping is not so common, and yet prejudice continues to exist. It is important to remember that America did not spring from one nationality or one tribe or one country. The most dramatic identification Americans have with one another is not the similarity in their backgrounds, but rather the variety represented. Respect for our heritage will diminish prejudice.

In a democratic society it is our responsibility to become more understanding in our thinking and in our interactions with all people, regardless of racial or national origin or religious belief, and thereby prove to other nations that we believe in democratic friendships and making the human brotherhood a reality.

COMMUNICATIONS

To communicate means to convey some thought, to make something known to someone else. Language, of course, is the principal medium of communication among human beings. We shall discuss certain aspects of language in this section. However, as you doubtless are aware, a great deal can be communicated from one person to another without recourse to either spoken or written language. We might call this "nonverbal communication," meaning that it does not involve the use of words but rather relies on the actions that express our feelings, attitudes, and thoughts.

Using All Your Senses

The art of communication involves the exercise of all five senses (taste, touch, smell, sight, and hearing), in many cases several of them simultaneously. For instance, imagine the person who compliments you verbally, but whose eyes tell you that she may not really mean what she is saying. In such a case you have received two conflicting messages—a conscious affirmation and an unconscious denial—and you must exercise both intelligence and experience to find out exactly what was being communicated. Did you ever find yourself drumming your fingers in impatience while listening politely to a long-winded person? This unconscious gesture communicates your real feelings more eloquently and simply than words. Did you handle patients roughly because you disliked them, yourself, your supervisor, or the world at large? There is something almost magical about the touch of a human hand, particularly a nurse's. If you are overly brisk, believing that briskness is a sign of efficiency, you are impressing nobody, and your jerky, hasty, and agitated manner will communicate to the patient many unfavorable things about you—impatience and callousness among others. If you concentrate on being smooth and gentle with your hands, you will find yourself concentrating on your patient's feelings as well—one leads to the other.

Ineffective communication between you and your patient may occur for various reasons, for example, if you state your personal opinions, give inappropriate reassurances, change the topic, jump to conclusions, belittle their feelings, or disapprove of or disagree with them. In developing effective technics you must be able to evaluate the individual situation, recognizing the need to be objective and observant. This will come with experience and time. Your faculty will also assist you in developing your own potential and the use of various therapeutic technics.

In nursing practice the importance of observation is emphasized constantly. One reason for this is that it enables the nurse to be a more sensitive "receiver" of nonverbal communications from the patient. In our society a traditional form of behavior is to suppress as much as possible any show of emotion; therefore, you will find that even though patients may be hesitant to tell the nurse anything about their fears, worries, or physical discomforts, they may communicate them to the alert nurse unconsciously. For example, the quiet, withdrawn patient may communicate fear of impending surgery by refusing to discuss it.

Being A Good Listener

A nurse is nothing if not a good listener. Listening is one aspect of observation; it is also a means of encouraging the development of complete confidence between nurse and patient, which is an essential therapeutic measure.

Listening is an art in itself. There is a difference between listening and merely hearing. Hearing is largely the physiological process of receiving sound waves, but listening is the *interpretation* of the spoken words; therefore, it demands conscious effort on your part. If you listen carefully to a patient, you not only will be attentive to everything verbalized but also, with some experience, you may hear many things not spoken. This is part of the process of "reading between the lines."

Perhaps the most immediately practical reason for listening well is that it enables the patient to feel more at easy by releasing emotional tension. If patients are encouraged to talk, they are certain to gain some relief, because talking is in itself an active process. Remember, though, that encouraging patients to talk does not entail probing into their personal lives. Be as receptive as possible, but remember your limited role. Once a patient suspects you of "snooping," all communication with you may be severed.

Bear in mind that listening to a patient is not the same thing as the give-and-take of social conversation. If the patient recounts some significant experience, do not feel impelled to counter blithely with a similar one of your own. Probably, the patient is not interested in your personal life. Listen quietly, not letting your attention stray (even if you are bored), and practice concentrating on what is said. If you must express agreement, nod your head, smile, and respond to cues, but do not interrupt. At the end, indicate to the patient that you have listened carefully, perhaps by asking questions, but never probe. Be sure that the questions that you ask do not arise from inattention on your part. To pay attention is a compliment, but to feign it and then give yourself away by unnecessary questions is an insult. If you must ask someone to repeat what has been said, use the expressions "Pardon me?" or "Please repeat what you have said," and not, "Huh?"

The saying, "It is better to remain silent and be thought dumb than to speak and remove all doubt," has a lot of merit. If you listen carefully and silently, you will find out what people want, what they need, and very often what they are.

Speaking

Speech is the most highly developed means of communication between human beings; it conveys not only words but also much of your personality. Therefore, any discussion of speech should be from two rather obvious standpoints: what to say and how to say it.

Naturally, very little advice can be included here on *what* to say to your patients. In this and other texts in nursing you will find hints and suggestions for saying the correct thing to a patient in various circumstances. Whatever you do, avoid little set speeches in the manner required of telephone operators and airline stewardesses. They sound wooden, and patients feel that they are trying to reason with a recorded message. If you come across a phrase in a book that may be useful, keep the thought and discard its words in favor of your own. Try to accumulate enough of a working vocabulary to explain technical points to patients in simple English.

Repeating or restating the patients' words as a means of continuing conversation is called *reflecting,* one of the most effective technics in verbal communication. Asking the patient"what do *you* think?"or "what is *your* opinion?" or "How do *you* feel about it?" will give the patient an opportunity to verbalize and express feelings and ideas. As an example, Mr. Jones, who is worried about his surgery, asks you "do you think I should tell the doctor . . . ?". Your response should be "do *you* think you should?" rather than some other comment such as "why are you afraid?" or "don't worry, everything will be fine."

In large measure, courtesy to your patients will determine your choice of words in conversing with them. Whenever you can, give simple explanations; most of the medical vocabulary that you take for granted is meaningless to the layman. Clear and complete explanations do wonders for the patient's peace of mind.

Address your adult patients by title (Mr., Dr., Mrs., Miss, and so forth), and do not resort to such terms as "dearie," "dear," "honey," "mother," and "grandma." Such endearments should be reserved for members of your family and for friends. Using them with patients will communicate one thing to them—disrespect. Always try to sound cheerful, even though you may not feel particularly cheery at the moment; your patients and coworkers will note your efforts and appreciate them. Eliminate all forms of sarcasm and teasing, because nobody really appreciates this type of humor.

The subject of cheerfulness brings us to the second aspect of speech: the *manner* in which a thing is said. It is true that the most accomplished speaker in the world is quite useless if there is nothing worthwhile to say. It is also true that a poor delivery can nullify the effect of a statement, however important. Therefore, it will pay to devote some attention to the improvement of your manner of speaking.

No two voices are exactly alike. The particular quality of your voice is determined by the size and the shape of your vocal cords and resonators, but it is your personality that gives your voice that individuality that sets it apart from everyone else's. As you speak, your words convey only half the story; other variants, such as tone, pitch, inflection (changes in pitch or tone), rhythm, stress, and timing, communicate subtler meanings. Because your voice tells so much more about you than you probably suspect, you should concentrate on controlling it. We all know how irritating a raspy or whiny voice can be, how nerve racking a voice is that is too loud, and how exasperating it is to listen to someone who does not bother to pronounce words in their entirety. Practice speaking before a mirror, and as you do, remember the little jingle: "children's speech should always be plain to hear and clear to see." This applies equally well to adults. Pronounce your words as distinctly as possible, without skipping any syllables, and watch your lips as you do so. Most of us tend to be lazy and slur over parts of words; the visual check will help to prevent this. As you speak, your audience not only listens to you but also watches you. Because lip movements are a confirmation of what our ears tell us, it is necessary that speech be "plain to see."

If you feel self-conscious about speaking to strangers and are not sure of your ability to initiate and sustain a conversation, practice the art of conversation with your classmates. Use the warm-up technic of asking simple questions or making timely observations. Encourage others to talk about themseves and their personal interests. Here again, listen attentively. There are two reasons for this: first, it is a compliment to the other person; and second, it will take your mind off yourself, and your self-consciousness will vanish mysteriously. When you feel more sure of yourself, deliberately practice the technic of conversation with your patients and then be bold enough to experiment with total strangers. Conversation is a fascinating exercise and a game calling for the highest degree of skill. Remember that the way you express yourself may form the basis for your patient's evaluation of you. Thus skill in oral presentation can greatly affect the relationship you achieve with your patients.

Reading

Perhaps the most important tool in furthering your education and keeping up to date in your nursing career is reading. To read is not only to absorb information but also to become exposed to ideas. The habit of reading is one of the most valuable ones that you will ever acquire. In the course of your career you will discover that books are no substitute for practical experience, but, conversely, you will find that much of human experience is meaningless without the sort of analysis that can be found only through reading.

Reading is a technical skill that, like any other, improves with practice. You should read with two purposes in mind: speed and comprehension. Of course, your reading speed will vary with the nature of the material. A newspaper article may be scanned rapidly, but an assigned lesson will have to read more slowly with a great deal more mental effort on your part. The rate of reading depends on the number of pauses that your eye makes as it travels across the page. If you read word by word, your reading rate will be slower than if you read in whole phrases, since your eye makes only a few stops as it takes in entire sentences. Lip reading, whispering, reading aloud, and pointing to the words with your finger as you read will slow down your reading speed. It is usually easy to increase reading speed, but somewhat more difficult to improve your comprehension. Every word must have an immediate, and correct, meaning to you; the only way to achieve this is to build up your vocabulary.

You should own both a general and a medical dictionary. If you come across an unfamiliar word while reading, take the time to look it up, preferably at the moment that you encounter it. When you learn a simple definition of the new word, restate it in your own words. After you have learned the correct pronunciation, begin using your new word as soon as you can. In this way you are more likely to retain it.

When you encounter new medical terms, pay particular attention to the prefixes and the suffixes (usually of Greek or Latin origin). These are retained very easily. Armed with them, you will be able to dissect most unfamiliar medical terms as they come up, without the need of the dictionary.

Most nurses will acquire a personal library of nursing and medical books to augment their professional training. It cannot be stated often enough that you should be selective in building your library. In reviewing your nursing journals, you will be able to remain up to date on the new books available to you. It should always be remembered that what you choose to read could prove to be the difference in a "life or death" patient crisis.

Writing

During your nursing career you must write clearly and legibly. There is the note-taking in classes, in in-service programs, or in your day-to-day reading. There are patients' charts, requisition forms, application blanks, and numerous other forms that not only test your penmanship but also your ability to put your thoughts (or someone else's) into words and on paper. Since (unfortunately) not everyone writes legibly, printing or a manuscript form of writing has become the acceptable method of recording observations and findings on official papers. Regardless of whether your employer wishes you to print or write in script, the important point is that what you record must be legible and neat. Your signature should also be easily decipherable and not a matter of guesswork.

Note-taking in class is not only useful in recording the essence of a lecture, a discussion, or a passage from a book; it is also excellent writing practice, because it forces you to compress the most information into the fewest words. If you fail to choose the right words, you will pay the penalty later on in notes that are illegible, incomplete, ambiguous, or meaningless. Since writing tends to interfere with listening and thinking, it is best to record only the essential words and phrases. Avoid long notes. Keep your attention free for thought, and make your notes as brief as practicable.

More and more hospitals are adopting standard procedures of problem-oriented charting in patient care. Undoubtedly this will become the norm in the near future. Thus skilled charting, like note taking, is an invaluable addition to your nursing skills. Your observations are recorded on paper, and your ability to communicate these observations in writing is vitally important to the welfare of the patient. In charting, abbreviations may be used, but these must be standard within the hospital or other establishment in which you work. Each hospital usually has its own list of abbreviations.

When recording your observations on the patient's chart, think carefully and try your utmost to use the most precise and descriptive words and phrases possible. Avoid the use of such vague expressions as "morning care" (specify what actually *was* done); "patient cooperative" (does this mean simply that the patient did not make any trouble for you?); "patient worried" (about what?); "patient resting" (sleeping? entertaining visitors? reading? under sedation or not? Or does this mean that the patient simply has not buzzed the call bell for some time? The night nurse recording ''sleeping'' should check frequently in order to record total hours of sleep); ''patient ate well'' (specify amount, quantity, and type of food). The point is *be specific and concise.*

Gossip, Rumor, and "Happy Talk"

Although to many people gossip may seem like an innocent pastime, it can actually be as powerful, and as unpredictable, as dynamite. Leading scientists, spurred by the havoc created by gossip and rumor during World War II, have proved that ''innocent gossip'' is not merely small talk but can wreck people's homes and lives. Gossip and rumors have ruined businesses, driven famous and successful people to commit suicide, and forced innocent teachers, nurses, ministers, and others to give up their jobs in disgrace. What if some unpleasant gossip suddenly touched you or a member of your family? What would you do? How can *you* stop gossip? Most people gossip and spread rumors because they need to give themselves a feeling of importance. Most of those who listen and take gossip seriously do so because they *want* to believe it.

Dr. Gordon Allport, Harvard scientist, made this statement: ''Sex interest accounts for much gossip and most scandal. Anxiety is the power behind the macabre and threatening tales we so often hear. Hope and desire underlie pipedream rumors. Hate sustains accusatory tales and slander.''

Dr. Hadley Cantril of the Princeton University Psychology Department offers a three-part formula for dealing with gossip.

(1) Don't try to stop gossip by answering it. A frontal attack upon gossip calls attention to the false stories that are being spread, thus bringing them to the attention of more and more people. If an angered father punches a man in the nose for gossiping about his daughter, he merely starts more gossip.

(2) Go on performing—doing your job, living your life—in a suitable manner. Frustrating as this may seem, it is the best way to hasten gossip out of existence. Friends rally round a man or woman who goes on with the job, business as usual, while the bitter tongues wag. By carrying on you are showing in a concrete way that you are not the kind of person characterized by the gossip.

(3) Stage a demonstration. By analyzing gossip it is often possible to kill it off indirectly. When a couple are dogged by gossip of a marital split-up, they can demonstrate their accord in numerous ways. It gives tongues something else to wag about.

In talking with others have you ever used the expression ''they said''? Did you identify the ''they''? Would you have been able to if asked? Have you ever taken the opportunity to question the person who is using ''they'' as the voice of authority or source of ''they said'' or ''they claim''? Often ''they'' represents an unknown source, which, upon closer investigation turns out to be the invention of gossipers and rumor spreaders.

As a reminder to all gossipers, remember that no gossip is ever harmless. It will damage not only the person at whom it is directed but the gossiper as well. Friends will not confide in those who gossip, and very often will not believe the truth when it is told by gossipers.

"Hospital happy talk" (the conversational jargon you hear in the hospital) is often frightening to those who overhear it—primarily your patients and their visitors. Discussing their work and patients seems natural for most nurses and doctors. Most people are not deeply interested in the new surgical procedure Dr. Scalpel has perfected, the infectious hepatitis case on 5 North, and the demanding patients that may be encountered. Be selective in your conversational topics, and remember that a "well-rounded" nurse must have other things to talk about besides school, hospital, patients, and nursing. (See Chapters 5 and 7 for sections on shop talk.)

APPEARANCE AND GROOMING
Cleanliness

In nursing, both men and women should follow similar guidelines for cleanliness, the importance of which is obvious. No patient will feel comfortable in the presence of a nurse whose lack of cleanliness is noticeable. In addition, there is always the risk of contamination or cross-infection by patients and nurses who are not clean. Cleanliness is related to one's self-image. The nurse who feels clean and attractive will generally convey an attractive image to patients. The nurse who has body odor, or obviously unwashed or unkempt hair, or whose hands or fingernails show dirt cannot possibly maintain the maximal positive relationship with a patient. Standards of cleanliness and appearance must by nature be higher for nurses than for people in most other professions, and every nurse should make an effort to achieve perfection in this area.

Clothing

Clean clothes go hand in hand with personal cleanliness. It is absolutely essential that every nurse wear clean clothes every day. Uniforms, shoes, and all external wearing apparel should be aired out after each wearing, if washing or brushing are not yet indicated. All personal items of clothing should obviously be washed after each day's wearing. Clothing is a very important aspect of the nurse's appearance. Often a patient will see only the white of the uniform that enters the room, so that the more attractive an image you establish in your uniform, the more positive will be your image as a nurse.

Makeup

Makeup is no longer as commonly used as it once was; however, nurses who do use it should apply it subtly and effectively, and never to excess. An effective and moderate use of makeup will make many women more attractive, not only to patients but also to themselves.

Uniform and Cap

Uniformity in dress for nuns and others working in convents probably began in the early Middle Ages, when the weaving of cloth was one of the duties of convent women. Also, it is presumed that the veil, which, by ancient custom, represents obedience and service, was adopted as a headpiece. As time went on, the customs pertaining to the wearing of veils and robes were influenced by religious and lay organizations, each of which prescribed the length of the veil, the color and the materials of the robes, and the manner of their use. The Sisters of Charity wore a gray blue gown of rough woolen cloth, a blue apron, and a spreading headdress. In the early 19th century, the Deaconesses of Kaiserswerth wore a dark blue uniform, a bibbed apron, a white collar, and a hoodlike cap with ruffle and broad strings that tied in a bow under the chin. In 1876, at Bellevue Hospital the first complete uniform for student nurses was introduced by Miss Van Rensselaer, who wore a blue and white striped long dress with white apron, collar, and cuffs. The cap, which was designed to cover the hair, was referred to by many Bellevue students as the "birdcage" and is still worn today.

Each school has always been interested in designing its own uniform and distinctive cap. In modern times many schools have turned away from delicate fabrics with frills, fluting, ruching, and other decorative items because of ironing problems. Instead, they are using cotton and wash-and-wear fabrics, which are simpler and therefore easier to launder and maintain. School bands, which are worn on the cap, often may be black for professional nurses and gray for practical nurses, although other colors can be used by these graduates as well. The popular belief that a graduate professional nurse wears a black band to signify that she has passed State Boards, or that she is in mourning for Florence Nightingale, or for some other such reason, has no basis in fact; each school of nursing sets its policy for the design of the school cap. A nurse who, for some reason, is unable to obtain her school cap may wear another type, provided that she does not pretend to be a graduate of some school other than her own. Therefore, one cannot always tell what school the nurse is from by the cap that she wears. Males nurses do not wear caps.

Most state-licensed practical nurse associations do recommend that their members identify themselves by wearing the letters LPN on the left wing of the cap or on the uniform sleeve. Many organizations have their own state insignias, which are available to the members. Alumnae associations as well as schools of practical nursing also have their own distinctive insignias.

Nurses should wear uniforms only when on duty. If lockers or a dressing area are not available, it has been generally accepted that nurses may travel to work in uniform, and add their cap, pin, and other items when they are ready to work. Most employers will encourage nurses to wear their state pin and sleeve emblem, and if they are graduates, they will be asked to wear their school cap, pin, and sleeve insignia. Usually, no other accessories may be worn except engagement and wedding rings.

Here are some "do's" and "don'ts" for wearing the uniform:

DO

Wear the uniform and the cap in accordance with your school's or employer's personnel policies.

Have your uniform spotlessly clean, ironed, properly buttoned, and the proper length.

Wear proper shoes that are polished and have supporting and straight heels that are in good repair.

Have a watch with second hand, a pen, scissors, and other articles that you need constantly in the performance of your duties.

If you wear a cap have it stiffly starched, without wrinkles, and make doubly sure that your "band" or emblem is affixed properly, without using visible clips, bobby pins, and so forth; and fastened so that there is no excess material showing.

Wear your uniform with pride and dignity. Be proud of it and set an example to others by being immaculately groomed and dressed as what you are—a nurse.

DON'T

Don't wear your cap in public places or on the street (except at official functions approved by your school or employer). Carry it in a plastic bag to protect it.

If you use perfume, makeup, jewelry, or fingernail polish, choose these with care to complement your uniform and general appearance.

Don't let the tobacco odor linger on and become a part of your uniform if you smoke. Never smoke in the presence of a patient, around inflammable and explosive mixtures such as anesthetics or oxygen, or in public places.

Don't chew gum or drink alcoholic beverages while in uniform.

Don't bring disgrace on your uniform or the vocation you are a part of by wearing the uniform in places of questionable reputation.

YOUR HEALTH

Nurses must not only look and act healthy but should also be healthy. Most of us will consult a physician if we are seriously ill or have some obvious symptom that needs medical attention, but very few nurses see their physician regularly once a year, or as often as recommended, for a physical examination—this should be considered mandatory. If the physician has your records and knows your health status, it will be easier to diagnose and determine the nature and the extent of your illnesses. Additional examinations may be needed to arrive at an early diagnosis to correct or treat any minor ailments. Medical as well as dental check-ups are "musts" for every nurse. If your employer does not offer a routine physical examination as part of the personnel policies, it should become a personal responsibility to have such an examination done on your own, not only to safeguard your health but also for the sake of your family, patients, and co-workers. If you desire personal medical advice, remember that it is undesirable and against good professional judgment for you to approach physicians while on duty with questions pertaining to your health problems or those of your family. Seek their advice through their offices, and be sure to offer to pay for the services rendered If the physician wishes to adjust the usual fee as a courtesy to you, or will accept your insurance coverage as total payment, it is important that you acknowledge this kindness.

If you are hospitalized, remember that your hospital bill must be paid like any other patient's. Sometimes nurses think that they need not pay their employers or those agencies with which they are affiliated, but unless personnel policies clearly state otherwise, the financial obligation is yours. (Herein lies the reason for considering a hospitalization insurance plan.) Many hospitals may offer certain courtesies to their employees in this regard; here again it is polite to thank them and not to expect these favors as a matter of course.

Diet

A balanced diet is important to the general well-being of the body. Regularity of mealtime, as well as eating in a relaxed atmosphere, is conducive to good nutrition. you should start the day with a good breakfast, because food provides energy; unless you keep your body supplied with the proper foods, you will tire easily and lack the energy to do your best in whatever you have undertaken. Your weight control depends on intelligent eating habits. It all adds up to the calories you did or did not have. To gain weight, your caloric intake must exceed the amount lost in normal energy expenditure. If you wish to lose weight, you simply reverse the process. Although eating between meals may be sociable and fun, it can add up in your caloric intake. You can eat quite adequately and still lose weight if you choose your foods wisely from the basic groups. A nurse who practices poor eating habits will certainly not set a good example to those cared for. Can you imagine a 210-pound nurse telling a patient how to reduce or to stick to a diet? Are you the one who does not drink milk and then turns around and insists that your child does?

Here is an eight-point guide to assist you in understanding the new concept about dietary moderation for improving health:

1. Eat a variety of foods.
2. Maintain your ideal weight.
3. Avoid too much fat and saturated fats and cholesterol.
4. Eat foods with adequate starch and fiber.
5. Avoid too much sugar.
6. Avoid too much sodium.
7. If you drink alcohol, do so in moderation.
8. Avoid crash diets and change your eating habits and include more exercise instead.

Alcohol

Alcoholism, one of today's major public health problems, affects more Americans than any other form of drug addiction. Once viewed essentially as a moral issue, it now has the attention of the physician, the nurse, the sociologist, and others interested in the health and welfare of our society. In the past few years there has been an enormous increase in alcoholism among women. An increase in the death rate of alcoholics as well has been noted.

Although alcohol initially produces a feeling of exhilaration, it is a nervous system depressant, acting on the brain and spinal cord. The effect of alcohol depends on one's sensitivity to it and the amount consumed. Excessive amounts produce dependence and may lead to confusion, stupor, and gradual mental and physical deterioration. Alcoholics can never be cured; if they take even one drink, they are unable to resist the desire to take more.

Alcoholism is an illness that not only causes human suffering but also costs a great deal in terms of crime, accidents, and medical care. You, as a nurse, must be aware of your responsibilities in the prevention and treatment of this illness. You may be asked to take care of an alcoholic in the home or the hospital, or you may be associated with an alcoholic in visiting or industrial nursing. Always approach the patient with an understanding of the illness and at all times show sincere respect and interest in the problem. It would be wise always to remember that alcoholism is more than just a psychological problem; it is an incurable disease that normally is the direct result of personal stress or frustration. In the fast pace of today's living, alcoholism has become so rampant that many of us have or will encounter it within our own families.

Human Sexuality

Sexuality—an important dimension of being a person—is a modern topic of discussion. Unfortunately, many health care professionals have not kept up to date with the needed information for patient teaching and counseling. Hang-ups on sexual matters have kept many nurses, social workers, and physicians from being effective counselors on sexual matters. Abortion, family planning, homosexuality, sex education, transexualism, and venereal diseases are the main topics that fall under this broad subject. Your objective knowledge in these areas, as the sexual revolution continues, will have a very specific impact on your personal attitudes and behavior toward your patients. Your patients will have their own sexual beliefs and self-determination based on sexual mores and practices that may be different from yours.

Sexually Transmitted Diseases

Sexually transmitted diseases (STD) is the new term for venereal diseases (VD). As infectious diseases, they are surpassed in incidence only by the common cold. In 1979, primary and secondary syphilis was provisionally reported at 25,210 with an estimated 80,000 to 85,000 cases occurring. Gonorrhea was provisionally reported at one million cases, with an estimated 1.6 to two million cases occurring annually. There were more than 10 million visits to physicians and clinics for sexually transmitted disease problems.

An epidemic of these diseases is creating a vast number of sterile women in the

United States. It has been estimated that 80,000 women become sterile every year because of failure to get treatment for pelvic inflammatory diseases. Table 4–1 depicts the cases of venereal diseases for 1948, 1958, 1968, and 1978; Table 4–2 depicts the other sexually transmitted diseases as they were estimated in 1977.

One of the best ways to control STD is through education, which must start with you. As a nurse armed with adequate facts, you will be able to speak to groups and individuals about the causative organisms, incubation periods, modes of transmission, methods of diagnosis, and principles of prevention and treatment. Because STD has no respect for anyone, contact investigation is part of the education and treatment program. As a nurse, you must not sit in moral judgment of the patient or anyone seeking your advice on this important topic. The spread of STD is always related to sexual relations; therefore you must be as honest, frank, and objective as possible in talking to your patient. It is imperative that the sex partner or contact also seek medical attention, or reinfection will result. Many state and local health departments offer free services and will accept minors for free STD diagnosis and treatment without parental consent.

In the last few years television programs such as public television's "VD Blues" have been shown with regularity in an attempt to educate the public about STD. However, the fact remains that in many American homes STD is not even allowed as a topic of conversation. Since education always starts in the home, an enormous percentage of young Americans are either misinformed or uninformed about STD and methods of prevention, protection, and cure. As a practical nurse you will be able to work for a reversal of this situation. STD is everyone's business, and only when education on this subject reaches every American home will we be able to foresee a method of controlling it.

Drug Abuse

In response to the widespread misuse and abuse of dangerous drugs (depressants, stimulants, and hallucinogens), the Bureau of Drug Abuse Control was organized as part of the Food and Drug Administration in 1966 (see Chapter 8). Drug addiction, like alcohol addiction, is the result of the habitual use of a drug and the establishment of a physical dependency. Many addicts start by smoking marijuana and than graduate to heroin and other potent addictive drugs.

The problem of drug addiction is acute among young people, particularly the teenager. A high percentage of preadolescents and adolescents smoke marijuana regularly and use other drugs such as pep pills. Because you are a nurse and sometimes have access to drugs, you may be asked for a supply of "barbs," "goofballs," "peanuts," "yellow jackets," or "red devils,"—some of the names given these drugs by the user. You must be aware of your legal responsibilities in this situation and under no circumstances make the drug available to any person unless it is prescribed by a physician. The use of marijuana has now become so commonplace that in some states marijuana users are for the most part not arrested. Many states have voted against proposals to legalize marijuana, but it is possible that in time such a resolution may pass.

According to a most recent National Institute on Drug Abuse (NIDA) survey,

TABLE 4–1.   CASES OF VENEREAL DISEASE REPORTED BY STATE HEALTH
DEPARTMENTS, AND RATES PER 100,000 POPULATION
United States Total (Known Military Cases Excluded): Calendar years
1948, 1958, 1968, 1978

			Syphilis					
Year	All Stages*		Primary and Secondary		Early Latent		Late and Late Latent	
	Cases	Rates	Cases	Rates	Cases	Rates	Cases	Rates
1948	314,313	218.2	68,174	47.3	90,598	62.9	123,312	85.6
1958	113,884	66.4	7,176	4.2	16,556	9.7	83,027	48.4
1968	96,271	48.7	19,019	9.6	15,150	7.7	58,564	29.6
1978	64,875	30.0	21,656	10.0	19,628	9.1	23,038	10.6

(Compiled from available data. Source: CDC 9.688, HEW-PHS-CDC-BSS-VD Control Division, Evaluation
and Statistical Services Section, Atlanta, Georgia)
* Includes stage of syphilis not stated.
† Rates less than 0.05 are shown as 0.

over nine million teenagers smoke pot. The NIDA has found that the percentage
of ninth graders using marijuana has risen from 16.9% of the class of 1975 to 25.2%
of the class of 1978. New research concludes that smoking marijuana may indeed
be hazardous to a person's physical and mental health. Dr. Ingrid L. Langer, a
pediatrician at the Erieside Clinic in Willoughby, Ohio reports alarming symptoms
among marijuana-smoking children—fatigue, decreased school performance, and
decreased performance in sports, irritability, sudden mood changes, paranoid
thinking, depression, and hallucinations. The most striking symptom is the loss of
short-term memory. Research also indicates that smoking marijuana affects the
reproductive processes and the immunity systems of the lungs. Dr. Robert Heath
of Tulane University, who specializes in the study of marijuana and its effects on
the brain, claims that there is no similarity in the way tobacco, alcohol, and
marijuana act on the brain. He states that "there is much more profound influence
induced on the brain functioning and on the brain structure by marijuana."

The more serious illegal drugs include the hallucinogen, LSD-25, a lysergic acid
derivative that may have totally unpredictable effects from person to person,
sometimes recurring weeks or months after it is taken; methedrine, better known
as "speed," which accelerates the metabolism, stimulates the nervous system,
and is often known to be fatal after extensive use; cocaine, heroin, and any of the
new substitute drugs invented to replace drugs about to become unavailable (an
example of which is "liquid hashish" created as a substitute for heroin, found
mainly in New York City and said to be even more powerful than heroin). All of
these drugs must be considered deadly, and every nurse should be able to recognize as many of their side effects as possible. You must be well informed about
both legal and illegal drugs, as drug abuse has become a problem so common that
it cannot be ignored.

The conviction of a felony (illegal possession of drugs in most states) in the
courts of a state, territory, or country, may be sufficient evidence for disciplinary

Congenital		Gonorrhea		Chancroid		Granuloma Inguinale†		Lympho-granuloma Venereum	
Cases	Rates	Cases	Rates	Cases	Rates	Cases	Rates	Cases	Rates
13,931	9.7	345,501	239.8	7,661	5.3	2,469	1.7	2,429	1.7
4,866	2.8	232,386	135.6	1,595	0.9	314	0.2	434	0.3
2,381	1.2	464,543	235.1	845	0.4	156	0.1	485	0.2
434	0.2	1,013,436	468.3	521	0.2	72	0.0	284	0.1

action by the Board of Nursing and Nurse Examiners. This would prevent you from writing the licensure examination or if you have passed, your license could be denied, suspended, or revoked.

It is, for example, both tragic and ironic that one of the most popular drugs available "on the street" is methadone, which was created as a nontoxic substitute for the killer drug heroin. Originally methadone was administered only in limited doses in special clinics for heroin addicts. It was and is a legal drug (if prescribed by a doctor), but now any addict can buy it on the street more easily than heroin.

The tragedy of drug abuse is one of the real dilemmas of our time. Just as sexually transmitted diseases can be controlled through education, so can drug abuse. As a nurse you must be prepared to answer questions about drugs and also to do what you can to help young people avoid the trap of drug addiction.

Smoking

In a sense, cigarette, pipe, and cigar smoking are both addictive and contagious. Your friends and parents may smoke, and you are constantly exposed to subtle and sophisticated advertisements. The decision of whether to smoke or not is a

TABLE 4–2. OTHER SEXUALLY TRANSMITTED DISEASES, 1977 *

Disease or Condition	Estimated Annual Incidence
Trichomoniasis	600,000-1,000,000
Genital *Herpesviris hominis*	150,000- 200,000
Pediculosis pubis (crab louse)	100,000- 200,000
Condyloma acuminatum (genital warts)	200,000- 400,000
Nongonococcal urethritis (NGU)	800,000-1,000,000

* (STD Fact Sheet, 34th ed, p 3. Atlanta, Center for Disease Control, 1979)

personal matter, but remember that "cigarette smoking may be hazardous to your health." Your image as a health teacher and a nurse should also be considered.

It has been established that smoking is directly connected with serious conditions such as heart disease, lung cancer, and emphysema. Health authorities are especially concerned about the increasing number of young people who smoke. In an attempt to prevent students from developing the habit, films are being shown in many school health programs, depicting the physical body changes caused by smoking.

In smoking withdrawal clinics, the first step is usually to analyze *when* and *why* a person smokes. Some of the reasons for smoking are tension, anger, and habit. Once the reason is determined, a personal program to eliminate the habit can be formulated. For many, a series of deep, slow inhalations and exhalations or physical exercise helps release tensions and ease the craving for a cigarette. The real addict may first have to learn to inhale less to avoid nostalgic feelings and to lessen his dependence on smoking.

The American Hospital Association was one of the many organizations that endorsed the Bill of Rights for Non-Smokers in 1974. The bill states that non-smokers have the right to breathe clean, unpolluted air, the right to speak out in public places, and the right to take action through legislative and other legitimate channels.

The rights of nonsmokers must be protected! "GASP" (Groups Against Smoking & Pollution) is being organized in many communities. Perhaps you would like to join or organize a chapter. Your involvement is needed.

No one can prevent you from drinking alcohol, using drugs, or smoking cigarettes. However, remember too that no one can *force* you to develop any of these potentially habit-forming activities. These are decisions that individuals must make for themselves.

Your Eyes

Since so many of your nursing skills will depend on keen vision, you should take good care of your eyes and preserve your eyesight. If you wear glasses or contact lenses, be sure that you have them with you and do not hesitate to use them whenever they are indicated. Your ophthalmologist will have given you specific instructions, and this advice must be followed. If your eyes need attention, and through heedlessness or vanity you fail to get glasses or to have your eyes checked, you penalize not only yourself but also others. Because you cannot see as clearly as you should, your safety and comfort as well as your job or study performance will be hindered; also, your body will tire much more quickly, and even your disposition may be affected. Save your eyes from unnecessary strain. When you read, hold the printed page about 45 centimeters (18 inches) from your eyes, with a good light coming over your shoulder to avoid your own shadow.

Rest and Sleep

Because of the heavy demands of study and practice, you may find that you need more rest than you did before you entered this vocation. Inadequate sleep and rest are most often indicated by fatigue, general lassitude, an indifferent or unpleasant disposition, and a colorless appearance. The recognition of these symptoms in the early stages of fatigue should lead to changes in your pattern of living. Although the amount of sleep necessary varies with the individual, it is generally believed that you need between seven and eight hours each night. One way to tell if you are getting enough sleep is to ask yourself, "Am I rested when I wake up?". You may have slept for hours but still wake up tired and tense if you were without fresh air in the room, a comfortable bed, or did not have a relaxed disposition when you went to bed. If you do not have enough rest (and remember, you cannot store up sleep), your efficiency and your general appearance will suffer. That "fatigue slump" will give you away, even if the circles under your eyes are hidden.

Posture and Body Mechanics

Good posture, the proper arrangement of body parts, adds to your appearance, provides physical comfort to you, and helps to promote the normal functioning of your body organs. It is essential, whether you are standing, lying down, sitting, stooping, or bending. Although most of your functional spinal curvatures began many years ago, and are rather well set as habits, you can always take steps to improve your posture. Good posture is not only attractive but also minimizes fatigue, because the muscular strains are imposed where nature intended.

Your nursing activities will include many kinds of complex bodily movements, such as moving, lifting, and turning patients. It is most important that you be familiar with the principles of good body mechanics, which is the science of using your body efficiently, safely, and without undue fatigue.

Dental Care

Your health and appearance will be influenced by the care that your teeth receive. An unclean mouth is offensive, and the "smile of good health" will not be effective unless good dental care is given. Frequent and proper brushing of your teeth and regular cleanings by your dentist will help to prevent tooth decay; however, your diet (particularly the foods eaten while you were a youngster) will determine to a great extent the number of dental cavities that you have or will have. Starches and sugars affect not only the waistline but also your teeth and gums. Cut down on those sweets and you will also save on your visits to the dentist. Regular visits to your dentist should be made at intervals of about six months, and even if you wear dentures, their fit and effect on the gums should be reviewed at scheduled intervals. Remember that many serious diseases can originate in infections of the mouth and the teeth.

Questions

A. Select the correct answer and circle the number that answers the question best.

1. Desirable qualities for practical nurses include (A) honesty, (B) a liking for people, (C) originality, (D) neatness.
   1. All of these
   2. All except C
   3. All except D
   4. All except A

2. Prejudices are (A) based on realistic judgment, (B) based on preconceived ideas, (C) characteristics of well-adjusted people, (D) overcome by those who desire to do so.
   1. A, B
   2. A, D
   3. B, C
   4. B, D

3. Mentally healthy people will (A) accept their shortcomings, (B) feel they are part of a group, (C) accept responsibilities, (D) set realistic goals.
   1. All of these
   2. All except A
   3. All except B
   4. All except D

4. Mature nursing students (A) derive satisfaction from nursing, (B) recognize patients as individuals, (C) follow orders, (D) face reality.
   1. All of these
   2. All except A
   3. All except B
   4. All except C

5. Habits are (A) good or bad, (B) easily broken, (C) related to personal interests, (D) hereditary.
   1. All of these
   2. A, C, D
   3. A, C
   4. A, D

6. "Culture" includes (A) food preferences, (B) language, (C) type of shelter, (D) religious observances.
   1. All of these
   2. All except B
   3. All except C
   4. All except D

7. Defense mechanisms include (A) fantasy, (B) regression, (C) compensation, (D) stereotyping.
   1. All of these
   2. All except B
   3. All except C
   4. All except D

8. The hierarchy of needs include (A) physical, (B) safety, (C) transactional, (D) self-esteem.
   1. All of these
   2. All except B
   3. All except C
   4. All except D

9. Physical needs include (A) food, (B) water, (C) oxygen, (D) shelter.
   1. All of these
   2. All except B
   3. All except C
   4. All except D

10. If convicted of a felony, your license could be (A) suspended, (B) revoked, (C) denied, (D) renewed.
    1. All of these
    2. A, B, C
    3. D
    4. A, B

B. Complete the following statements.

1. The first complete student nurse uniform was introduced by Miss Van Rensselaer at _____ Hospital.

2. Repeating or restating the patient's comments to him is called _____

_____

3. The superego is called our _____

4. The relationship between mind and body is accepted as the basis for_____

_____

5. Although sleep needs vary with the individual, student nurses should have _____
_____ hours every night.

6. When you replace a "guilt-producing" activity with a socially accepted one you use
the defense mechanism known as _____

7. A person with "good mental health" is considered to be emotionally _____

_____

8. The hierarchy of needs was developed by _____

9. P stands for _____

10. A stands for _____

11. C stands for _____

C. True or False. Write *T* or *F* in answer space.

_____ 1. The id controls the ego.
_____ 2. Black bands on the nurse's cap are worn by all RNs.
_____ 3. Weight control depends primarily on eating habits.
_____ 4. Regular visits to the dentist are not necessary once you have dentures.
_____ 5. A mature person is usually one with good mental health.
_____ 6. Prejudices are usually inherited.
_____ 7. Communication can be verbal or nonverbal.
_____ 8. Nurses should "listen" rather than "talk" to patients.
_____ 9. "Set speeches" are good in building patient relationships.
_____ 10. Conversion and compensation are identical.
_____ 11. Syphilis outranks gonorrhea in incidence among the sexually transmitted
diseases.
_____ 12. Sensitivity group participation for all people is highly recommended by leading
authorities for developing self-awareness.

Answers (3⅓ points each)

A. Multiple Choice	B. Completion	C. True or False
1. 2	1. Bellevue	1. F
2. 4	2. reflecting	2. F
3. 1	3. conscience	3. T
4. 1	4. psychosomatic medicine	4. F
5. 3	5. seven to eight	5. T
6. 1	6. sublimation	6. F
7. 4	7. mature	7. T
8. 3	8. A. Maslow	8. T
9. 1	9. parent	9. F
10. 2	10. adult	10. F
	11. child	11. F
		12. F

5

Health Care Facilities and You

Health Systems Agencies • Comprehensive Health Services • Kidney Dialysis Centers • The Hospital of Today • Nursing Homes • Home Health Services • Hospices • Community Mental Health Centers • Acupuncture Clinics • Health Maintenance Organizations • Pharmacies • Health Insurance • Health Care Providers • Health Quackery • Getting Along in Your Institution • Questions and Answers

Objectives

Upon completion of this chapter you should be able to

1. list health care facilities by classification,
2. identify ten inpatient and ten outpatient health care facilities,
3. explain the educational preparation and major responsibilities of at least 15 health care providers,
4. diagram the table of organization for the nursing department in one of your affiliating agencies,
5. summarize the health insurance benefits obtainable from Medicare,
6. discuss the problems of health quackery,
7. review your obligations and responsibilities when working in a health care facility,
8. explain your relationship with colleagues, physicians, and registered nurses in a health care setting.

   The United States Department of Health and Human Services conducts annual studies on health care manpower and facilities. The health care agencies are designated as "inpatient health facilities" and "outpatient and nonpatient health services."
   In 1976 there were an estimated 34,199 hospitals and nursing care and related homes facilities. Of these, 20,185 were in the nursing care and related homes

category, and 7,271 were hospitals. There were an estimated 3.2 million beds distributed as shown in (Table 5-1).

Other inpatient facilities included residential schools or homes for the blind or deaf, homes for the emotionally disturbed, facilities for the physically handicapped, homes for unwed mothers, homes for dependent children and orphanages, facilities for the mentally retarded, institutions for alcoholics, sheltered care homes, and boarding homes.

Outpatient health services such as those provided by a hospital outpatient department, emergency room, and clinic are increasingly being used to meet community needs. In 1976 there were about 273 million such visits, of which one third were of an emergency nature. In 1976 there were over 77 million visits. Emergency treatment facilities existed in 5,087 hospitals, and 1,914 hospitals conducted outpatient departments.

Additionally, there were 13,883 ambulance services, 100 ambulatory surgical centers, 6,820 blood banks, 13,626 clinical (medical) laboratories, 11,500 dental laboratories, 4,660 family planning clinics, 841 kidney dialysis centers, and 654 poison control centers. Other health services offered in 1976 included 8,500 group practices by three or more physicians, 2500 home health care agencies, 5,900 opticianary establishments, 244 psychiatrist and mental health outpatient services, 3,000 rehabilitation centers, and 189 suicide prevention centers.

HEALTH SYSTEMS AGENCIES

The National Health Planning and Resources Act of 1974, or Public Law 93-641, was signed into law in 1975 and oversees health planning provisions of previous legislation. This law provides for the creation of health systems agencies (HSAs), the designation of state health planning, and the development of agencies on local levels within the states. The state and local agency must certify the need for new institutional and health services within that state and implement the health system plan devised by these agencies. The health system agency has the primary responsibility for effective health planning and identifies needed health facilities, health services, and health care personnel.

On all health systems agencies, the board of directors must be a representation from the consumers within that area as well as the providers of health care.

COMPREHENSIVE HEALTH SERVICES

A complete range of all services directed toward the promotion of positive health is embraced by comprehensive health services. This includes preventive measures and early detection of disease as well as prompt and effective treatment of the physical, social, and vocational rehabilitation needs of the patient. Comprehensive health services are provided by several establishments within the community, including hospitals that have facilities for home care programs, health care facilities that have personal care and residential centers, community health programs that are public, and voluntary and personal services of physicians, dentists, and other health professionals. Comprehensive health services are primarily directed to the special needs of the people. The most generally known comprehensive health care services include those for the poor, mentally ill, and migrants.

KIDNEY DIALYSIS CENTERS

Hemodialysis treatment is now available in Kidney Dialysis Centers or End-Stage Renal Dialysis (ESRD) facilities, also known as Artificial Kidney Centers, hemodialysis centers, or dialysis centers. These centers may be part of a hospital's inpatient or outpatient services or may be under private auspices. It is expected that about 50,000 to 60,000 patients will receive treatment in these centers.

THE HOSPITAL OF TODAY

With its improved facilities for patient care, the hospital of today is a technological marvel. Intercommunication systems between patient and nurse, electrically operated beds, automatically controlled oxygen and suction pipelines, monitoring devices, computers, disposable and prepackaged sterile equipment, and numerous other innovations have dramatically and efficiently improved patient care. High-level patient care is becoming a reality because of improvements in medical and nursing technics.

Hospitals have steadily improved, but not until now has the rate of progress seemed so impressive. In the last 10 years there has been a much better use of hospital beds. Shorter hospitalization periods have probably made this feasible, since no notable increase in the physical number of hospital beds has been reported.

From the standpoint of investments, personnel employed, and services rendered, hospitals are among the top 5 industries of the United States. Their total assets are more than $47.3 billion. Over 3.2 million people are employed in hospitals, and a total of $37.1 billion is spent for payroll expenses. The operational costs of hospitals are almost $70.9 billion annually. It has been estimated that hospital employees represent about 375 different job classifications of professional and vocational workers; it is easy to see that with increasing expansions in the fields of health and medicine, more and more specially skilled and trained employees will be needed.

One thinks of a hospital as an institution designed to meet the needs of the sick. The average person is seldom aware of the many other responsibilities and lesser known activities of hospitals that occur both within and outside of the institution. The modern hospital not only takes care of the sick and the injured but also provides facilities for the education of physicians, nurses, technicians, and other personnel. It runs clinical and research laboratories and takes an active role in the prevention of disease and the promotion of health through its clinics and outpatient departments. In 1978 more than 3,250,000 babies were born in hospitals. On an average day there were almost 1.1 million patients hospitalized, with over a half million of these in nonfederal short-term hospitals, where more than 2,662,000

TABLE 5–1. INPATIENT HEALTH FACILITIES 1976

	Facility	Beds	Per 1,000 Population
Total	34,199	3,200,920	14.9
Hospitals	7,271	1,381,267	6.4
General medical and surgical hospitals	6,361	1,069,828	5.0
Specialty hospitals	910	311,439	1.5
Psychiatric	502	244,358	1.1
Chronic disease	63	19,933	0.1
Tuberculosis	21	3,546	0.0
Other*	324	43,602	0.2
Nursing care and related homes	20,185†	1,406,778†	6.6†
Nursing care	13,312	1,173,519	5.5
Personal care home with nursing			
Personal care home without nursing	6,873‡	223,259‡	1.0‡
Domiciliary care			
Other inpatient health facilities	6,743†	412,875†	1.9†

(Compiled from U.S. Department of Health, Education, and Welfare: Health Resources Statistics 1976–77, p 302. Source: Unpublished data from the National Center for Health Statistics Master Facility Census)
* Includes eye, ear, nose, and throat hospitals; epilepsy hospitals; alcoholism hospitals; narcotic addiction hospitals; maternity hospitals; orthopedic hospitals; physical rehabilitation hospitals; and other hospitals.
† Preliminary data.
‡ Includes personal care homes with nursing, personal care homes without nursing, and domiciliary care homes.

employees took care of them. About 323 employees are needed to care for every 100 patients in these voluntary general hospitals, also called community hospitals.

A partnership designed to offer patients in an acute short-term hospital the benefits of extended care and nursing home care has been achieved under the Medicare program. Extended care facilities often have transfer agreements with the general short-term hospital, with staff participation in coordinated educational and teaching activities.

A bold new approach to the prevention and treatment of mental illness was authorized by the United States Congress in 1963. Comprehensive community health centers are being built and developed separately or in conjunction with general hospitals, whereas state mental hospitals are being phased out. General hospitals are adding psychiatric screening and acute treatment facilities. They are also providing inpatient and outpatient services, with partial hospitalization for night care when suitable home arrangements are not available.

To bridge the gap between hospital and home care, a new pattern has evolved to bring continuity of care to patients in their homes. The development of new rehabilitation technics, better home care concepts, the demand for hospital beds, and the lack of skilled personnel in the hospital have necessitated a cooperative venture between the hospital and community health and welfare agencies. The coordinated home care program usually involves the nursing and social work staff of the hospital, the Visiting Nurse Association, Home Health Services, and other vocational rehabilitation agencies. A home care team representing these disciplines and others works cooperatively through the referral system. Such cooperative efforts may be initiated by the physician or an alert nurse when the patient's discharge plans from the hospital are discussed. Interdisciplinary planning involving therapeutic and nursing specialists determines the best procedures for the individual patient and family, or meaningful others, so that the doctor's orders may be followed in the home under the supervision of qualified visiting nurses and home health aides.

Size of Hospital and Length of Patient Stay

All hospitals are categorized according to the number of available beds. There are those with less than 25 beds, 25–49 beds, 50–99 beds, 100–199 beds, 200–299 beds, 300–399 beds, 400–499 beds, and 500 beds and over. The largest category of nongovernment not-for-profit hospitals falls into the 100–199–bed capacity, with the 50–99–bed capacity next. The greatest number of official federal and state operated hospitals are those with 500 beds and over, whereas county and city hospitals are predominantly in the 50–99–bed capacity, with 25–49 beds next in frequency.

Hospitals are also classified according to the average length of stay of their patients. Those hospitals caring for patients who usually stay less than 30 days are called short-term, whereas those hospitals housing patients who stay more than 30 days are called long-term institutions. Short-term institutions far outnumber long-term ones.

Service and Control

Hospitals are arbitrarily grouped into four major classifications: general, tuberculosis, psychiatric, and other specialized fields. The ownership and the type of organization controlling the institution makes up the next category. The terms voluntary or private, nongovernmental not-for-profit, investor-owned (for profit), or governmental or official, generally are used. Governmental institutions are those operated and owned by federal, state, city, or county governments. This includes those hospitals that fall under the auspices of the United States Armed Forces (Army, Navy, and Air Force), the Veterans Administration, the Bureau of Indian Affairs, and the United States Public Health Service. In 1978 there were 370 federal and 1,843 local and state-operated government institutions.

The private or voluntary institutions are those owned and operated by churches and religious orders, labor unions, business and industrial corporations, or by individuals or partners. If the institution is organized and administered to make a profit for the services rendered, it is called "proprietary" or investor owned. However, most hospitals are nonprofit in nature. The American Hospital Association reported that in 1978 the total average daily expense per patient in a short-term voluntary not-for-profit institution was almost $200, which was several dollars per day less than it actually cost to render patient care. *The Wall Street Journal* reported that in September 1980 a semiprivate room ranged in cost from a low of $78 per day in Lexington, Kentucky, to a high of $270 per day in New York.

Organization and Functions

At the head of any hospital organization there is usually a governing body known as the Board of Trustees, or Directors, who see to it that the hospital renders adequate service to its patients at as low a cost as possible. The Board also defines the functions of the institution as well as the philosophy of the administration under which these functions are carried out. Every hospital has three primary functions. The first centers around patient care. Most hospitals have "inpatients," or those who occupy beds; others have "outpatients" as well, who receive treatment only in the emergency room and the clinic areas. Outpatients may become inpatients; some inpatients may become outpatients as well, after their discharge from the hospital, for followup treatment in the clinic or the outpatient department. Teaching is the hospital's second major function, including the education of nurses, physicians, and other hospital personnel, and, to a lesser degree, patients. Research programs for the prevention and treatment of disease, as well as any active community program to promote health and prevent illness, may round out a hospital's total range of responsibilities, as approved by most Boards of Directors.

Administration

The Board delegates the administration of the institution to a director or superintendent (usually called the administrator, discussed more fully under The Hospital Team), who is responsible for managing all hospital affairs. This administrator, along with other department heads (depending on the size of the institution), will oversee the professional care and the business matters of the hospital. The business manager, or comptroller, functions under the administrator and is usually responsible for all financial aspects of running the hospital, which include the administration of various departments such as payroll, cashiering, storeroom and purchasing, maintenance and information, or a grouping of these under different divisions. Professional care is usually administered by a medical director or a group of staff physicians who, with other department heads, will supervise the medical staff, interns, residents, and the diagnostic and therapeutic departments as well. The nursing service and nursing education departments include all those professional and nonprofessional workers who render nursing care and participate in the teaching programs of the schools of registered and practical nursing. Medical records, social services, physical therapy, the dietary division, the pharmacy, the clinical laboratory, and the admitting office are classified as professional departments. Hospital organization varies with each institution. Although some features are almost universal, the amount of financial support and the size of the hospital will determine the number of departments rendering service. Medical care is becoming more and more complex every day. The table of organization in most institutions is kept current by careful coordination and by adding service departments as they are needed.

The Hospital Team

It takes all types of skills to operate a hospital or medical center efficiently. Some of the responsibilities of nurses were discussed in Chapter 3. However, there are many other people who make up the hospital team, contributing to the *total* care of the patient. Following is an alphabetical list of some of the individuals, briefly stating their major responsibilities and the preparation needed for their positions. (It should be understood that despite efforts to standardize educational and training programs, there is still considerable variation in the preparation and duties of hospital personnel.)

Administrator   A person with leadership skills appointed by the Board of Directors to be responsible for all hospital affairs. May be a physician, a professional nurse, or a business executive, and is a college graduate who has majored in business and has been prepared for a career in hospital administration.

Anesthesiologist   A physician who has qualified as a specialist by spending additional years of study and training in the field of anesthesia (the loss of feeling or sensation) and anesthetics (drugs or agents used to abolish feeling or sensation). The *nurse anesthetist* is a graduate of both a professional nursing school and a school of anesthesia for nurses, and is prepared to administer anesthetics.

Dentist (DDS)   The holder of a state license to practice dentistry, who has completed undergraduate study (usually four years) and has graduated from an approved four-year dental school. *Oral surgeons* have had additional training and are prepared to perform surgery in and around the mouth.

Dietitian   A graduate of an approved college program with a bachelor's degree, specializing in foods and nutrition. For professional recognition, most dietitians complete the one-year dietetic internship recommended by the American Dietetic Association (ADA).

Electrocardiograph Technician   A technician trained on the job to use the electrocardiograph (EKG) machine. No special formal education is required, and the training program varies in length.

Laboratory Assistant   A person who performs many of the simpler diagnostic tests and procedures in the laboratory. Most laboratory assistants are high school graduates who have completed a one-year course in an approved hospital or laboratory school under medical auspices.

Medical Doctor (MD)   A physician who graduated from an approved four-year medical school after having completed three or four years of undergraduate study. Usually serves a one- to five-year hospital internship for clinical and practical experience. A certified specialist must have an additional three years of residency practice. A board-certified specialist must complete the full residency requirement followed by two years of full-time specialty practice and pass the oral, written, and practical examinations in the specialty field. As of December 31, 1976, there were an estimated 410,600 doctors of medicine in the United States. Specialists outnumber general practitioners by more than three to one. Medical specialties include allergy, cardiovascular disease, dermatology, gastroenterology, internal medicine, pediatrics, pediatric allergy, pediatric cardiology, and pulmonary disease. Surgical specialties include anesthesiology, colon and rectal procedures, neurology, obstetrics and gynecology, opthalmology, orthopedic surgery, otolaryngology, plastic surgery, thoracic surgery, and urology. Some other fields of specialization are psychiatry, child psychiatry, neurology, aerospace medicine, preventive medicine, occupational medicine, pathology, physical medicine and rehabilitation, public health, and radiology. Unlike the full-time specialist, the general practitioner (GP) practices medicine and surgery on a general basis and serves as a family physician to provide routine health maintenance care. The present trend indicates that in the future, the family physician will also specialize, through advanced preparation, and will be qualified to coordinate the total health care of the family.

Medical Technologist (MT—ASCP) A person working in the medical laboratory under the supervision of the *pathologist,* a physician specializing in laboratory methods used to diagnose and treat disease. The medical technologist has had at least three years of college and one year of training in a school approved by the AMA. After passing an examination, is certified by the Registry of Medical Technologists of the American Society of Clinical Pathologists (ASCP).

Occupational Therapist A college graduate of an accredited program that has met the requirements of the AMA and the American Occupational Therapy Association. The occupational therapist is concerned with alleviating a patient's physical and emotional problems, modifying functional ability, and encouraging adaptation to meet the activities of daily living, work, and recreation. The occupational therapist who has had supervised clinical practice may qualify to take the national examination conducted by the American Occupational Therapy Association and become registered (OTR occupational therapist registered). Occupational therapy assistants and technicians work under the supervision of the OTR and are eligible for certification (COTA).

Optometrist (OD, Doctor of Optometry) A graduate of a school of optometry who has had preoptometry education in an approved college or university. Is specifically educated, trained, and licensed to examine the eyes and related structures for vision problems, disease, or other abnormalities. Also prescribes and fits eyeglasses and contact lenses and may fill personal prescriptions.

Osteopathic Physicians and Surgeons (DO, Doctor of Osteopathy) A person with an educational background similar to that of medical doctors, but with special emphasis on the importance of body mechanics, bone structure in illness, and the use of manipulation and massage of body parts as part of the treatment of illness. Some states have high standards in the education and training of osteopaths, whereas the standards of others are much lower than they are for medical practitioners.

Pharmacist A graduate of an accredited college of pharmacy (five to six years of professional college education) with a Bachelor of Science degree, who is licensed and registered by the Board of Pharmacy in the state where employed. Compounds and dispenses medicine, abiding by the state regulations as they affect all drugs.

Physical Therapist A graduate of an accredited program with a minimum background of a bachelor's degree who works under the supervision of the physician in providing the patient with therapeutic exercises, massages, and various applications of water, cold, heat, light, ultrasound, traction, and electricity. Usually registered in the state where employed and a member of the American Physical Therapy Association (APTA), the therapist may be helped by the physical therapy assistant, a graduate of a two-year program accredited by the APTA.

Physician's Assistant (PA) An assistant to the physician, qualified by education and practical training to provide selected patient care. May also be known as associate, medex, or medic, and is directly responsible to the physician for the performance of duties. The legal status of the physician assistant is still being defined by a number of state legislatures. At present there is no uniform standard for national recognition; however, the AMA and collaborating organizations have accredited some of the programs that meet their standards.

Podiatrist A graduate of a school of chiropody or podiatry (about six years of professional college education), who treats disorders of the feet. Licensed by passing the state board examination. Colleges of podiatry grant the degree of Doctor of Surgical Chiropody or Podiatry (DSC or PodD).

Psychologist A university graduate who usually has a doctor of philosophy degree (PhD) with an internship in supervised clinical experience. May assist in treating, diagnosing, and counseling individuals with mental or emotional problems or physical illnesses.

Radiologic Technologist (RT) A person who has completed a two-year training program in a hospital approved by the AMA and has passed the certifying examination given by the American Registry of Radiologic Technologist (ARRT). Assists with diagnostic x-rays and fluoroscopy, radiation therapy, and the use of radioisotopes. There is a college- or university-affiliated course for this specialty, which offers a bachelor's or associate degree in radiologic technology.

Respiratory Therapist One who administers, under medical supervision, gases, drugs, and equipment to restore normal functioning of the body's cardiopulmonary system. Trained on the job in the past, and called inhalation technician, the therapist is now a graduate of an American Medical Association (AMA)–approved program two years in duration. The American Association for Respiratory Therapy conducts oral and written examinations for those who wish to become registered with the National Board for Respiratory Therapy (NBRT) and certifies those who meet their educational and experience requirements in addition to passing the written examination. A one-year program prepares technicians who assist the ARRTs (American registered respiratory therapists).

Social Worker (Medical, Psychiatric, and so forth) The holder of a bachelor's degree from an accredited college or university who has had two years of graduate education at an accredited school of social work, leading to the master's degree. The social worker is skilled in helping patients and their families handle various personal problems resulting from illness or disability. Graduate schools of social work are accredited by the Council on Social Work Education (CSWE). The National Association of Social Workers (NASW), the membership organization, administers a national certification program, through which social workers who meet the competency requirements are admitted to membership in the Academy of Certified Social Workers.

There are many other important members of the hospital team, but space limitations preclude discussing them in this section. Among them are the speech pathologist, the medical record librarian, the prosthetist (one skilled in the construction or application of artificial body parts), all of whom make a significant contribution to the patient's care and welfare.

Nursing Department

The department of nursing education and nursing service in a typical hospital is outlined in Figure 5-1. Not shown are the many committees, such as quality assurance, research, infection control, education procedures, policies, and scholarship and loan, that contribute to the successful administration of a department.

Most directors of nursing, assistant or associate directors of nursing (as they are sometimes called), as well as coordinators, supervisors, and head nurses in many teaching institutions have their bachelor's or master's degree in nursing. The importance of a well-qualified faculty and supervisory staff is stressed by State Boards of Nursing, the National League for Nursing, and the National Association for Practical Nurse Education and Service, Inc. in their accreditation recommendations and standards.

The Joint Commission on Accreditation of Hospitals pays special attention to the nursing services of a hospital seeking accreditation. These five standards are used as guides:

- The nursing service shall be under the direction of a legally and professionally qualified registered nurse. There shall also be a sufficient number of duly licensed registered nurses on duty at all times to plan, assign, supervise and evaluate nursing care, as well as to give patients the nursing care that requires the judgment and specialized skills of a registered nurse.

- The nursing service shall have a current written organizational plan that delineates its functional structure and its mechanisms for cooperative planning and decision making.

- Written nursing care and administrative policies and procedures shall be developed to provide the nursing staff with acceptable methods of meeting its responsibilities and achieving projected goals.

- There shall be evidence established that the nursing service provides safe, efficient and therapeutically effective nursing care through the

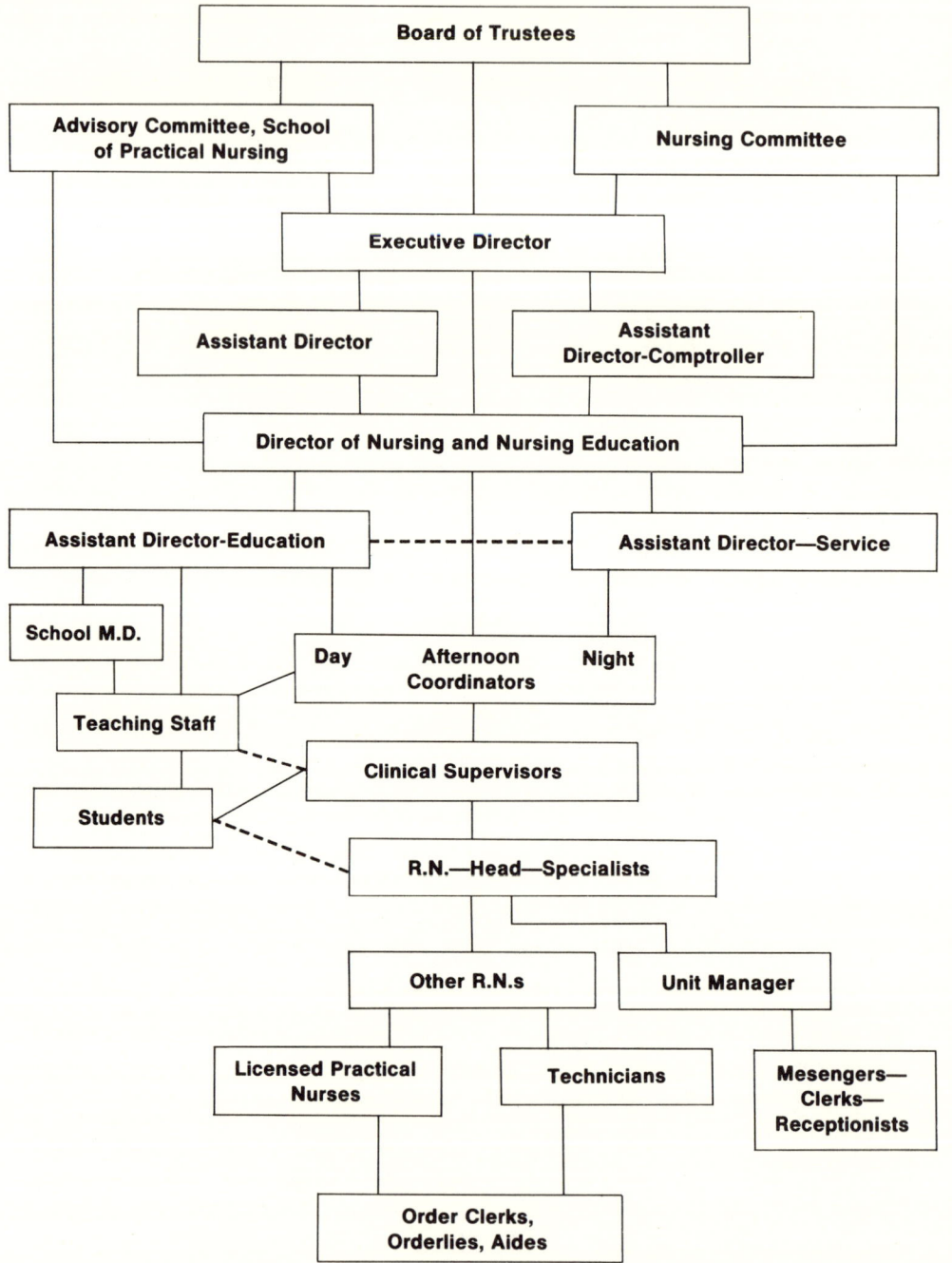

FIGURE 5-1. *Organizational plan of a nursing department.*

planning of each patient's care and the effective implementation of the plans.

- There shall be continuing training programs and educational opportunities for the development of nursing personnel.*

Every nursing department establishes its own lines of authority and delegation of responsibilities. Since this hierarchy also forms the basis for an official channel of communication, the practical nurse should be familiar with the plan of organization for nursing department personnel of the hospital, as well as for the school of nursing. From the Table of Organization, illustrated previously, the lines of authority are easily seen and must be followed. The director of nursing or nurses is usually in charge of the school of nursing and of nursing services and may appoint various assistants who act as representatives in administering nursing services and educational programs. These assistants may include an *educational director* for the school, who directs the faculty and plans class schedules and curriculum, and correlates the courses taught. The faculty includes instructors who teach classroom material as well as supervise the students in clinical practice. There may also be *clinical instructors,* specialists in certain clinical areas (who may be nursing service supervisors as well) to assist in teaching, although they are not full-time faculty members.

If a practical nursing school comes under the state vocational education system rather than the hospital, the students and instructors are subject to a different organizational setup. At the top, the *State Coordinator* or *Supervisor of Health Occupation* and/or *Practical Nurse Education* is responsible for the administration of this type of practical nursing program. Besides being a registered nurse with additional college work, the coordinator must also meet the requirements as set by the State Department of Education; these requirements are similar in nature to those for public school supervisors and principals. In each local school, registered nurses with additional preparation in teaching carry out the practical nurse classroom and hospital experience program. The student nurses travel to community hospitals (that is, they affiliate) for patient care experience, where their activities are supervised by clinical instructors. Even when students and instructors are under the jurisdiction of the vocational school, they should be familiar with the table of organization and administrative routines of the hospital nursing service.

You may meet several groups of hospital nursing staff members. One consists of *supervisors,* in charge of one or more departments or special clinical divisions, such as obstetrics, operating and recovery rooms, outpatient clinics, central service, communicable disease sections, psychiatric services, and so forth. The functions of the supervisor are varied and all-inclusive. They involve responsibilities for developing and administering the nursing service rendered within the unit, accounting for supplies and equipment, arranging the time schedule for personnel, and maintaining the quality of patient care. Additionally, supervisors may be in charge of a specific tour of duty, such as day, afternoon, or night, and then are responsible for administering the entire nursing care program for the hospital

---

* JCAH: *Accreditation Manual for Hospitals*, pp 49–53 (Chicago, JCAH, 1970).

during these specific hours. Sometimes tour supervisors are called coordinators, assistant directors, or administrative supervisors.

Head nurses, are usually responsible for the administration of a single nursing service unit, such as emergency room, recovery room, medical or surgical unit, or specialities such as orthopedics, urology, or intensified nursing. the responsibilities of the head nurse usually include planning, supervision, and provision of nursing care in the unit, assisting in the orientation and the teaching of students and new personnel, and carrying out all procedures and regulations in conformity with the hospital's policies and practices. In large nursing units there may also be assistant head nurses or charge nurses who share the responsibilities of the head nurse on the day tour but are themselves in charge on the afternoon or the night tours if so assigned.

General duty or *staff nurses* are engaged in the general activities of the nursing unit, so that their functions will depend on the type of nursing care performed and the availability of the other nursing employees discussed in Chapter 3.

A 1976 estimate of employed nursing personnel showed that there were 961,000 registered nurses (RNs), 489,000 licensed practical nurses (LPNs), and 1 million nursing aides, orderlies, and attendants. More and more parttime employees are being utilized to help relieve the shortage of qualified personnel. There is a shortage of RNs in most community hospitals; most vacancies are primarily on the afternoon and night tours of duty, when more RNs are needed to provide optimum patient care and realistic supervision for LPNs and auxiliary personnel.

Accreditation of Hospitals

Accreditation gives the hospital recognition for the service it renders and also protects the patients by assuring them that the institution has met certain basic requirements, as set by the accrediting agency. The patient can feel far more secure when receiving care in an institution that is approved by the Joint Commission on Accreditation of Hospitals. This Commission is made up of representatives from the American College of Physicians, the American College of Surgeons, the American Medical Association, and the American Hospital Association. Surveys of hospitals are conducted by field representatives who review and evaluate the hospital's standards and report their findings to the Board of Commissioners of the Joint Commission on Accreditation of Hospitals. It is hoped that standardization in hospitals and, with that, better care will result from these accreditation programs.

In 1978 the 7,123 hospitals listed by the American Hospital Association had almost 1.6 million beds available for patient use, with an average occupancy rate of 77.5%. Only 5,124 of these hospitals were accredited by the Joint Commission on Accreditation of Hospitals (JCAH); more than 1,170 offered approved affiliations for residents, and 737 conducted programs for interns. Those with approved medical school affiliation numbered 866; 490 conducted approved registered nursing schools; and 196 had approved practical nursing programs. It must be noted that many hospitals have affiliates whose teaching programs are controlled by the educational institution, such as the vocational school, the college, or the university.

In addition to the Joint Commission there are other accreditation agencies for registered and practical nursing schools, intern and resident programs, medical school affiliations, and technicians' programs.

The *American Hospital Association* (AHA) was founded in 1898 by a group of hospital administrators "to promote public welfare through the development of better hospital care for all the people." It provides a meeting ground where hospital problems are reviewed and answers sought and stresses the hospital's many community service responsibilities. There are about 8,500 personal members and close to 9,000 institutional members, which include extended care facilities, dispensaries, hospitals and hospital auxiliaries, Blue Cross plans, area-wide planning agencies, and hospitals in the planning or construction stages. A library service is available at the national headquarters, located at 840 North Lake Shore Drive in Chicago. The AHA also makes available staff specialists for consultation in areas such as nursing, medical records, public health, accreditation, careers, and legislation. Each year it sponsors National Hospital Week during the week of Florence Nightingale's birthday (May 12th).

Osteopathic Hospitals

One specialized type of hospital is the osteopathic hospital. In 1979, 214 osteopathic hospitals located in 31 states provided a total of nearly 25,000 beds and 1,760 bassinets. An estimated 825,000 patients were admitted, resulting in some 6.3 million patient days of care. In addition, outpatient departments in these hospitals accommodated some 3.1 million patients each year for emergency and other ambulatory care.

The Federal government designated the American Osteopathic Association as the official accrediting agency for osteopathic hospitals that participate in Medicare and Medicaid programs. The Federal government, state governments, and private and public health agencies have also recognized osteopathic medicine as a separate but equal branch of American health care. As a result, osteopathic physicians, of which there are about 18,000, have the same rights and professional obligations as allopathic (MD) physicians.

Of 150 accredited hospitals, 83 were approved for internships and 69 for residencies. Nursing care in these institutions is similar to that of any other hospital.

NURSING HOMES

The nursing home is a relatively new institution in the United States. Social Security legislation, which made federal funds available for the needy and aged, helped to establish these homes in the 1930s; the 1965 Medicare amendments to the Social Security Act made them flourish. A nursing home is defined as an institution in which 50% or more of the residents receive at least one of the following nursing services: application of dressing or bandage, having blood pressure taken, bowel and bladder retraining, catheterization, enema, full bed bath, intravenous fluids, irrigation, medication, nasal feeding, oxygen therapy, having temperature taken, and pulse and respiration checks. The facility must have at least one RN or LPN employed full time. The level of care is protected by qualification and certification. "Extended care" represents a new level of patient care that provides medically supervised skilled nursing and related services on a continuing basis in an institutional setting.

A personal care home with nursing usually has less than 50% of the residents receiving nursing care. The personal care home provides personal services such as assistance with bathing, dressing, eating, and walking, but no nursing services. A domiciliary care home routinely provides less than three of the previously defined personal services and is primarily a sheltered environment for persons who are able to care for themselves.

Nursing homes require licensing in all states. Licenses are usually granted by the departments of health and/or welfare after the home has met certain minimal requirements. Nursing homes participating in the health insurance program for the aged must be certified by the designated state agencies and are surveyed periodically. Voluntary accreditation is available through the Joint Commission on Accreditation of Hospitals.

Other Inpatient
Health Facilities

Persons who are not necessarily ill or aged and are residents of schools or homes include deaf, blind, physically handicapped, alcoholics, drug abusers, emotionally disturbed, unwed mothers, orphans, dependent children, and mentally retarded persons. These hospitals, homes, or residence schools are listed under the "Other Inpatient Facilities." It is estimated that some 358,017 persons are housed in 6,743 such facilities. There is much variety in laws among the states regarding the standards and accreditation policies for these institutions.

HOME HEALTH SERVICES

Approximately 2,800 home health aide and homemaker service programs are provided by public and voluntary agencies now operating in the 50 states, the District of Columbia, and Puerto Rico. These services assist patients in their homes and prevent or postpone hospitalizaiton.

Home care varies and takes numerous forms, from "meals on wheels" to skilled nursing care. The coordinated home care program is physician-directed or -requested and provides medical, nursing, social, and other related services.

There are about 22,000 home health aides and homemakers who work under the supervision of a registered nurse or, when appropriate, a physical, speech, or occupational therapist. A home health agency may participate in the Medicare program if it is primarily engaged in providing skilled nursing care and other therapeutic services to patients in their homes. Agencies that have been certified under the Medicare program include the Visiting Nurse Associations, health departments, hospitals, group practice units, "retirement villages," religious nursing orders, neighborhood health centers, homemaker agencies, rehabilitation centers, and homes for the aged.

HOSPICES

A caring environment for dying patients and their meaningful others is provided by the hospice. The goal of hospice care is to assist terminally ill patients in achieving the highest quality of life possible, and the movement emphasizes that supportive emotional and spiritual care are as important as medical care. With an interdisciplinary team approach, an individualized plan of care is developed and followed.

"Hospice" is a medieval term and signifies that the doors are open from one life to the next. The most widely known hospice is St. Christopher's Hospice in London. Hospices in the United States may provide not only inpatient care but also home care.

COMMUNITY MENTAL HEALTH CENTERS

A community mental health center may consist of several types of health facilities that cooperate to provide inpatient and outpatient services, day care and 24-hour emergency services, and consultation and education for patients, community agencies, and professional personnel. In 1977, there were 649 federally funded community mental health centers, of which 570 were in operation. California led the nation with 42 centers and was followed by Pennsylvania with 32 centers.

ACUPUNCTURE CLINICS

Acupuncture is the ancient Chinese practice of piercing certain nerves to cure disease or release pain. Nine special metal needles are used to puncture the body at predetermined points for treatment of specific symptoms. There are 365 points, known as meridians, where these needles may be inserted.

According to some sources, this method was used as early as 106 BC. There is no accurate documentation, however, until 228 AD. Although the practice of acupuncture is based in antiquity, it has only recently been accepted by Western culture.

HEALTH MAINTENANCE ORGANIZATIONS (HMOs)

The concept of a federally supported HMO was first announced publicly during 1970 Congressional hearings on reorganization of Medicare benefits under the Social Security Act. Federal funds were authorized to stimulate HMO development in 1971 and the first experimental HMOs were under way by January 1972.

The HMO differs chiefly from traditional multispeciality practice of medicine by requiring prepayment for health care.

It is difficult to estimate how many HMOs are in operation. Surveys have reported somewhere between 500 and 800 independent plans. Thirty states have legislation allowing HMOs to operate. A survey in 1976 indicated that 185 HMO-type prepaid medical care plans served an estimated 6.1 million members. Perhaps the best known of the HMO prototypes is the Kaiser Foundation–Permanente system of regional health plans, which started in 1933 in southern California as a 10¢-a-day fee to prepay the medical costs of Kaiser Engineering workers.

This new concept in the delivery of comprehensive health care operates on a prepaid capitation basis for enrolled population groups. The payments (premiums, dues) are made in advance into a fund used to pay for health services that generally include emergency care, inpatient hospital care, physician care, ambulatory diagnostic treatment, and preventive health care and services.

PHARMACIES

Pharmacies differ widely both in their level of pharmaceutical services and in the products they make available. They may vary from the huge supermarket-type operation, which also stocks a wide variety of nonhealth-related merchandise, to the drug store that specializes in pharmaceutical service and dispenses medications and health-related supplies only. There are more than 50,000 community pharmacies in the United States. All states require these pharmacies to be licensed. Additionally, there are more than 5,000 hospital pharmacies that provide pharmaceutical services to the public. Five states—Connecticut, Iowa, Maine, New Hampshire, and Wyoming—do not require the licensing of hospital pharmacies by the State Board of Pharmacy but rather by the State Board of Health.

HEALTH INSURANCE

Today, three out of four persons in the United States carry some type of health insurance to be able to meet some of the expenses of medical care and hospitalization. On July 1, 1966, the health insurance plan under the Social Security Act went into effect and Medicare benefits, including basic hospital benefits and voluntary supplementary medical insurance, were available for 19 million citizens 65 years of age and older. Since then, new Social Security legislation has been enacted and the benefits of the Medicare program have expanded. Some states, in conjunction with the Federal government, offer other programs to help defray medical expenses for residents with low incomes or recipients of welfare assistance or relief. This program is known as Medicaid, and requirements for eligibility vary in different states.

There are two parts to Medicare—A and B. Part A, or hospital insurance, is financed by special contributions from employees, employers, and self-employed persons, which are collected along with the amount regularly deducted for social security during a person's working years. Part B, medical insurance, is financed jointly by the federal government, which pays half, and by the basic medical insurance policies of those who enroll voluntarily when they became eligible.

A large share of private health insurance for Americans is provided by life insurance companies. They paid more than $18.7 billion of the health insurance benefits to Americans in 1978. Of these payments, $14.6 billion was for medical expenses, including hospital and surgical expenses, $3.1 billion was for loss of income, including accidental death and dismemberment payments, and $1 billion was for dental policies. These statistics do not include disability payments, which are under life insurance policies, or health insurance policy payments by casualty and other health insuring companies such as Blue Cross/Blue Shield and similar organizations.

More than 1,800 private insuring agencies offer their services to the public through individual or group plans. The largest single supplier of hospital insurance is Blue Cross. Their plans usually provide room and board, general nursing care, use of operating and delivery rooms, pathology and laboratory services, drugs, dressings, casts, special treatments, electrocardiograms, the taking of x-ray pictures, and many other hospital services. A reciprocal agreement covers members in one plan who move into another area, to which the membership must be transferred. Hospitalization insurance should be considered as a part of the family budget, since hospital care has become a part of modern life.

Although Blue Cross and Blue Shield policies are the generally accepted ones in many areas of the country, various other types of protection are designed to help one meet the costs of sickness and accidents. Some policies encourage the use of preventive care and will cover medical costs for the insured even when there is no hospitalization. The size of the benefits, including length of time covered, hospitalization, surgery, general medical expenses, major medical expenses, loss of income because of disability, and nursing care, may vary with each policy; therefore, you should know and understand the policy before you purchase it. If you are a member of a group plan, you have reasonable assurance that the sponsoring group has checked the reliability of the company. Very often, embarrassing moments with physicians and employers will be prevented if you can say, "My insurance will cover the expenses or at least part of them."

Within the last few years much has been said about the need for an effective form of national health insurance to benefit all Americans. Although several plans have been proposed (the latest one emanating from the White House in 1979), there seems to be no real consensus at this time as to what kind of plan is needed.

Effective health care calls for a partnership of the private sector and the government to meet the personal health needs of all citizens regardless of income or where they live. This goal could be achieved by action to

- Increase the supply, and improve the productivity and distribution of health manpower.
- Develop ambulatory health care services to promote health maintenance and reduce costly hospital use.
- Improve health care planning to distribute current and future health resources more equitably and effectively.

- Contain rising health care costs and upgrade the quality of health care.
- Establish national goals and priorities to improve health care.
- Improve the financing of health care for everyone, and protect against the costs of catastrophic illness.

Undoubtedly, a plan will be developed within the next few years that offers unlimited possibilities for new kinds of health care. Nursing could, for example, change drastically in the direction of preventive care and health education. It is very possible that you, the practical nurse, will be involved in the planning stages of these innovations. Make sure that you follow pertinent political developments closely through nursing journals and other available sources. After all, your future as a nurse will be affected.

HEALTH CARE PROVIDERS

About 5.1 million persons were employed in 1976 in the health professions, with occupations divided into about 717 primary and alternate job titles. About 30 occupations in the health field are licensed in one or more states. All states and the District of Columbia require that chiropractors, dental hygienists, dentists, environmental health engineers, nursing home administrators, optometrists, pharmacists, physical therapists, physicians, podiatrists, practical/vocational nurses, registered nurses, and veterinarians be licensed. Most states license psychologists, sanitarians or sanitary inspectors, midwives, and opticians.

In addition, states license clinical laboratory directors including bioanalysts and clinical laboratory personnel such as medical technologists or technicians, naturopaths and other drugless healers, and social workers. Physical therapy assistants are licensed in 22 states and Puerto Rico. A few states license or certify radiological technologists (x-ray technicians), hospital administrators, and health department administrators. Within some professions there are specialty and certification boards, or registries established by the profession itself. Persons who meet the requirements of education, experience, and competency, and pass an examination given by the board may use specific professional designations.

In order to standardize terminology as it relates to the level of training and education in the health occupations, the National Center for Health Statistics provides the following definitions:

Technologist ⎫ Therapist ⎭	Educational preparation at the baccalaureate level or above
Technician ⎫ Assistant ⎭	Educational preparation at the associate degree level (2 years of college education or other formal preparation beyond high school)
Aide	Specialized training of less than 2 years duration beyond high school, or on-the-job training*

---

* Department of Health, Education, and Welfare: *Health Resources Statistics, 1971*, p 405.

HEALTH QUACKERY

Unfortunately, today there are thousands of quacks who promise quick cures for almost every disease. They have extorted millions of dollars from their gullible patients, but a greater danger is that they will delay patients from seeking legitimate medical attention during the early period of disease when prompt, efficient, and accurate diagnosis can often make the difference between life and death. State and Federal law enforcement agencies are usually summoned whenever frauds are committed. it has been stated reliably that health quackery costs more lives in the United States each year than all crimes combined. It is estimated that over $50 million a year is wasted by patients pursuing nonexistent cancer cures and treatments. An Arthritis Foundation survey estimated that 14 million arthritis patients in the United States waste more than $310 million each year in their fruitless effort to achieve bodily comfort and freedom from pain.

If you or your patients come in contact with a quack be sure to report this to the proper law enforcement agencies. The AMA has a Department of Investigation that informs the public about these exploits and warns:

> Quacks generally are well dressed, neat, healthy, kind, patient, and sympathetic to the people with whom they deal. They give the patient sufficient time to tell his troubles. Simple indicators for spotting a quack are:
>
> 1. He uses a special machine or formula he claims can cure disease.
>
> 2. He guarantees a quick cure.
>
> 3. He advertises or uses case histories and testimonials to promote his cure.
>
> 4. He clamors constantly for medical investigation and recognition.
>
> 5. He claims medical men are persecuting him or are afraid of his competition.
>
> 6. He says that surgery, x-rays, and drugs will cause more harm than good.
>
> 7. He uses high-sounding titles easily confused with qualified scientific professionals and organizations.*

GETTING ALONG IN YOUR INSTITUTION

Honesty

Success in your career will depend to a large extent on your attitude toward your coworkers and the institution that employs you. Perhaps the most indispensable attribute you will need is honesty. There is no place for the nurse whose integrity is questionable. The nurse who charts something before it is done, records a temperature without actually taking it, does not admit mistakes, makes unauthor-

---

* American Medical Association: *Health Quackery* pp 2–3 (pamphlet) (Chicago, Illinois).

ized substitutions, is habitually late and gives shifty excuses, "borrows" equipment and supplies for home use, or ignores patients' or physicians' requests, is undesirable, regardless of any compensating virtues. Although some of these characteristics are attributable to slovenliness rather than dishonesty, they are no less serious.

Conserving Hospital Supplies

A chronic problem in all hospitals, which is caused largely by thoughtlessness and neglect on the part of the employees, is wastage of hospital supplies and equipment. Hospitals are usually nonprofit in nature, and there is a continual increase in their operating expenses, especially in the care of part-paying or free patients. Very often a nurse may reason, "What's the difference—the hospital pays for it." However, who is the hospital? You are part of it! By being economical and not wasting or abusing equipment and supplies, you are able to contribute toward caring for more patients, purchasing new and needed equipment, or possibly even promoting better salary scales. The extravagant or uneconomical use of supplies and equipment by one nurse and then another and finally by a group of nurses can make a large difference in the operational costs of the institution. In wasting supplies and equipment you are doing the equivalent of throwing away someone else's money. If you are to receive a bonus or a part interest in the money saved by being economical, preventing breakage, and being conservative in the use of supplies, would certain of your working habits change?

Understanding Hospital Charges

Although you have no control in setting fees pertaining to patient charges, you should understand their meaning. One reason is that you are in a strategic role to explain costs to your patients. On the surface, the hospital charges may appear to be exorbitant, but when your patients consider that there are very valid reasons for these costs, they will realize that they are getting a lot for their money. Hospital room charges usually include room (maintenance, housekeeping, all the linen that is needed) and meals (special diets, nourishment, and diet instruction) as well as 24-hour nursing care and the attention of other hospital personnel on duty to meet the needs of the patients as prescribed by the physician. A $96-a-day room charge comes to $4 an hour. Where else would such highly trained personnel be readily available at a pull of the call bell or at the physician's order? What does the patient pay the TV repairman, cleaning woman, electrician, or plumber? All these, plus many other technically skilled employees, are on duty for the patient's benefit.

Medical costs are certainly rising. Advances in science have necessitated more skilled personnel. The standard of the 40-hour work week means that extra employees are needed, since the hospital must remain open 24 hours a day, seven days a week. Although salary scales in hospitals are lower than in industry, hospitals must compete in order to attract and retain competent employees; therefore, salaries cannot drop below a certain level. In addition, drugs, equipment, and diagnostic procedures that did not exist previously are used today—at increased costs. Food, maintenance, general supplies, and all the other items for public consumption that have risen in cost also add to the patient's bill. However, individual incomes have risen correspondingly, so that medical costs may not be disproportionately high. Also, it should be taken into consideration that the shorter average hospital stay reduces the number of productive days lost by the patient and therefore, the income lost.

Perhaps the best way to reassure the patient regarding charges is to make sure that billing occurs only for what is really used in the patient's care. Unused drugs, equipment, or supplies should be returned promptly for proper credit.

Courtesy

Courtesy is the expression of respect for others. Because courtesy is so essential to harmonious human relationships, every society has evolved formal expressions of it that are observed in spirit, if not to the letter. These might be called rules of accepted behavior, or etiquette. They are exercised impartially; whether or not we feel any particular affection or respect for the person to whom they are directed is beside the point. We follow these formed rules simply because it is the proper thing to do.

Much more significant are the spontaneous, informal expressions of courtesy. Unlike formal rules of etiquette, which are more ritualistic than heartfelt, informal courtesy is an extra effort made freely on behalf of another. Because the omission of small courtesies usually entails no direct penalty, ordinarily it will not occur to an indifferent person to exert one's self. For this reason the habitual—virtually automatic—observation of small courtesies is an almost infallible index to a person's character.

Some people refer to courtesy as a lost art, but it is not lost, it has merely been misplaced by some people. Courtesy is something that comes from within. An unknown author once wrote:

> I am a little thing with big meaning. I help everybody. I unlock doors, open hearts, dispel prejudice, I create friendship and good will; inspire respect and admiration. Everybody loves me. I bore nobody, violate no law, cost nothing. Many praise me. I am pleasing to those of high and low degree. I am useful every moment. . . . I am COURTESY.

Nurses are expected to be courteous, not only because it is worth doing for its own sake but also because it has the practical result of winning for you the respect and the cooperation of patients and colleagues. One reason that small courtesies are so effective is that they have all the charm of the unexpected.

Frequent use of the simple expressions "please" and "thank you" will go a remarkably long way in smoothing human relationships. The importance of such words lies mainly in the fact that you care enough to use them. Consciously and deliberately keep an eye out for opportunities to thank people (not overdoing it, of course). Did you ever thank the physician for writing orders so completely and legibly? Did you show your appreciation to the charge nurse for taking time out to explain a procedure or to correct you? The next time someone does something for you, acknowledge your appreciation of it; it will be encouragement to do even more.

Courtesy is really the essence of the nurse/patient relationship, because it is an acknowledgment of the basic worth of the individual. For instance, it is not only unwise but also terribly discourteous to burst into a patient's unit and briskly begin preparation for some procedure without first explaining what is happening and why. The frightened and upset patient will conclude rightly that you are uncaring by not explaining the procedure or its purpose.

Here are some other points of common courtesy that you should remember. If you see that someone is in a hurry, step aside to make room. If you find people conversing together in the hall, do not break up the group by dashing through them but walk around them instead. If you are late for a meeting or a class, excuse yourself and offer an honest and brief apology. Another point to remember is that closed doors are never opened without knocking and then waiting for an acknowledgment. Do not enter a private room if the person it belongs to is absent, unless you have special permission to do so—and then only if you really must.

You will find as nurses that the increasing costs of operating hospitals has been responsible for increased work loads for every member of the nursing team. You may find that you will not have as much time with your patients as you would like. Therefore, make the most of every minute spent with a patient. In this light, courtesy becomes more a matter of sensitivity and compassion than an impersonal attitude.

One should not expect rewards for courtesy. I should like to emphasize to you that hospital personnel are hired to help those who are sick, and therefore tips and gifts from patients should not be expected, hinted at, or accepted. (See Chapter 7 for more details.)

Etiquette

Rules of etiquette, the formal expressions of courtesy, are designed to be used in specific situations—for instance, at the table, at parties, or in certain professional relationships. One reason for their existence is that they furnish everyone concerned with a common standard of behavior and therefore are valuable in preventing misunderstanding and the possibility of awkward incidents. If only for this reason, rules of etiquette are a necessary adjunct to a civilized society.

Not only do rules of etiquette differ from one society to another but there will also be many variations within a society. Furthermore, the rules are changing constantly. Some institutions, such as schools and hospitals, have retained certain formal rules of etiquette; others have modified them or let them lapse altogether. Much depends on tradition. You should be prepared to adapt yourself to your work situation. The following few points of etiquette have more or less universal acceptance.

Greetings and Introductions

It is a generally accepted rule of etiquette that a younger person, or one with less authority, offers respect and courtesy to an older person or to one of superior rank. When you meet such a person, it is customary that you extend the greeting. Be cordial and dignified, and if you know the person's name, use it. Your friendly manner will not be misinterpreted, but do not become overbearing. In introducing two people, first you name the person *to whom* the introduction is being made. The words "introduce" and "present" are equally acceptable. Avoid the use of surnames or given names only, unless your employer or school condones this.

Telephone Manners

A smile in your telephone voice is as attractive as a smile on your face. Your telephone personality will enhance the impression you make on others. Always be conscious of your speaking voice. It will carry most clearly when you speak directly into the mouthpiece in a natural tone of voice. Your speech should be neither too fast nor too slow, and above all it must be clear. The next time the telephone rings, pause for a moment and think before you answer it, so that you may remind yourself to speak properly.

Since it is easier if the caller knows who is answering, it has been generally accepted that you identify yourself by saying, for example, "Fourth Floor, Miss Jones, LPN" or "Recovery Room, Miss Smith, Student Nurse." If it is necessary for you to leave the telephone to obtain information, explain that you must leave, and on your return thank the person for waiting. If you anticipate a long delay, it may be best to offer to call back instead of keeping the caller "dangling." If the call must be transferred, tell the caller this, and then contact the operator. It is a good rule to be brief and courteous, to end all calls graciously, and to hang up the receiver gently.

Shop Talk

There is nothing unethical about discussing your work with your colleagues, so long as you do not bandy names and personalities about. Be especially careful when discussing patients and their attending physicians. If you seem to be able to do nothing but indulge in aimless chatter about the job, it is time to curb yourself. Do not talk shop in public places, such as the elevators, halls, cafeteria, bus, or nurses' residence. The dangers of careless shop talk are discussed more fully in Chapter 7.

Your Co-workers—The Cooperative Spirit

In your daily work you will come in contact with scores of different categories of workers, all of whom contribute either directly or indirectly to the patient's welfare. They include not only the physician and the nurse but also the laboratory technician, the orderlies and nurse's aides, the dietetic aide, the clergy, the x-ray technician, and many others. Cooperation among all these people is absolutely vital to the smooth running of a complex healing institution. A willingness to adopt the give-and-take approach pays personal benefits in terms of job satisfaction.

The first step in cooperation is to learn the rules. In every institution there is usually an administrative manual with explanations of the duties and responsibilities of each department. In order to promote efficiency, standing orders pertaining to administrative routines and policies are usually included. Every nurse should be familiar with the precedents and the procedures advocated by the supervisor or department head and then abide by them.

Cooperation implies loyalty to the institution in which you work. It may not have occurred to you that the public opinion of your institution will be based largely on the reports of patients, so remember that your efforts to be a good nurse will pay double dividends. By contrast, if you are dissatisfied with conditions in the hospital and must air your dissatisfaction, keep it "in the family" to as limited an audience as possible. Do not broadcast information that could possibly make the public fearful of hospitalization.

Another expression of your cooperative spirit is in acknowledging the value of those with whom you work. Refrain from being overly eager to assume anyone else's responsibilities. Do not make your career one of winning race after race; give the other student or nurse a break. Although competition can be contagious, cooperation and courtesy can also be. By giving the other person a chance you will usually be making it easier for yourself. Do not try to achieve perfection in everything. Admirable as this may be, it is often impracticable and may even be an invitation to failure. No one can be perfect in everything. Put your major efforts into those things you can do right and well, and derive your satisfaction from performing to the utmost of your ability.

Working with Colleagues and Subordinates

Do not stress the fact that you are perhaps better prepared or more skilled than others with whom you are working; rather, assist them in developing better technics. If you feel that your coworkers will benefit from constructive criticism, discuss possible deficiencies or faults with them *privately* and allow them the courtesy of being the first to know. If they still do not improve, you might have to report their inadequacies to those in higher authority.

Whenever you must work with personnel other than nurses, you must realize that they also have a supervisor who is responsible for them; therefore, before you attempt to correct a situation it might be wiser for you to report the incident to your immediate charge nurse, who would then follow through using the proper channels. The only time you would have the right to act against another hospital employee would be in case of emergency, when common sense would dictate the policy.

The best way to win the respect of those you work with is by demonstrating skill in your profession (by doing, not by talking about it), a cooperative manner, an understanding nature, and courtesy.

Relationships with the RN

You are responsible, in one way or another, at all times to an RN. However, because both of you work closely together and need one another, ordinary courtesy and mutual respect should bring about a harmonious relationship. You may resent it if your charge nurses are many years younger than you. You may feel contemptuous of them if they are less experienced in human relations than yourself, or less emotionally mature, or lacking in the "common sense" that comes with experience. However, you should rise above these petty considerations, be as cooperative and helpful as you can be, and remember the responsibilities that they have been given. Remember, too, that the RN's educational preparation and qualifications are more extensive than yours and imply the right to be "boss" in planning and supervising patient care.

You may encounter some RNs who will not readily accept you as an important member of the nursing profession, but you should make the effort to accept them first, and then try to analyze the reasons for their feelings and behavior toward you. If their attitude still does not make sense, do not brood about, but put every effort into your work. Competence is still the best way to earn respect.

If you are studying or working in an institution in which there are registered nursing students, remember that even though your educational programs differ in scope and content, your objectives are the same—good nursing. There is only one way to do a procedure—the right way, regardless of who carries it out. If you see an RN or a student perform some duty that you know is not being carried out in the best interests of the patient or institution, report this to your instructor or charge nurse for follow through. If a patient complains to you about any incompetent nurse, do not discuss the nurse's inadequacies further with the patient, but report the matter to the charge nurse or supervisor in order that proper measures may be taken. Always follow the "chain of command."

Put yourself out to be helpful to the RN. A registered private duty nurse who turns to you for advice regarding the newer trends in nursing, or who would like some help in a procedure that is unfamiliar, should be given all the help possible. The patient always comes first, regardless of your personal feelings, and as long as the nursing care is good, you have done your share.

Relationships with the Physician

One of your most important vocational relationships is with the patient's physician. At all times you must inspire the patient's confidence in the physician. You should never advocate the dismissal or replacement of a physician or consultation with another physician. If you believe that the physician, intern, or resident is not competent (and there are very few such cases), you should bring this to the attention of your supervisor, who is responsible for the patient's welfare.

The best way to prove to the physician that you are a capable nurse is to carry out orders to the letter; when in doubt about how to do this, find out by asking pertinent questions. At all times be loyal, respectful, and cooperative. Do not impose upon the doctor by asking for free medical advice. Do not discuss personal problems while on duty, and do not become overly familiar. Physicians are never called by their first names while they are on duty, regardless of how friendly you may be with them. Fraternization with interns, residents, and medical students while on duty is frowned on in some schools of practical nursing and hospitals; it might be wise to check the institutional policies pertaining to such a situation.

There may be times when you are consulted by a physician about a particular patient. This will happen more frequently if you are an outstanding practical nurse, and as your reputation for solid nursing practice and judgement becomes known throughout the hospital.

Questions

A. Select the correct answer and circle the number that answers the question best.

1. Hospitals are usually classified as (A) official, (B) clinical, (C) proprietary, (D) specific, (E) general, (F) voluntary, (G) non-profit.
   1. All except A
   2. All except B
   3. All except C
   4. All except D

2. An official hospital (A) may be supported by taxes, (B) has civil service employees, (C) never charges patients, (D) may be subsidized by federal funds.
   1. All of these
   2. All except B
   3. All except C
   4. All except D

3. A voluntary hospital (A) has only volunteers, (B) may be supported by donations, (C) is supported by patient charges, (D) has civil services employees.
   1. A, B, C
   2. B, C
   3. B, C, D
   4. C

4. A nonprofit voluntary hospital may be operated by (A) labor unions, (B) the United States Public Health Service, (C) religious orders, (D) industrial or private corporations.
   1. All of these
   2. All except A
   3. All except B
   4. All except D

5. The Joint Commission on Accreditation of Hospitals has representatives from the (A) NLN, (B) ANA, (C) AHA, (D) AMA.
   1. All of these
   2. B. C. D
   3. A, C, D
   4. C, D

6. A hospital, privately owned and operated, taking care of all types of patients regardless of age, sex, or condition would be classified as (A) voluntary, (B) general, (C) specific, (D) official.
   1. A, B
   2. A, C
   3. B, C
   4. B, D

7. Functions of a modern hospital include (A) treatment and prevention of disease, (B) research and rehabilitation, (C) education of patient and personnel, (D) custodial care of the aged.
   1. All of these
   2. All except B
   3. All except C
   4. All except D

8. If a patient complains about an incompetent employee, (A) forget about it, (B) report it to the team leader, (C) agree with the patient, (D) argue with the patient.
   1. A, C
   2. B, C
   3. A, D
   4. B

9. The health insurance plan that is under the Social Security Act   1. A
   is called: (A) Blue Cross, (B) Kaiser, (C) Medicare, (D) HMO.   2. B
        3. C
        4. D

10. Health systems agencies' functions include (A) health plan-   1. All of these
   ning, (B) identifying needed health facilities, (C) certifying the   2. All except A
   need for new hospital beds, (D) ascertaining health care per-   3. All except B
   sonnel needs.   4. All except C

B. Complete the following statements.
   1. A federal, state, or local government operated hospital would be classified as
   _____
   2. Hospitals are accredited by the_____
   3. A psychiatric tax-supported hospital would be classified as a/an _____
   hospital.
   4. When answering the telephone, you should state your name, status, and_____
   5. Home Health Aides usually work under the supervision of_____
   6. Nursing Homes developed under_____legislation.
   7. A technologist or_____usually have education on the baccalaureate level.
   8. Health insurance under Social Security is called_____
   9. Inpatient hospital benefits under the Social Security Act include_____
   10. Hospitals administered for profit are classified as_____

C. True or False. Write *T* or *F* in answer space.
   ____ 1. Hospitals operate at about $1 billion annually.
   ____ 2. All hospitals are accredited by the JCAH.
   ____ 3. The average hospital patient stay is about three weeks.
   ____ 4. The VA Hospital is an official hospital.
   ____ 5. A younger person extends a greeting to an older one.
   ____ 6. If a patient complains about a fellow nurse, agree with the patient.
   ____ 7. DO are the official initials for the degree of the optometrist.
   ____ 8. Home health benefits, after hospitalization, are not covered by Medicare.
   ____ 9. Home Health Services and Health Maintenance Organizations have the same
   functions.
   ____ 10. Osteopathic physicians and chiropractors are identical.

Answers (3⅓ points each)
A. Multiple Choice   C. True or False
   1. 2   1. F
   2. 3   2. F
   3. 2   3. F
   4. 3   4. T
   5. 4   5. T
   6. 1   6. F
   7. 4   7. F
   8. 4   8. F
   9. 3   9. F
   10. 1   10. F

B. Completion
1. official
2. Joint Commission on Accreditation of Hospitals
3. official or specific (can be used interchangeably)
4. station or location
5. an RN
6. Social Security
7. therapist
8. Medicare
9. semiprivate room, nursing services, meals, drugs, laboratory tests, and so forth.
10. proprietary or investor-owned.

6

Your Patient

Economics of Health Care • Transcultural Nursing • Understanding the Patient as an Individual • The Hospital from the Patient's Point of View • Patient Safety • The Patient's Religion • Death • Visitors • Questions and Answers

Objectives

Upon completion of this chapter you should be able to
1. understand the economics of health care,
2. describe transcultural nursing and identify the four ethnic/racial minorities,
3. explain what understanding the patient as an individual means to the nurse in giving care,
4. compare the National League for Nursing's and the National Hospital Association's Patient's Bill of Rights,
5. review the importance of the nursing care plan and problem oriented record in giving patient care,
6. identify specific needs of the following patients: abortion, children, elderly, homosexual, mentally ill, suit-prone, and vegetarian,
7. summarize the spiritual needs of Jews, Catholics, Protestants, and other denominations,
8. arrange the five stages between a serious illness and death that Dr. Elizabeth Kubler-Ross has identified,
9. describe your role as a nurse in dealing with the patient's family and visitors.

ECONOMICS OF HEALTH CARE

Every patient or client in the health care program is faced with rising health care costs. These problems are well documented. From 1965 to 1976 national health expenditures increased from $39 billion and 5.9% of the gross national product (GNP) to $139 billion and 8.6% of the GNP. Nearly half of this increase can be contributed to inflation and the prices of medical goods and services with the other

40% to greater per capita use of health services and 10% to population growth. By the late 1970s, national health expenditures were more than $162,627 billion (Table 6–1) or an average of $737 per person. Undoubtedly, this figure will continue to increase substantially every year.

Twelve reasons are generally given for the increase in health care costs. These include advances in medical technology, rising age of the population, increased demand for health care services, demand for the highest possible quality of care, defensive medicine techniques, reimbursement systems, inefficiency in the health care industry, government regulations, duplication of available services, numbers and training of health care professionals, reliance on acute care, and the inflation factor. The impact of recent medical expenditure is even more impressive when we realize that in 1977 American consumers spent about $245.2 billion on food; $95.6 billion on clothing, accessories, and jewelry; $81.2 billion on recreation; and $184.6 billion on housing (Table 6–2).

Both public and private sources pay the personal health care bill. The private share has always been by far the largest, but with the addition of Medicare and Medicaid programs in recent years a shift to more public financing has occurred. In fiscal 1977, $68.4 billion was spent for health and medical programs at all levels of government. Increased public spending for health services has done much to ease the financial burden of health care for the nation's poor and elderly.

In 1978, 37.2 million patients were admitted to hospitals, and 263 million out-patient visits were made. On an average day almost 1,042,000 patients received nursing care. More than 80% of these patients were admitted to community hospitals defined as nonfederal short-term general and special hospitals, where they occupied more than 980,000 beds—each patient expecting individualized and patient-centered care.

The prospect of a national health care plan will probably assure massive expansion in health care expenditures within the near future. In fact, it has been estimated that in the year 2000 the total economic costs of illness will exceed $3 trillion and will account for 11 to 12% of the GNP.

TRANSCULTURAL NURSING

Transcultural nursing focuses on the scientific and humanistic study of persons of all cultures and how the nurse can assist with their daily health and living needs. It has been estimated that there are 2,500 cultures and subcultures in the world. Each of these reflects a set of values, beliefs, and practices that influence the delivery of health care. Health care practices and beliefs, therefore, are determined by culture, and the quality of care is based upon perceptions of the people. The health value system of a specific culture should guide the decision-making process for the delivery of health care (see Culture, Chapter 4.) Receivers of health care must be actively involved participants in decision-making concerning their care.

The population of the United States in the 1970 census was 203,212,912. Whites composed about 87.64% of the population, or 178,107,190 people. The ethnic racial minorities constituted about 17% of the population. This included Asian

TABLE 6–1.   NATIONAL HEALTH EXPENDITURES FISCAL 1977 BY TYPE OF EXPENDITURE AND SOURCE OF FUNDS (000,000 omitted)

Type of Expenditure	Total	Private*	Public
Personal Health Care	$142,586	$85,465	$57,121
Expenses for Prepayment and Administration	7,572	5,829	1,743
Government Public Health Activities	3,729	—	3,729
Research	3,684	284	3,400
Construction	5,055	2,607	2,448
Total	$162,627	$94,185	$68,442

(Sources: U.S. Department of Health, Education and Welfare, Health Care Financing Administration, *Social Security Bulletin,* July 1978; and *Book of Health Insurance Data 1978–1979,* p. 43.)
*Includes spending by philanthropic organizations.

Americans, Black Americans, native American Indians, and Hispanic Americans. The Black American population was more than 25 million, the Hispanic American population was more than 9 million, the Asian American population was about 1.5 million, and the native American Indian population was 798,119. It is generally felt that census data are not accurate and it is believed that the greatest numbers of uncounted people exist in ethnic minority groups.

Asian Americans include Koreans, Filipinos, Chinese, Japanese, and Hawaiians. The Hispanic American population comprises all Spanish-speaking people, including those of Cuban, Central and Southern American, Puerto Rican,

TABLE 6–2.   PERSONAL CONSUMPTION EXPENDITURES FOR 1977 IN THE UNITED STATES (in billions of dollars)*

Type of product	Personal consumption expenditures (billions of dollars)	Percent of total
Food (including alcohol)	$245.2	20.3%
Housing	184.6	15.3
Household operation	176.9	14.7
Transportation	172.1	14.3
Medical care*	115.6	9.6
Clothing, accessories and jewelry	95.6	7.9
Recreation	81.2	6.7
Personal business	59.3	4.9
Private education and research	18.8	1.5
Personal care	16.7	1.4
Tobacco	16.5	1.4
Religious and welfare activities	15.4	1.3
Foreign travel and remittances—net	5.1	.4
Death expenses	3.5	.3
Total	$1,206.5	100.0%

Sources: U.S. Department of Commerce, Bureau of Economic Analysis, *Survey of Current Business,* July 1978; and Health Insurance Institute, Book of Health Insurance Data 1978-1979 p. 5.
*Includes all expenses for health insurance (except loss of income type).

and Mexican origins. The native American Indian population comprises Amerindians, Aleuts, and Eskimos.

It was also estimated as part of the 1970 census that more than 33% of native American Indian families had incomes below the poverty level. This group was followed by Black Americans, with 29.9% below the poverty level, Hispanic Americans, with 21.2% below the poverty level, Asian Americans, with 8.8% below the poverty level, and White Americans with 8.6% below the poverty level. All these income levels have specific implications for health care and the maintenance of health.

UNDERSTANDING THE PATIENT AS AN INDIVIDUAL

You must remember that no two patients are alike. A patient is a person who, in addition to everyday problems, has the added burden of illness. It is up to you as a nurse to not only give the maximum benefit of your technical skill but also to do your utmost to minimize the patient's distress. Illness is a lonely business. It weakens the will as well as the body. The patient's ordinary defenses are down, and the emotional self-sufficiency of the well person is usually absent. The patient is dependent on the physician and nurse for both physical and emotional support; under normal circumstances the greater part of the responsibility for providing emotional support is yours.

Holistic care emphasizes personal responsibility for balancing the body, mind, spirit, and environment in order to achieve and maintain a high level of wellness. It includes all safe modalities of diagnoses and treatment, including drugs and surgery, emphasizing the necessity of looking at the whole person, including analysis of physical, nutritional, environmental, emotional, spiritual, and life style values. It focuses a great deal upon patient education and patient responsibility for exerting personal efforts to achieve balance.

Before you are able to render holistic or comprehensive care (emotional as well as physical support) to your patients, you must understand how normal people behave. The real key to having an ideal nurse/patient relationship is to learn about human nature as it is, and not about human nature as you think it should be. Patients have biological and cultural differences that make them individuals just as much as you, as the nurse, are an individual.

It is impossible to remove stress in hospital situations. However, its effect on the patient can be reduced greatly by an understanding nurse (Figure 6–1). Some nursing measures and patient care procedures are painful or embarrassing for the patient. No one likes to receive injections, use the bedpan, or be catheterized. Besides physical discomfort, the patient's privacy is violated, possibly causing anxiety for both the patient and you. Being able to understand your patients as individuals, and caring for them, despite, or perhaps because of, their individual behavior, will be rewarding.

The sick person is dependent upon others for care. This dependence usually leads to frustration for the patients and for the caretakers. Too many nurses want their patients to be "grateful" and "obedient," and do not take time to listen to

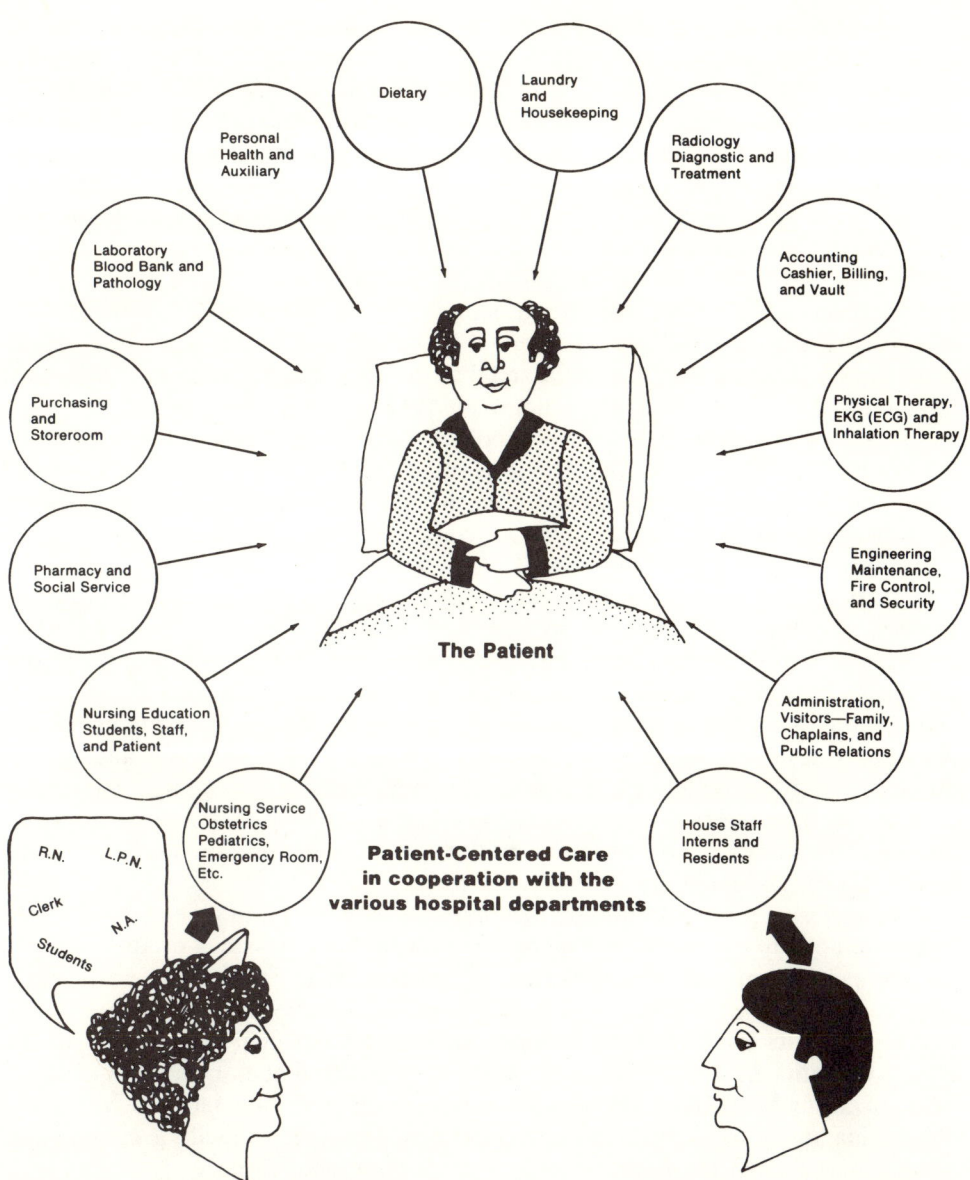

Dietary

Laundry and Housekeeping

Personal Health and Auxiliary

Radiology Diagnostic and Treatment

Laboratory Blood Bank and Pathology

Accounting Cashier, Billing, and Vault

Purchasing and Storeroom

Physical Therapy, EKG (ECG) and Inhalation Therapy

Pharmacy and Social Service

Engineering Maintenance, Fire Control, and Security

The Patient

Nursing Education Students, Staff, and Patient

Administration, Visitors—Family, Chaplains, and Public Relations

R.N.   L.P.N.

Clerk   N.A.

Students

Nursing Service Obstetrics Pediatrics, Emergency Room, Etc.

Patient-Centered Care in cooperation with the various hospital departments

House Staff Interns and Residents

Team leader as coordinator of health care

M.D.—prescriber of medical care

FIGURE 6-1. *The nurse, in a coordinating role with various hospital departments, is responsible for seeing that effective patient-centered care is rendered. The physician prescribes the necessary and desired care, but only through smooth coordination can various departments schedule the diagnostic tests and procedures ordered without upsetting the necessary nursing and total care routines. Since personnel other than nurses sometimes fail to focus their attention on the patient as an individual, you may find yourself in the role of a "security guard" or a "traffic director" to protect your patients from unnecessary interruptions and confusion.*

reasonable requests or justified complaints. If the patient is dependent on you, you should not become annoyed with an "uncooperative" attitude until you have determined the causes. Patients may become "difficult" for valid reasons. The following situation illustrates this point. A maternity patient, in active labor with ruptured membranes and some bleeding, was being admitted to the labor room. While being prepped and examined she kept insisting that she must use the telephone. Since there were no phones for patient use in the labor room, the nursing staff told her she could not use one, labeled her "most uncooperative," and told her to relax and to be cooperative. When the student nurse entered the room with the injection to sedate her, the patient knocked it out of her hand and dashed out of the room toward the elevator, where she was stopped by the instructor and the head nurse. Hysterically, she screamed that she must call her neighbor, who must have returned by now from shopping, to advise her of her whereabouts, since her son had to be picked up at nursery school and her husband was in another city on a business trip. The instructor wrote down the neighbor's telephone number and reassured the patient that she would make the call, after which the patient willingly let herself be wheeled back to the labor room.

Patients are not isolated individuals. They are part of a family unit. Remember that most people, moving from an environment of customary comfort to one of possible discomfort, are subject to fears and anxieties. Try to provide an atmosphere that helps the patient to feel comfortable and secure. The secret of your success is acquiring a knowledge of human nature. This can be done by constant self-scrutiny—not the infantile kind of preoccupation with self, but constructive self-appraisal in which you recognize your strengths and weaknesses and are not afraid to call these by their right names. An emotionally mature person can do this despite the uncertainty that necessarily goes along with a ruthless examination of oneself. The more you come to terms with yourself, the freer you are to give your best to those who most are in need of you.

In considering your patients, realize that their behavior in a given situation can be predictable up to a point, but recognize as well that illness can produce temporary or permanent alterations in the personality, or at least exaggerate weaknesses. You can be fairly sure that patients will be relatively helpless, supersensitive to elements in their surroundings, and will be especially vulnerable to the effects of criticism (real or fancied), neglect, or indifference on the part of those who are caring for them. Everyday worries, particularly financial ones, will probably be magnified to overwhelming proportions. In short, you will be called on to share a burden that the patient simply cannot cope with alone.

The Human Element

Patients need nothing so much as an understanding and compassionate person to give them the strength they are unable to summon for themselves—that person is you. What you have to give might be called the human element, and it is impossible to overemphasize its importance. The demands that this will make on you are formidable, because you are expected to have a reserve of friendliness, courtesy, and sympathy, even though you may be rushed and weary and especially prone to overlook small courtesies that mean so much to patients. "Difficult" patients exact even more from you, but that does not mean they deserve less consideration.

Understanding your patients means you will recognize their individuality and acknowledge it. Get to know them—their backgrounds, their families, their special interests, and their ambitions and goals. The more you know of your patients as individuals, the more accurately you can tailor your services to them. Recognize that even though large institutions such as hospitals have certain routines that are necessary for good management, patients must not be allowed to feel that they have fallen onto a therapeutic assembly line. Recognize that a sick person lives in fear, day and night. To acknowledge your patients' individuality is to let them know indirectly that you understand they are afraid. A newly admitted patient experiences a special fear—that of the unknown. Most patients come to the hospital, the doctor's office, or the clinic with preconceived ideas about illness, physicians, hospitals, and nurses. Many of these prejudices are based not only on ignorance but also on fear, and it is important that we recognize that the patient has a *right* to be afraid. Fear is a powerful emotion and can give rise to behavior over which the patient may have no control. Because many patients attempt to cover up their apprehensions, it will take considerable insight on your part to sense an unspoken fear in order to help them face reality and be relieved of anxieties. The best way to help patients unburden fears is to let them "talk it out" with a maximum of listening and a minimum of talking on your part.

TLC

You have heard about TLC (tender loving care). I also think of TLC as tactful loyal care, since I feel that tact and loyalty are essential for fulfillment in all human relationships. Tact and courtesy go together. Saying and doing the right thing at the right time, regardless of how small or unimportant it may seem, may be your first step in improving your relationships. A good example of the exercise of tact in nursing is in securing the patient's cooperation. Many patients are pleasantly surprised to find that they are not being treated like laboratory guinea pigs. Instead, the patient is approached as an intelligent human being, enlisting personal efforts for recovery. The modern concept of healing is to work with the patient toward this end. This method calls for more teaching on the part of the health team, but it is worth it. Furthermore, it does wonders for the patient's self-respect. We cannot expect people to be familiar with procedures and cooperate unless we offer assurances and explanations and are courteous and tactful. Understand the patients' position, and look at them as special people to be accepted for themselves. Do not insist that they be perfect in your estimation. Be friendly to your patient, never forget the value of a sense of humor, and be able to take a joke as well as tell one. Develop your smile; keep saying to yourself that patients will be friendly and reasonable once you get to know them.

Practice the art of remembering names and faces. Calling your patients by name, will make them distinct individuals in your mind.

From the patient's viewpoint, the "dedicated" nurse is reliable and responsive to personal needs. Many patients are apprehensive about possible mistakes in their care that may be caused by neglect and confusion in the unit. Therefore, checking "identabands," calling the patients by their names, reassuring them regarding "what their physician has ordered," and carefully explaining their therapy will be comforting. If the patient's room is not a private one, introduce the new patient to the roommates, and make them feel at home; the more secure you can make patients feel, the easier it will be for them to adjust.

Rights of Patients

In 1959, the National League for Nursing, in attempting to define the patient's needs as well as to reassure the public regarding their care, published the "Patient's Bill of Rights." According to this statement, every patient has the right to expect that

> He will receive the nursing care necessary to help him to regain or to maintain his maximum degree of health.
>
> The nursing personnel who care for him are qualified through education, experience and personality to carry out the services for which they are responsible.
>
> The nursing personnel caring for him will be sensitive to his feelings and responsive to his needs.
>
> Within the limits determined by his doctor, the patient and his family will be taught about his illness, so that the patient can help himself, and his family can understand and help him.
>
> Plans will be made with him and his family, or if necessary for him, so that, if possible, continuing nursing and other necessary services will be available to him throughout the period of his need. These plans will involve the use of all appropriate personnel and community resources.
>
> Nursing personnel will assist in keeping adequate records and reports and will treat with confidence all personal matters that relate to the patient.
>
> Efforts will be made by nursing personnel to adjust the surroundings of the patient so as to help him to maintain or to recover his health.

This "Patient's Bill of Rights" was reviewed and discussed by National League for Nursing state and local constituents, nursing services in hospitals, and voluntary and official public health nursing agencies, and schools of nursing in universities, colleges, and hospitals in almost all the states; it was an effective statement for more than a dozen years.

In 1972, the American Hospital Association, issued another "Patient's Bill of Rights" which was circulated to more than 7,000 member hospitals across the nation to promote more effective patient care and more satisfaction among patients with the physician and the health care agency. It states

> It is recognized that a personal relationship between the physician and the patient is essential for the provision of proper medical care. The traditional physician-patient relationship takes on a new dimension when care is rendered within an organizational structure. Legal precedent has established that the institution itself

also has a responsibility to the patient. It is in recognition of these factors that these rights are affirmed.

1. The patient has the right to considerate and respectful care.

2. The patient has the right to obtain from his physician complete current information concerning his diagnosis, treatment, and prognosis in terms the patient can be reasonably expected to understand. When it is not medically advisable to give such information to the patient, the information should be made available to an appropriate person in his behalf. He has the right to know by name, the physician responsible for coordinating his care.

3. The patient has the right to receive from his physician information necessary to give informed consent prior to the start of any procedure and/or treatment. Except in emergencies, such information for informed consent, should include but not necessarily be limited to the specific procedure and/or treatment, the medically significant risks involved, and the probable duration of incapacitation. Where medically significant alternatives for care or treatment exist, or when the patient requests information concerning medical alternatives, the patient has the right to such information. The patient also has the right to know the name of the person responsible for the procedures and/or treatment.

4. The patient has the right to refuse treatment to the extent permitted by law, and to be informed of the medical consequences of his action.

5. The patient has the right to every consideration of his privacy concerning his own medical care program. Case discussion, consultation, examination, and treatment are confidential and should be conducted discreetly. Those not directly involved in his care must have the permission of the patient to be present.

6. The patient has the right to expect that all communications and records pertaining to his care should be treated as confidential.

7. The patient has the right to expect that within its capacity a hospital must make reasonable response to the request of a patient for services. The hospital must provide evaluation, service, and/or referral as indicated by the urgency of the case. When medically permissible a patient may be transferred to another facility only after he has received complete information and explanation concerning the needs for and alternatives to such a transfer. The institution to which the patient is to be transferred must first have accepted the patient for transfer.

8. The patient has the right to obtain information as to any relationship of his hospital to other health care and educational institutions insofar as his care is concerned. The patient has the right to obtain information as to the existence of any professional relationships among individuals, by name, who are treating him.

9. The patient has the right to be advised if the hospital proposes to engage in or perform human experimentation affecting his care or treatment. The patient has the right to refuse to participate in such research projects.

10. The patient has the right to expect reasonable continuity of care. He has the right to know in advance what appointment times and physicians are available and where. The patient has the right to expect that the hospital

will provide a mechanism whereby he is informed by his physician or a delegate of the physician of the patient's continuing health care requirements following discharge.

11. The patient has the right to examine and receive an explanation of his bill regardless of source of payment.

12. The patient has the right to know what hospital rules and regulations apply to his conduct as a patient.

No catalogue of rights can guarantee for patients the kind of treatment they have a right to expect. A hospital has many functions to perform, including the prevention and treatment of disease, the education of both health professionals and patients, and the conduct of clinical research. All these activities must be conducted with an overriding concern for the patient, and, above all, the recognition of the needed dignity as a human being. Success in achieving this recognition assures advocacy in the defense of the rights of the patient.

The main difference between these two "Bills of Rights" is that the National League for Nursing's is directed toward nursing personnel and the one issued by the American Hospital Association stresses the physician/patient relationship.

Understanding the Patient's Illness

Many nursing responsibilities in patient care start from the time of admission to the hospital, or when a diagnosis, even of a tentative nature, is made in a primary health care setting. The nurse must observe the patient for any symptoms that may be significant to the physician and must be prompt and accurate in reporting and recording them. The patient must be properly prepared and be on time for any diagnostic tests. If certain instruments or equipment are needed, they should be easily available and ready for use. Throughout diagnostic workups and laboratory tests the patient will need emotional support. Simple instructions and explanations should be given, preferably from the physician, but certainly from the nurse if asked (and if there are no orders to the contrary). In addition, there may be the need for reassurance and clarification. If possible, a patient should always be accompanied by a nurse or another qualified person during diagnostic tests.

Once therapies have been ordered, the nurse must make sure that they are carried out according to the physician's wishes. Medications must be checked, prepared, and administered as ordered, and recorded promptly. Adverse reactions to a drug should be brought to the physician's attention immediately. In carrying out treatment orders, such as irrigations, changes of dressings, suction, and drainage, the nurse must be aware of appropriate precautions, and, as in the checking and administration of medications, must be prompt and accurate in recording all necessary information. The proper preparation of the equipment, the solutions, and (most important of all) the patient, is the direct responsibility of the nurse. The physician will probably explain the treatment or procedure to the patient in order to gain cooperation, but the rest is up to the nurse. In attending to the patient's comfort the nurse must consider personal habits and preferences: for instance, personal standards of physical cleanliness (is there something that you can teach here?); elimination habits; need for privacy; and environmental considerations, such as sensitivity to odors, noise, and room temperature.

If preventive measures can be instituted through nursing care, you should discuss them with the physician so that they can be ordered. Such measures include the maintenance of proper nutrition, fluid balance, muscle tone, elimination, and rest. In these preventive aspects of nursing care, you will have an excellent opportunity to teach the patient principles for maintaining good health. Be sure to give reasons for everything that you do or recommend; the more patients know, the more enthusiasm they will have for their therapeutic regimens, and more likely to protect future health. In your teaching remember what you learned about communication. Make sure that you are being understood. You must define every term carefully as you go along.

When your patient has or will have any physical limitations, you must be able to recognize their significance. Patients who are blind, deaf, or unable to speak English will probably have a more difficult time adjusting to illness, since it will be harder for you and their physician to communicate with them. Patients who require major or radical surgery that will mar their bodies will need your understanding and sympathy; you can give them the emotional support that they must have.

The Nursing Care Plan

In 1970, with the revised standards of the Joint Commission on Accreditation of Hospitals (JCAH), nursing care plans came into their own. The JCAH Standard IV states, "There shall be evidence that the nursing service provides safe, efficient and therapeutically effective nursing care through the planning of each patient's care and the effective implementation of the plans." The interpretation of Standard IV reads as follows:

> A brief and pertinent written nursing care plan should be developed for each patient; this nursing care plan must be coordinated with the patient's medical plan of care. The nursing care plan should give evidence that planning has been done to make sure that the patient receives appropriate nursing care; it should also serve as an effective method of communicating pertinent information to all nursing personnel concerned with the patient. The plan should indicate what nursing care is needed, how it can best be accomplished, what methods and approaches are believed to be most successful and what modifications are necessary to ensure the best results. It may include:
>
> Medication, treatment and other items ordered by individuals granted clinical privileges and by authorized house staff members;
> Nursing care needed;
> Long-term goals and short-term goals;
> Patient and family teaching programs;
> The socio-psychological needs of the patient.
>
> The nursing care plan should be initiated upon the admission of the patient and, as part of the long-term goal, should include discharge plans. The medical staff and nursing service may find that active liaison with agencies or facilities in the com-

munity is necessary in order to accomplish the successful transition of patient care from the hospital to another facility or to the patient's home. The nursing care plans should be available to all nursing personnel and should be reviewed and revised as necessary.

Nursing records and reports that reflect the patient's progress, and the nursing care planned, must be maintained. These records and reports should demonstrate adherence to the objectives of the nursing service. To contribute to continuity of patient care, the nursing notes on the patient's medical record should be significant, accurate and concise. . . .*

The best way to start a nursing care plan is to use a "Nursing History" or interview. This initial evaluation should avoid the duplication of information that is already available from other patient records and reports such as the admission's office data, the physician's history, and the physical examination. The nursing history interview usually takes about 15 minutes and is the foundation on which the patient's individual care is based.

In many institutions only registered nurses (RNs) do the interviewing; however, more and more licensed practical/vocational nurses (LP/VNs) are expected to admit patients to the hospital, nursing home, or extended care facility. Therefore, you must know the proper procedure for interviewing patients and members of their families. Make sure that the patient is comfortable, at ease, and able to participate in an interview. Observe appearance, behavior, communication skills, and answer questions to the best of your ability. Ask for help from other team members when it is needed. Be a listener, not a talker and "hear the patient out." The history form, sometimes called the patient admission record, will vary from institution to institution, as will the nursing care plan.

The plan usually is kept in two parts. The first section often includes the admitting diagnosis and those diagnoses established thereafter; operation(s) and date(s) of surgery; height, weight, age, and religion; and the physician's orders pertaining to diet, intake and output, activity, vital signs, frequency of medications, and diagnostic studies. The second section is intended for recording special approaches to meet the total needs of the patient as seen by the nursing team leader. Here, team members may include notations such as: "Keep door closed"; "Offer warm milk by 11 PM"; "Hot water with lemon at 6 AM"; "Discuss grandchildren"; "Yankee fan"; and so forth. These are strictly nursing orders and comments and may be carried out unless they contradict orders prescribed by the doctor. Any pertinent information that will assist you in modifying hospital routines to accommodate the day-to-day needs of your patient usually will make the difference between a satisfied and happy patient and a frustrated, complaining one.

Problem-Oriented Record

The problem oriented record (POR) is based on the scientific problem-solving process just as the nursing process is. This type of charting and record keeping is relatively new and was introduced by Dr. Lawrence Weed as the problem-oriented medical record or POMR. It encourages the identification of all the patient's problems and uses a systematic approach with written documentation as part of the patient's permanent record. The POR components include the data base (sum total of patient's admission information), problem list (observable or nonobservable unmet need), initial plans (doctor and nurse's orders), and the progress note (followup).

The SOAP format is used in documenting. The four elements in this type of charting are *subjective* (problem from patient's point of view), *objective* (clinical observation including laboratory data), *assessment* (conclusions after evaluating objective and subjective findings), and *plan* (course of action for resolving this problem). Each problem has separate SOAP notes. The patient problems are usually identified as physical, psychological, or socioeconomic, whereas the plan for nursing care is written in relation to the diagnostic, therapeutic, and patient education plans.

Quality Assurances, Professional Standards Review Organization, and Audit

Quality assurance has been one of the major issues facing the health care industry. In 1972, the Professional Standards Review Organization (PSRO), was established by Federal law, mandating that all health care programs, in order to receive federal funds, must be evaluated by specific criteria. Since health care evaluation involves value judgement and objective decision making, health care institutions have a quality assurance committee and a program director to carry out the patient-care audit. To audit means to verify by examination. This process may include all or any of the following: patient interview and inspection, open or closed chart review, staff interview and observations, and group conferences. From the collected data, a conclusion is drawn based upon the pre-established patient-care standard, and these conclusions are shared with the health care providers.

Empathy

As we saw earlier, a large part of the nurse's job consists of giving the patient emotional support, that is, offering encouragement and understanding. We might sum up this attitude in one word—sympathy—but this is not exactly the right word. To feel sympathetic means literally that you are a cosufferer with your patients. To be sympathetic in this exact sense might be dangerous to you and detrimental to your career, because it means that you personally would experience a great part of each patient's misery. If you were to do this, it would drain you physically and emotionally.

The ideal attitude for the nurse to assume is called empathy, which is the ability to place yourself in the patients' position and to understand for the most part their thoughts and feelings, yet not to become emotionally involved. This is the only practical attitude to adopt in nursing, because, ironically enough, the more susceptible you are emotionally to your patient's plight, the less able you are to give him necessary help.

Empathy helps you maintain a certain emotional distance from your patient, so your mind can be clear and free of irrelevant considerations evoked by strong feelings. You will be able to think a situation through and take appropriate action. Your patients will not think you callous—quite the contrary. They will appreciate (probably more than you realize) your self-control, your coolheaded objectivity, and your intelligent awareness of their feelings. When empathy is at work, a certain air of mutual confidence and trust is present in the nurse/patient relationship.

An empathic person is always distinguished by the *interest* that is taken for its own sake. There is no substitute for the feeling conveyed to the patient (and his family) that, "This nurse is *really* interested." It is easily observable in many ways: by physical contact—the way you place your hand on a child's head, or cuddle a baby while teaching the mother child care; by waiting tactfully for a patient to learn how to do something, rather than hurriedly doing it because it is easier; by commenting about the drawing that the grandchild sent; by asking about the picture on the nightstand or the greeting cards; and most of all by "feeling with the patient"—enough to understand the problems. Thinking how you would feel if this were your problem may help to develop empathy; you must think also of how you can make this patient consciously aware of your feelings in the care that you render. Can you say, "Yes, I know you are worried about that operation tomorrow," and really show that you mean it?

When you first learned various nursing skills, you possibly did not welcome, or may even have objected to, the thought of cleaning bedpans and urinals, giving a bath to a patient of the opposite sex, or taking care of an incontinent one. To be a successful, interested nurse you must be able to accept these tasks as part of your nursing care routines and not as unpleasant duties. It requires very little common sense or understanding to remember not to turn on the overhead light at 4 AM, if the task to be performed can be done by flashlight, or to know that once patients are asleep, they should not be awakened for a sleeping medication, or to proceed to fluff up the pillow when they are apparently quite comfortable.

The patient's behavior always means something. How you interpret this may depend primarily on what you see and hear. However, your reaction to your observations should also be based on additional information about the patient that might be found in the nursing care plan, the physician's progress notes, and the observations of others. It is strongly recommended that before you reach any definite conclusions, or decide on specific actions, you explore your thoughts and reactions with the patient and your team leader or instructor. Let us examine two nursing situations:

> While feeding your patient, Mr. White, who is on absolute bed rest, you find that he rejects the meat (which happens to be pork chops) and refuses to eat the vegetables if some meat remains on his fork. You insist that meat is good for him and will help him to get better. In fact, his doctor has ordered a high-protein diet, and therefore you point out that he *must* eat the meat. You become more annoyed as the patient still refuses to do so. He tells you that he would rather be left alone,

and does not want you near him. You leave the room and report this incident to your instructor, who in turn, checks with the patient and learns that he is a Seventh-Day Adventist, and that members of this denomination do not eat pork products and usually are vegetarians. The instructor will then report this to the patient's physician and also to the hospital dietitian so that proper arrangements can be made for his diet.

You offer an elderly patient, Mr. Black, his medication. He takes a good look at it and states that he will not take *that* pill. You coax him and try to explain that it has been ordered by his doctor and will help him to get well faster. He still stubbornly refuses to take it. You report this to your team leader, who talks with the patient, trying to find the reason for his refusal. In discussing his illness, family situation, and background, the patient sheds some light on his anxieties. The particular pill that he was expected to take happens to be the same size, shape, and color as the pills that his wife had taken prior to her death. The sight of them has brought back painful, unhappy (and perhaps fearful) memories.

From these two illustrations you can readily see that a great deal of insight, patience, and understanding are needed to establish good nurse/patient relationships and to prevent such problems from occurring.

Good nurses do not necessarily always use the most efficient technics, nor are they always "master brains." However, good nurses are invariably courteous, realistic, sensible, and empathic.

Rehabilitation

You will be caring for patients of all ages—from newborn to geriatric, who may have physical handicaps. Rehabilitation begins at the time of the patient's admission, continues throughout hospitalization, and involves arrangements for follow-up care after discharge. Therefore, the need for nurses to know rehabilitation technics—such as preventing and correcting deformities; teaching self-care, crutch walking, or other methods of ambulation; and assisting other members of the rehabilitation team—has become an important aspect of total patient care. Although most of the emphasis is placed on the prevention of illness in rehabilitation, special consideration should be given to restoring the physical and the mental health of the patient. The hemiplegic patient, the amputee, the patient with severe coronary disease, the patient with arthritic disabilities, as well as many others, may be beyond complete rehabilitation and therefore must be taught how to make adjustments and must discover how to live with their handicaps.

There is nothing more frustrating to a patient than the loss of verbal communication. The aphasic patient needs frequent reassurance to prevent complete withdrawal. Since the aphasic patient usually comprehends all that is said but cannot effectively respond, realistic rehabilitation goals must be undertaken that consider personality structure as well as medical diagnosis.

Rehabilitation is usually a two-way process. Patients must be motivated to help themselves and must realize that being taught self care is for their own benefit. You, as the nurse, must practice patience; you must realize that the patient may not be thinking clearly at this time and may not be able to communicate properly.

You will be taught specific rehabilitative nursing technics in your program; proper bed positioning, transfer technics, and the prevention of joint stiffness, muscle weakness, and decubiti are all part of good nursing care. You usually do not need a doctor's order to carry out these preventive procedures.

THE HOSPITAL FROM THE PATIENT'S POINT OF VIEW

To most patients the hospital world is a strange and difficult place. There are some specific adjustments that you, as the nurse, must make to the differing needs of patients. Patients bring to the hospital certain attitudes and modes of behavior that reflect individual or group standards. For example, some may find the hospital a haven of refuge from certain hardships at home. Perhaps some have no home and enjoy the comfort and the protection afforded by their hospitalization.

A vast amount of research has been done for the purpose of improving patient/nurse relationships. In one report the authors* revealed certain attitudes on the part of hospitalized patients that every nurse should keep in mind when planning individual care. Patients do not feel in a position to object to hospital routines that conflict with their mores of privacy and modesty. For example, very few patients make any comment when asked to share a room with a stranger. Patients realize their dependency on others and are afraid deviation from expected standards of behavior may not result in good service. The researchers were impressed with the patient's continuous efforts to cope with the demands involved in being not only a patient but also a "good patient."

What is a "good patient"? Usually, it is one who is reluctant to seize initiative, who tries not to be too demanding or to "make trouble" for the staff. Such patients do not disturb the equilibrium, in the hope that they will obtain services without having to ask for them. In various interviews it was clear that patients had real concern with being a "good patient" in order to earn those vital services that otherwise might be withheld. This attitude is not always beneficial; in fact, it can be dangerous to the patient. It should not be necessary for patients to be "good" to receive the care due them.

Patients sometimes have a stereotyped image of hospitals. They believe that most hospitals tend to suffer from a shortage of personnel, that nurses are rushed and very busy, and that physicians are inevitably overburdened and deserving of special consideration. Patients reveal a strong moral commitment to other, sicker patients in the hospital; they rarely consider themselves as sick as others in the same room or in the same department. Conversely, it was found in this report that those who demanded more than their illness seemed to justify were criticized by the other patients for being too demanding and inconsiderate.

The researchers explored the attitudes and reactions of patients concerning the nursing service. The nurse who brought a touch of humor into the sickroom without causing undue excitement was the one whose service was sought. Patients

* Hans Mauksch and Daisy Tagliacozzo, *The Patient's View of the Patient's Role* (Chicago, Ill.: Institute of Technology, 1963).

feel grateful to the nurse with a ready smile, a hearty handshake, and a generally optimistic attitude. Most patients commented that the "nice" nurse with the "pleasant personality" made it easier for them to express their feelings without embarrassment or fear of unknown consequences. This nurse made the task of being a "good" patient less difficult. From the point of view of many patients, mistakes are less likely to happen if nurses know their patients, and take a personal interest in them. Many emphasized that their confidence increased when they could observe such attitudes. Patients appear to rely heavily on first impressions, which can cause them to relax or , conversely, to become anxious and distrusting for the rest of their stay in the hospital.

Nurses may feel that "good patients" have no problems. This is not true. This study suggests that the problems of "good patients" often are hidden behind a cloak of conformity. The "good patient" needs and deserves attention, even when not demanding it. The patient's individual or group standards must be considered. Those who work with the hospitalized patient will have to be sensitive to "cultural bias."

Children

Hospitalization to most children is a frightening experience. Young children normally have fears, and when they are separated from familiar faces and surroundings, they may be terrified. Most of all, they fear pain and injury, especially if their previous experiences with doctors and nurses have not been pleasant ones. The youngster less than three years of age cannot even verbalize properly and "talk out" fears. You may therefore encounter frightened children in the pediatric unit who especially need your reassurance and approval. You can demonstrate these qualities by holding a child, talking softly, and offering praise whenever possible. If the child is to have elective surgery, you can also help the parents prepare the child for hospitalization. Recommend that the child bring along familiar objects such as a "security blanket" or favorite toy. Things of this nature help to build positive feelings about hospitalization. Even though in the hospital you may be a "parent substitute," include the parents in the care of their child. Be patient and understanding and accept them as members of your team.

Even though it is normal for ill children to regress to earlier patterns of behavior, this regression can be modified by allowing them to do as much for themselves as possible. It may be easier and faster for you to do the tasks yourself, but your patience in limiting yourself to supervision will be many times rewarded. If a playroom is available, and if the physician permits it, let children eat and play together. They learn readily from each other. Consistency in disciplinary measures is important and should be observed by all personnel around the clock. This is even more important in long-term illnesses when "spoiling" may become a habit.

The use of foster grandparents, especially grandmothers, has been instituted in some hospitals, providing a trained substitute to offer emotional support to hospitalized children whose own parents, for one reason or another, cannot offer this. This has been most helpful for children who are deprived, "battered," depressed, homesick, or frightened, who have feeding or sleeping problems, or who fail to thrive as expected. Hospitalized children usually are happier when parents visit regularly and can be called on the telephone.

The Abortion Patient

With the liberalization of abortion laws in the United States, a substantial number of women have had unwanted pregnancies legally terminated at approved medical facilities. In 1973, the United States Supreme Court eliminated almost all statutory barriers to abortions, and abortions are now a legal method of birth control. However, state abortion laws vary greatly. These differences are created both by the medical interpretations given state laws by doctors and hospital boards and the legal interpretations given by state attorney generals and legal counselors. (For information about your state's laws, consult your legal officer.)

In 1978, 29% of pregnant women chose to terminate their pregnancies by abortion. Almost 3% of women of reproductive age in the United States obtained an abortion. The total number of abortions may have been 1,456,000. There were about 406 abortions for every 1,000 births. Additionally, it was estimated that 479,000 women were in need of but were unable to obtain abortion services. From 1967–1978, approximately 6 million women obtained about 8 million legal abortions; about one in eight women of reproductive age has had a legal abortion. About one in three abortions were obtained by teenagers, and three in four were obtained by unmarried women.

Contraceptive services were provided to about 4.5 million women through various organized family planning services. Besides hospitals these included health departments, Planned Parenthood affiliates, community action groups, neighborhood health centers, and women's health programs. One third of the patients availing themselves of contraceptive services were teenagers.

As abortion becomes more and more an accepted practice in our society, your attitude may need to change. Patients undergoing abortions need a great deal of psychological support and acceptance by the personnel who care for them. If you are going to care for these patients, be aware of your feelings. If for one reason or another, you cannot offer kindness and understanding, discuss your attitudes honestly with your superior. Learn to cope with these patient-care situations so that you may give realistic nursing care based on maturity and understanding of the many social, cultural, emotional, religious, physical, and medical aspects involved. To help you do so, the Nurses Association of the American College of Obstetricians' (NAACOG) Statement on Abortion has set up appropriate guidelines for members of the nursing team.

NAACOG STATEMENT ON ABORTION

The Nurses Association of the American College of Obstetricians and Gynecologists recognizes that current knowledge of human behavior, population pressure and changes in medical technology challenge the position traditionally held regarding interruption of pregnancy.

We are aware of our nursing role in relation to cooperating with team members in meeting the health care needs of the woman seeking an abortion or sterilization.

Genuine concern and compassion for this woman is strongly urged. However, there may be concern regarding nursing practice and participation in this particular area of health care. It is, therefore, our aim to recommend that an individual's rights must be maintained and safeguarded by written policies.

The 5,000 member Association recommends the following principles and guidelines:

Nurses have the responsibility to provide nursing care.

Nurses have the right to refuse to assist in the performance of abortions and/or sterilization procedures in keeping with their moral, ethical and/or religious beliefs, except in an emergency when a patient's life is clearly endangered, in which case the questioned moral issue should be disregarded. This refusal should not jeopardize the nurses' employment nor should they be subjected to harassment or embarrassment because of their refusal.

Nurses, in dealing with such patients, should not impose their views on the patients or personnel.

Nurses have the right to expect their employers to describe to them the hospital's policies and practices regarding abortions and sterilizations.

Nurses have the obligation to inform their employers of their attitudes and beliefs regarding abortions and sterilizations.

The Unmarried Mother

Although all babies have mothers and fathers, not all women who have children have husbands. Becoming pregnant out of wedlock is not something that "just happens." Some of the reasons for such pregnancies are pentup emotions and frustrations, loss of inhibition resulting from alcohol and/or drugs, naïveté and lack of proper information, religious and family differences that prevent marriage, and, perhaps most important of all, the need to feel wanted, loved, and cared for. Additionally, many couples that do not believe in formalized legal marriages have planned children. Even though society has become more tolerant of the unmarried mother, many student nurses have difficulty accepting her and cannot relax when caring for her, because of their personal beliefs.

There was a dramatic increase in pregnancies among unwed adolescents in the early 1970s. Many of these young mothers are keeping their out-of-wedlock babies. It is important for you to know about the local community resources, such as homes for unwed mothers, social casework agencies, and family counselors. There may be a time when someone in this situation will turn to you, her friend, for advice and guidance. Your understanding and ability to refer her to a qualified agency is the first step in helping her find proper medical care and counseling for her problems.

During her hospital stay, the unmarried mother needs particular understanding and supportive care from the nursing and social service department personnel. In fact, you have a greater responsibility toward this mother than to other maternity patients. She is usually hospitalized in the same room with married women who are inquisitive about the absence of visits from her husband or friends. There may be no telephone calls, greeting cards, or gifts for her or the baby. Often she may be assuming a deceptive role; details of hospital routine such as requests for birth certificate information, breast feeding, or having the baby brought in to the mother all keep her focused on the conflict with which she is faced. Be sure you do not add to her discomfort by giving uncalled-for opinions or advice. Be a good listener and, whenever possible, seek more qualified professional help for her if she has not already received it.

The Mentally Ill Patient

Almost every physical illness is accompanied by some emotional problems. Psychiatric nursing concepts are an integral part of all nursing, and every nurse should be able to use them. The dynamic nursing approach—looking for the reasons behind your patient's behavior—is the key to good patient care. Once you are aware of these reasons and have also developed an understanding of your own behavior, you will be able to establish therapeutic nurse/patient relationships.

You will encounter patients in every hospital unit who show signs of depression, anxiety, stress, and other symptoms that may lead to suicide. Since the "breaking point" varies so greatly among individuals, your powers of observation, recording, and reporting are vital and are often the first line of prevention. The patient who unexpectedly settles personal affairs and straightens out the dresser and night stand, giving away belongings and valued possessions, may unknowingly be offering clues that your help is needed: Statements like "no one needs me," "I'm only a burden," "I'd be better off dead," and so on should not go unheeded. These should be charted and referred immediately to the team leader.

Almost half of all the hospital beds in the United States on any given day are occupied by psychiatric patients. Current thinking and planning for the care of the mentally ill focuses on prevention and early diagnosis and treatment. Progress has been made in establishing special day-care and night-care centers, halfway houses, foster family care, and clinics for the mentally ill, (often taking the place of psychiatric hospitals).

The National Institute of Mental Health reports that the number of patients in state and county mental hospitals is declining annually. In some states such as California practically all mental health care is now given in community clinics and hospitals. Since President Kennedy in 1963 called upon Congress to stop neglecting the critical health problems of mental illness and mental retardation, community resources have improved and many more are being created. As the public begins to realize that mental illness can be cured, and treatment has become increasingly more effective, former patients are being accepted back into family and community life. It is a well-established fact that mental illness alone does not bar successful job placement.

Crisis Intervention

What is a crisis for one person may not be a crisis for another. As long as you are able to handle stressful events and emergency situations, you will not experience a crisis. However, if you are unable to handle stress and it overwhelms you, crisis results. The crisis intervention movement has become part of the delivery of mental health services. It assists people who have difficulty in managing their feelings, have suicidal or homicidal tendencies, are drug or alcohol abusers, and/or have problems adjusting to the laws of society. Special services for individuals and groups are also available when unexpected situations occur, such as death, natural disasters (earthquakes, fires, hurricanes), loss of a job, or prolonged illness.

The Homosexual Patient

It is estimated that there are at least 20 million homosexuals in the United States and that every tenth patient the nurse comes in contact with is homosexual. These patients may be frightened of being rejected because of their sexual orientation. They may hesitate to talk about their sexual preference in order not to alienate the nursing staff. Your personal feelings should not compromise your nursing practice. Take an inventory of your feelings and eliminate the stereotyped image of the homosexual. Make an effort to meet homosexuals and you will discover that most homosexuals lead rather normal lives. The Gay Nurses Alliance has been involved in providing speakers and materials on this topic. Feel free to contact them to assist you and your colleagues in becoming more knowledgeable about this topic. The American Psychiatric Association removed homosexuality from its list of diagnostic categories in 1973 because there was no valid research that provided evidence that homosexuality was a mental illness. These patients, just like all your other patients, have the same rights to quality nursing care. The ''Patient's Bill of Rights'' includes all patients in the hospital.

The Elderly

The field of geriatrics is now considered a specialty. It encompasses medical, surgical and psychiatric disorders. Many of us tend to generalize about the ''older folks'' and feel that they are often demanding, critical, and unreasonable. Older patients, especially those who are senile, require more of your time and understanding; their feelings of loneliness, depression, helplessness, rejection, insecurity, and confusion, as well as their mental deterioration, must be considered. A family quarrel, fear of a crippling disability, physical impairment, or other illness often dominate the thoughts of the elderly. The physiological changes of aging involve impairments of the senses and often cause psychological maladjustment. In addition, the aging person's response and reaction-time may be slowed and psychomotor abilities may decline, making it difficult for solving problems and carrying out everyday activities. Although personal independence is to be encouraged, the nurse must be aware of the normal changes in the aging process and, with understanding patience, help the patient maintain dignity by resuming as active a life as is feasible. In addition, the nurse must be fully aware that older adults have many of the same physical and psychosocial needs as younger people. Thus, always remember to treat your geriatric patients not as relics but as human beings who just happen to be older.

As the average life-span increases, families face more problems with elderly relatives who insist upon living alone under conditions that endanger their health and safety. Unfortunately, many aged persons react adversely to physical changes in their environment and resent being placed in nursing homes or senior citizen housing developments, wanting to remain in their familiar surroundings as long as possible. However, there are many who readily accept such a change of environment, which offers diversional activities and a chance for new friendships with people of the same age.

The Suit-Prone Patient

Lawsuits against physicians, hospitals, and even nurses are brought much more readily than ever before for real or imagined negligence. Legal authorities, juries, and the general public are more aware of the legal responsibilities of these practitioners. You, therefore, have the obligation of knowing how to prevent malpractice claims.

A suit-prone patient is usually defined as a person who is generally unhappy, resentful, and dissatisfied with life and, therefore, because of the psychological makeup, is more likely to bring suit for malpractice than other patients when something goes wrong.

Good nursing practice, based on sound knowledge, skill, and an understanding of the principles of human behavior will make you less vulnerable to such charges. Studies also have shown that the personality of the nurse or other hospital employee involved was often the deciding factor of whether or not the patient sued. Most nursing malpractice suits can be traced to the patient's general dissatisfaction with nursing care. Your early interactions will influence the decision. If you assess individual needs, listen, explain your actions, and remain attentive, patient, and understanding, chances are that you will not antagonize patients.

If you are aware of a suit-prone patient, do pay special attention to the psychological needs while giving personalized care so that the patient feels secure and important. Indifference to this type of patient will often lay the groundwork for a later lawsuit. Do alert others, keep very accurate records, and report as well as record all incidents promptly according to the employer's policy. (See Chapter 7, Negligence and Malpractice.)

Vegetarians

Nurses working with patients on vegetarian diets must explore the nature of their personal diet patterns, since there are at least four basic types of vegetarians. Each demands different approaches. The lacto-ovo-vegetarian diet is an all-vegetable diet supplemented with milk, cheese, and eggs. There is no problem in securing adequate protein with this diet, since only wheat is omitted. The lacto-vegetarian diet is an all-vegetable diet supplemented with only milk and cheese. Here, too, the patient receives an adequate supply of amino acids, since only meat and eggs are omitted. Pure vegetarian, or "vegan" diets, are all-inclusive vegetable diets without any animal foods, dairy products, or eggs. Very careful planning is required here to achieve the intake of the essential amino acids. This is also true of the fruitarian diet. These diets are usually based on Eastern religions. The Zen Buddhists believe that one's health and happiness depends on a proper balance between the Yin and Yang foods. To many this is known as the Zen Macrobiotic diet.

PATIENT SAFETY

The importance of knowing about fires and their prevention, electrical hazards, and other safety factors in the care of your patients cannot be overemphasized. Four potentially serious hospital fires occur every day, not counting the many minor and unreported ones. The modern hospital may be built with fire resistant materials, but there is no fire proof hospital.

Hospital and nursing home fires occur for many reasons, some of which include careless people (visitors, patients, and personnel), combustible materials (paper, cloth, wood, trash, mattresses, linen, and curtains), flammable liquids and gases (gasoline, paint, oil, and anesthetics), and electrical equipment (beds, lamps, TV sets, and faulty wiring).

Upon discovering a fire, seeing flames or thick smoke, remain *calm,* save lives in the immediate area, and confine and fight the fire. Follow the fire action procedure where you are. Be familiar with it and do not ever attempt to "outguess" a fire situation. TURN IN THE ALARM!

Since most hospital fires are class A, B, or C, you should be familiar with types and proper use of fire extinguishers (Table 6–3). Familiarize yourself with the directions usually found on the extinguisher. Be sure you also know where extinguishers are located as well as the location of fire alarm boxes.

Providing a safe electrical environment for the patient is another important aspect in patient safety. Ralph Nader's investigation revealed that about 40% of hospital equipment is electrically hazardous and that approximately 1,200 patients have been electrocuted.* Electrical hazards are also dangerous to the personnel using or touching electrical equipment. Be sure you report frayed power cords, broken plugs, faulty lamp sockets, and any instance when you are "shocked," no matter how minor. All electrical hazards have the potential of allowing contact with lethal voltages. There is no simple or small shock for the patient on monitoring equipment with internal electrodes or catheters. Use only equipment grounded with a three-wire plug and cord. Multiple electrical equipment for one patient should be plugged into the same wall power receptacle and grounded properly. Report all electrical problems immediately and become familiar with "electrical isolation" procedures. Safety for the patient begins with you.

THE PATIENT'S RELIGION

The large majority of Americans identify themselves as Catholics, Jews, or Protestants. There are many people who are members of other religious sects that may not be as well known.

Conversely millions of Americans do not claim membership in any religious

---

* Editorial: *Modern Hospital,* vol. 111, no. 31 (March 1969).

TABLE 6–3.   CLASSIFICATION OF FIRES AND COUNTERACTION REQUIRED

Class	Combustible Material	Counteraction
A	Ordinary combustibles	Cooling and soaking by water
B	Flammable liquids	Smothering, flame interruption and cooling by foam, carbon dioxide, or dry chemicals; or shutting off air supply
C	Electrical components	Shutting off power source and saturation by carbon dioxide or dry chemicals
D	Combustible metals	Saturation by special dry chemicals

group. The nurse should never assume such patients are antireligious. In many instances quite the opposite is apparent: these individuals are truly "religious" and show it in their thoughts and actions. As John Lovejoy Elliott put it, "I have known many good men who believe in God. I have known many good men who did not believe in God. But I have never known a human being who was good who did not believe in man."*

Religion is a dominant force in the lives of a large number of people, and many an indifferent person has found a new meaning in religion during illness. It is one of the primary duties of the nurse to see to it that the patient's spiritual life is administered to. Very often the nurse is the sole link between patients and their religious representatives.

In the modern concept of therapy, assisting patients in spiritual welfare is considered a part of total or holistic care. In some institutions there are routine visits by the chaplain. Pastoral training in hospitals is becoming more and more common, so that theological students and clergy may learn firsthand what patients and their families experience in the hospital.

Because patients' attitudes toward religion vary so widely, the nurse must handle this subject tactfully. For example, if with no preliminary inquiry you suggest that the chaplain pay a visit, the patient may conclude that death is imminent, but if, in getting to know your patient, you throw out a few unobtrusive "feelers" and find out something of the religious attitude (and observe any changes in it that may occur), you will be able to offer intelligent assistance. The first step is to know something about the major faiths. These will be discussed briefly.

When clergy are called to visit the sick, they should be extended every courtesy. There may be definite times when they ask for your assistance, and you must be understanding and help them in every way, regardless of your own attitude or religious affiliation. Although you may not be in agreement with your patient's religious beliefs, you must respect personal wishes, ensure privacy whenever the cleric visits and otherwise be conscientious and understanding about religious practices.

Judaism

Judaism is the religion of the Jewish people based on the Torah (the five books of Moses), which teaches the Fatherhood of God and the brotherhood of man.

* Leo Rosten, *Religions in America*, p. 214 (New York: Simon and Schuster, 1963).

Since Judaism is also a way of life, and since its adherents have developed different patterns of living, three divisions have emerged through history. The Orthodox group, oldest in tradition, resists ritualistic changes and is strictest in its devotion to the ceremonies, the teachings of the rabbis, the laws, and the observances. The Conservative group is less rigid and strict in following the traditions and the interpretations of the Torah, believing that Judaism is based on the evolving religious character of the Jewish people. The most modern is the Reform group, who have adjusted the Jewish observances to the conditions of modern living. Religious customs that are commonly observed by those of the Jewish faith include:

Celebration of the Holidays.   All holidays begin at sunset on the evening before the holiday and end after sunset the next day. Some holidays are celebrated for two days by the Orthodox and the Conservative groups. The most important holiday is the Day of Atonement (Yom Kippur), which is celebrated 10 days after Rosh Hashanah, or the Jewish New Year. This most holy day usually is marked by fasting and prayer and ends the 10-day period of penitence. The Jewish religious year is based on the lunar calendar. New Year, 5742, falling in the autumn of the year 1981, is based on the traditional date of the creation of the world. The Jewish Festival of Thanksgiving (Succoth) celebrates the final gathering of the harvest, and it is believed that the Pilgrim Fathers derived the American observance of Thanksgiving Day from this occasion. Hanukkah, the Feast of Lights, is celebrated for eight days in honor of the victorious struggle of the Jewish people under the leadership of Judah Maccabeus against the tyranny of the Syrian King Antiochus, who had restricted their freedom of worship. Candles are lit on each of the eight nights, songs are sung, games are played, and gifts are exchanged in recognition of religious liberty. Since this holiday occurs in December and often falls around Christmas time, it has gained in popularity and observance, more than other, more traditionally sacred holidays. The Festival of Freedom and Independence (Passover or Pesach) is the celebration of Israel's deliverance from Egyptian bondage. The festival lasts for eight days, and matzoh (unleavened bread—similar to crackers) is eaten. The seder, a family dinner with special readings and observances, is celebrated the first night, and in some homes for two nights. The family and the home usually are specially prepared for this occasion, which falls in early spring.

Dietary Laws.   The laws of kashruth (kosher) are observed by Orthodox, Conservative, and a few of the Reform Jews. These laws regulate the food customs and, except on the advice of their physicians, patients will not violate these rules. Even when given permission to do so, some Jews will find it impossible to eat or to swallow a mixture of milk and meat, or snails, lobster, crabs, shrimp, or pork products. The basic dietary laws are that meats must come from cloven-footed, cud-chewing animals such as cows, sheep, goats, and deer, or from fowl (excluding birds of prey) such as chicken, duck, and turkey. The meats can be eaten only if they have been slaughtered in a prescribed manner (Shehitah). Fish that have scales and fins may be eaten with either meat or dairy products, provided that they are not prepared with elements of one or the other and then interchanged. The same is true of eggs. Dairy products are kept separate from meat and are not eaten with a meat meal or immediately after. All utensils for food preparation and serving are kept separate, according to whether they are used for meat or dairy products. They are not interchanged except for glassware, which may be, if cleansed in the prescribed manner.

Many food products today are manufactured in accordance with kosher dietary standards and are marked with a U. If the product is labeled "pareve" (neither meat nor dairy product), it may be used with meat or dairy foods. A Kosher Products Directory is published annually by the Union of Orthodox Jewish Congregations of America and lists a particular product as meat, dairy, or pareve. These lists are available free of charge. Kosher foods should be served in their original containers or paper dishes.

Even stricter than the common dietary laws are the Passover regulations forbidding the eating of any food containing leavened grain products. Therefore, the greatest care should be taken during Passover week that only foods sanctioned for Passover are served. Equally important to most orthodox Jews is complete abstention from all food and drink on the Day of Atonement. Even though observing the dietary laws is most important to the patient's psychological and spiritual welfare, it must be remembered that these, and similar, traditional religious laws, are suspended whenever human life is in danger. A critically ill patient may be given nonkosher food if kosher food is not available. If the physician feels that fasting would endanger the patient's life, the patient is excused from observing the fast.

Circumcision through Bar Mitzvah.   On the eighth day following birth, unless medical reasons make it inadvisable, male children are circumcised in a religious ceremony that follows prescribed rituals. At this time the boy receives his name. The ceremony is usually presided over by a rabbi or the spiritual leader, and the "mohel" performs the actual circumcision. The mohel is specially trained for performing this function and usually provides his own instruments. Reform Jews require either a mohel or a Jewish doctor to perform the circumcision in the presence of a rabbi who reads the appropriate prayers. Female children are named in the synagogue or house of worship, with appropriate prayers.

Many traditionalist Jews celebrate "Pidyon Ha-ben" (redemption of son) on the 30th day after the baby's birth in honor of the ancient practice that the first born male child become a priest. Bar Mitzvah ("son of duty") is celebrated primarily to mark the completion of one stage of religious education, to encourage mature religious attitudes, and to strengthen Jewish allegiance. It is celebrated on the Sabbath following the 13th birthday and the boy or girl (Bas Mitzvah) reads the weekly Torah portion and participates in the prayer service to signify the ability to assume religious obligations and duties.

Although neither the bible nor the Talmud specifies that Jews should pray with headcovering, Jewish people adopted the Eastern practice of donning headcover as a mark of respect; hence orthodox and many conservative Jews wear a "yarmulka" (skull cap) when praying at home, in the hospital, or in the synagogue. Beginning with Bar Mitzvah, devout orthodox Jews usually put on tefillin each morning (except Saturday). The tefillin or phylacteries are two leather boxes to which are affixed thin leather loops that are bound around the left arm and head in a prescribed fashion in accordance with the biblical directive to keep the teachings of God ever before one as "a sign upon they hand, and for frontlets between thine eyes." (Exodus 13.16)

Death.   The dying orthodox Jew should not be left alone and usually a member of the family or synagogue sits with the patient. After death has been ascertained, the eyes and the mouth of the deceased must be closed and a sheet drawn over the face. If possible, the rabbi should be called immediately so that he may notify the burial society who will care for the body in a prescribed manner. It is best not to touch the body or move it unless permission from the religious authority has been obtained. If the deceased was found with severed limbs, or with blood-stained clothes these should be kept with the body, since these must also be buried. Since the prohibition of autopsy is of a moral/religious nature for the Orthodox Jew, permission should be obtained only from the family if an autopsy is definitely needed. The family will usually consult an authority on religious law after consultation with the physician and nurse. The donation of eyes, heart, kidneys, and other organs is a very complex issue of medical ethics for the Orthodox Jew and is under rabbinic discussion. The laws of observance connected with death, burial, and mourning have been modified in Reform practice, and the basic consideration is to spare the feelings of the bereaved and to give as much consolation as possible. If no special burial or other ceremonies are planned or indicated, the body may be prepared in the postmortem care procedure prescribed by that institution or funeral home.

The doctrines of salvation and life after death do not affect Jewish thinking and beliefs as much as they do Christian ones. Judaism is more concerned with life and living "here" than in the "hereafter." Orthodox Jews are accustomed to burying their dead within 24 hours, or as close to that time as possible, except on the Sabbath and certain holidays. Nonorthodox Jews have no objections to embalming and, therefore, do not rush the burial of the dead. A "Seven Day" candle is kindled in the home of the mourner in memory of the departed. On the anniversary of the death, a "Yahrzeit" light is usually kindled by the next of kin and burned for 24 hours in mourning, and the Kaddish memorial prayer is recited.

The Sabbath.   Sabbath, the day of rest, prayer, and study, begins at sunset on Friday and extends until after sunset on Saturday. Since Judaism stresses the importance of worship and observance in the home, the Sabbath meal is regarded as one of the most important for the Jew. Special blessings are recited over candles, bread, and wine. The children and the home are blessed, and the entire family participates in this ceremony. Synagogue services are held on Friday evenings and Saturday mornings. Some of the Orthodox female patients may request candles for lighting purposes before sundown on Friday night. Candles are also kindled before sundown to usher in Jewish holidays. In most institutions candles are available through Central Supply or the service unit.

Catholicism

As with practically all Christians, Catholics attribute their faith and their Church to Jesus of Nazareth, whom they proclaim as the Christ. That faith flows from Judaism and is grounded in the belief that almost 2000 years ago God (in what is called the Incarnation) became a human being, known as Jesus. Jesus taught insights about God, for example, God is a trinity of personalities sharing the unique divine nature; God is love; God desires that all people be saved and live forever in heaven; God forgives all who are sorry for their sins. Jesus was eventually executed on a cross; his followers believe that after three days he arose to a new life, and this death and resurrection brought salvation from sin and death to all humanity.

According to the Christian scriptures, Jesus formed a group of 12 disciples (who came to be called Apostles) to spread his doctrine, and Peter was their leader. Catholics believe that their functions and authority are carried down through the centuries by the body of churchmen called bishops. And since Peter died as the leader of the local church in Rome, Catholics consider the elected Bishop of Rome to be his successor and, therefore, the head of all the bishops and Catholics throughout the world. In that function the Bishop of Rome has come to be known by the title of Pope.

It is the responsibility of the local bishop to preside over the performance of the seven symbolic acts, called sacraments. To assist him the bishop ordains priests to represent him in local parishes and institutions. Of these sacraments, baptism, confirmation, Eucharist (including communion), confession, and anointing of the sick may concern a nurse in caring for a Catholic patient.

Whenever a Catholic patient is admitted to an institution, this information should be made available to the priest of the local parish. In cases of emergency and danger of death he should be phoned immediately, at any hour, and preferably before sedation while the patient is still conscious.

Dietary Laws.   As the name Catholic implies, the Catholic Church is composed of many branches, each of which has its own customary laws concerning fasting and abstaining from meat on certain days. These rules do not apply if detrimental to the recovery of the patient. Within the capabilities of the institution, these penitential dietary restrictions are worked out between the patient and the priest, but the physician has the final word.

Baptism.   Baptism is absolutely basic to a Catholic. It is the sacrament by which he shares in the death and resurrection of Jesus and is initiated into membership in the Catholic Church. It can be done only once in a person's life. If a patient desires baptism a priest should be called. In emergency situations in which there is danger of death of an unbaptized child or baby (including a living fetus) of a Catholic parent, that parent would be anxious to have the baby baptized. Do not waste precious time calling a priest. Proceed to baptize. Preferably, this should be done by a Catholic, otherwise it may be performed by any attending nurse, regardless of that nurse's religious affiliation. It is done by pouring water over the head (or some other skin area if this is not possible) *while saying aloud:* ''I baptize you in the name of the Father, and of the Son, and of the Holy Spirit.'' This should then be reported to the family and the local priest.

Confirmation.   This sacrament is closely allied with baptism, and is ordinarily performed by the local bishop (in America). In emergencies any priest is authorized to do it. If aware that a Catholic patient (regardless of age), in danger of death, has never been confirmed, the nurse should make the local priest aware of this fact.

Eucharist.   This is the sacrament by which Catholics celebrate the death and resurrection of Jesus, made present to them in their assembly by means of a holy meal of bread and wine eaten and drunk at the altar—the Lord's table. Catholics believe that the bread and wine are really the body and blood of Jesus. They are obliged in conscience to join the community in this celebration every Sunday and on certain "holy days of obligation" (for example, Christmas) unless prevented by illness or other circumstances. To prepare for this communion in the body and blood of Jesus, Church law requires Catholics to abstain from food and drink for one hour preceding communion. However, medicine and water may be taken at any time. Catholics have a tradition of bringing communion to the sick in institutions or private homes when the sick cannot be present at the community Eucharist. Catholics often request this, especially before an operation. All such requests should be forwarded by the nurse to an available priest. Catholics who must spend Sunday in an institution might appreciate a nurse arranging for them to watch Mass on TV, or have some privacy for bible reading and prayer.

Confession.   This is the sacrament by which Jesus continues to forgive sins that have been committed since baptism. It is performed by the priest, to whom a Catholic (privately) confesses the sins committed, accepting a token penance, and being assured forgiveness. It is very important that the nurse assure the greatest possible privacy. Especially before a serious operation a Catholic will probably want this opportunity to "make peace with God" and if so, the nurse should notify a priest and do everything possible to see that the patient is conscious when the priest arrives.

Anointing of the sick.   In this recently revised sacrament the priest uses special oil to anoint the sick so as to help them regain physical and spiritual health. There is a misconception among many Catholics and hospital personnel that this is a "last rite" for surely dying patients. Nurses can help to dispel that false impression; it has been responsible for priests being called too late to communicate with the patient, and has led patients and their families to fear calling the priest for anointing. Church law restricts anointings to once for each sickness, and in many hospitals this sacrament is noted on the patient's information sheet, which should be checked before a priest is called. Since priests do not always go by the same definition of death as physicians do, a priest should be called in an emergency, even an hour or so after the patient's being pronounced dead.

Protestant and Other Denominations

Lutherans, Methodists, Presbyterians, Congregationalists, Baptists, Episcopalians, and some other denominations are classified as Protestants. This classification is general and is not to be considered an accurate description of common faith and practice. Although there are differences in the beliefs of these denominations, they hold many doctrines in common, and the spiritual needs are generally similar.

Not all denominations believe that baptism is essential for salvation. Some believe that individuals should have the right to choose for themselves the type of religion which they feel more nearly meets their own personal needs; furthermore, they teach that each person is competent to deal with God without the aid or intervention of another individual. Some denominations do not accept the interpretation of certain institutions as being "sacraments" and refer to them as "ordinances" (which are symbolic only). Some recognize only baptism and the Lord's Supper as sanctioned by the New Testament.

If the hospital has a Protestant chaplain, contact should be made if the patient so desires. Episcopalians normally desire the ministry of an Episcopal priest, or a Roman Catholic priest if the other is not available. Always try to call the clergy while the patient is still conscious and before sedation. If the patient is unable to express individual religious needs to you you might discuss with the family ways in which you might be of help in this regard.

A hospitalized *Baptist* does not consider the sacraments of baptism and communion as a means of salvation. Infant baptism is not practiced, since a person at baptism must be at the age of accountability and make a conscious response to God concerning salvation. Although the importance of confession is stressed in dealing with guilt, Baptists do not place the same emphasis on the need for the sacraments of reconciliation and the anointing of the sick as do Roman Catholics. In terminal cases every possible effort should be made, however, to notify the patient's minister, the hospital chaplain, or both, so that adequate spiritual preparations can be made.

Methodists believe in either infant or adult baptism by sprinkling or immersion and will accept baptism of all other denominations, including the Roman Catholic. The *Episcopalian* patient usually likes to receive Holy Communion. Holy Unction (anointing) is used not only for those who are in danger of death but also and more often, as a sacrament of healing. If death of an infant seems imminent, the child should be baptized.

All of these denominations stress the importance of individual and group study and devotional reading of the Bible, and private and public worship, with emphasis on prayer. They require that their members carry out in their everyday life and in their relationships with others the teachings of the Bible, as interpreted by the individual and also by the leaders and teachers.

If a patient belongs to a church or group that believes that baptism is essential to salvation, or if death is imminent, and there is danger that the minister may not arrive in time, the nurse may baptize an unbaptized person (adult or child), provided that another baptized person is present to act as a sponsor or a witness. The nurse must state the person's name while pouring water on the head, making sure that the water touches the skin, while saying, " .... (name), I baptize you in the name of the Father, and of the Son, and of the Holy Spirit, Amen." Most Protestants consider Baptism with water in the name of the Trinity (Father, Son, and Holy Spirit) to be valid when administered by a lay person.

Emergency baptism should be reported to the church, and the family should be informed as to what was done. This should be recorded also in the nurse's notes on the patient's chart.

There are various other Christian denominations and religious groups. For example, *Eastern Orthodox churches* follow many of the Roman Catholic observances, but it is always best to check with the patient or family as to which religous representative should be called. In addition, there are the *Friends,* or Quakers, who do not have ordained ministers, and in times of sickness or other trouble or for spiritual aid they turn to members of the Meeting to which the patient belongs.

A *Christian Scientist,* when confronted with sickness or disability, would turn to a Christian Science practitioner for treatment by prayer. If nursing care is needed, the patient would be admitted to a Christian Science Nursing Home or sanitorium. There are Christian Science nurses available for home nursing care. If the patient is admitted to a hospital without consent—for instance, as a result of an accident—only emergency treatment consistent with the hospital policy should be administered, and a Christian Science practitioner should be contacted. If the patient enters a hospital voluntarily, admitted by the physician, orders would be written accordingly.

Jehovah's Witnesses believe that God has revealed himself to mankind through his word, the Bible. They believe that Jehovah is the true God, the creator of heaven and earth. The bible teaches what they believe, and since Genesis 9:3,4 states: "Only flesh with its soul—its blood—you must not eat," transfusions of whole blood, blood plasma or blood fractions are forbidden, since this would violate God's laws. They will reject blood transfusions even if it is the only method left to maintain or to extend life. This obedience to God means the reward of everlasting life in God's new world.

Seventh-Day Adventist patients usually are vegetarians and will refuse any pork products. Some may eat clean meats as listed in Leviticus, Chapter 2. The other teachings are basically Protestant, and the church does not practice infant baptism.

Muslims do not eat pork or pork products and alcoholic beverages are prohibited. Black Muslims, especially, follow a specific diet that eliminates many of the traditional foods of Black Americans such as collard greens and cornbread. There is a carefully prescribed procedure for washing and shrouding the dead, and usually it is the family members who wash and prepare the bodies.

As a nurse, you must be very understanding and respect the wishes of your patients.

Pastors, priests, rabbis, or other spiritual leaders, physicians, nurses, and additional members of the hospital staff are all part of the health care team. You, therefore, should be familiar with the religous observances and the traditions of your patients. It is also most helpful if any rituals or rites performed are noted on the patient's chart. As stated previously, in emergency baptism, the local parish must also be notified.

When a chaplain or other clergy is not available it may be helpful to patients who have guilt feelings for sins of commission and omission and/or fears and anxieties, to find comfort and relief in reading (or having someone read to them) selected passages from the Bible. Passages that cover areas of concern such as *fear* are Psalm 23; Psalm 46; Psalm 27; John 14:1–6; 14:25–27; Hebrews 11; Romans 8:18–39; and John 20. Selections to help one who has *anxiety* might include 2 Timothy 3:10–17; Ephesians 3:14–21; Psalm 91; Matthew 5:1–13; 6:1–13; 6:19–34; Matthew 7:7–12; 7:24–29. For the patient who feels *guilt,* turn to such passages as Psalm 51; Psalm 56; Psalm 103; 1 John 1:5–10; Matthew 22:34–40; Luke 11:1–4, and 1 Corinthians 13.

DEATH

In recent decades, the overall death rate of the population in the United States has decreased because of medical developments, improvement in public health and job safety, and rising standards of living. The death rate continued to decline in 1978 to the lowest rate every recorded. Medical improvements and environmental changes have been more effective in reducing death from some causes than from others. There has been increasing success in identifying and controlling contagious diseases but very little success in controlling death from accidental causes. In 1978 the death of seven out of 10 life insurance policy holders resulted from two principle causes: (1) cardiovascular/renal diseases and (2) cancer. Since the 1950s, deaths attributable to cardiovascular/renal diseases have decreased slightly, whereas cancer has been an increasing cause of death. The percentage of deaths due to cardiovascular/renal disease declined to 48.8% of all deaths caused by ischemic heart disease. Chronic diseases of the endocardium and other myocardial insufficiencies were 31.7%. Cerebral vascular diseases also declined to 6.1%. The proportion of deaths due to cancer continue to increase to 22.4%. Motor vehicle death, another major cause of death, is currently at 3.3%. United States life insurance companies keep an accurate account of distribution of death by cause; Table 6–4 illustrates this for 1973, 1975, and 1978. Both natural and external causes of death are shown.

As a nurse, you will be taking care of dying patients, and your acceptance of death—what it means, not only to you but to the patient's family—is something that you must face and understand. Throughout history the idea of death has posed the eternal mystery that is the foundation of many religious beliefs and rituals. Because so many personal conflicts, fears, and emotions are involved, discussion of death usually is avoided.

Dr. Elisabeth Kübler-Ross, author of the renowned book, *On Death and Dying*, has researched this important topic by interviewing dying patients and studying their reactions as well as those of family members and of the hospital personnel caring for them. She states that patients go through five stages between their awareness of serious illness and death: denial, anger, bargaining, depression, and acceptance.

From Dr. Kübler-Ross's "Therapeutic Grand Rounds Number 36, On Death and Dying," Journal of the American Medical Association (July 10, 1972), pp. 174–179, the following has been excerpted for your information:

> Most patients respond with shock and denial when they are told that they have a serious illness. This may last from a few seconds to a few months . . .
>
> Patients begin to see, when they are seriously ill, that the family comes in and does not know what to talk about and becomes estranged. Someone may come in with a red face and smile. Others may change their conversation a bit; they may talk more about a triviality because of this discomfort. Patients accept quickly that things are not at all perfect. When the patient cannot maintain his denial anymore, he will become difficult, nasty, demanding, criticizing; that is the common stage of anger. How do you respond to one who complains and criticizes everything you do? You may tend to withdraw and not deal with him anymore. What else can

you do? You can avoid him, you can stick the needle in a bit farther—not consciously—but when you are angry you touch patients differently. We can measure some of these responses. In California some investigators measured the response time between patients ringing for the nurse and the nurse actually coming into the room. They showed that patients beyond medical help, terminally ill patients, had to wait twice as long as other patients for the nurse to respond. This behavior should not be judged; it should be understood. It is very difficult to remember that members of the helping professions, who work hard all day, may have a difficult job coming into the dying patient's room. In the first place, the professional is uncomfortable; second, she is worried that the patient may ask how long he has to live or all sorts of unpleasant questions, and if the nurse does something for the patient, he may begin to criticize her. The nurse comes in and shakes the pillow, and the patient says, "I just wanted to take a nap. Can't you leave me alone?" When you don't shake the pillow, the patient remarks, "Why can't you ever straighten up my bed?" Whatever you do is criticized. Such patients are very difficult to manage and the families suffer tremendously because, when they come in and visit, they are always too early, too late, or there are not enough people, or too many people. Someone has to do something for these patients, to facilitate life for everybody concerned. It is important to understand that these patients are not angry with the nurse or the family. The more vibrant the nurse is when she comes into the patient's room, the more energetic she is, the more she is going to get through to the dying patient. In a way she should be able to accept the anger as a compliment because what the nurse reminds the patient of is functioning health, ability to go to work, to go for a coffee break, all those things that the patient is about to lose. Because the nurse reminds the patient of all these things, and because he is desperately attempting to deny that he is dying, he becomes angry and says in effect, "Why me?" But he is also asking, "Why couldn't this happen to Joe Blow or somebody else?" If the nurse can put fuel into the fire, if she can help him to express this anger; if she can permit him to ask the question, "Why me?" without the need to answer it, then she will have a much more comfortable patient almost immediately. We interviewed a young patient who was dying. She was in my office and looked completely numb and I asked her if she felt like screaming. She looked as if she were on the verge of an explosion. She asked if we had screaming rooms in hospitals. I said no, we had chapels. "No, this is wrong," she said, "because in chapels we have to pray and be quiet and I need just to do the opposite. I was sitting out in the car yelling at God and asking him, 'Why did you let this happen to me?'" I encouraged her to express this in my office and to cry on my shoulders. They never scream as loud as they think they will.

If you can help patients express the question, "Why me?" you can help them express their rage and anger; then your patients become more comfortable and ring for the nurse less often and stop nagging and complaining. Sometimes they even quickly become more comfortable patients and we wonder what has happened to them.

That is often when they reach the stage of bargaining. In the bargaining they may pray for another year to live; they would donate their kidneys or their eyes, or they may become very good people and go to church every Sunday. They usually promise something in exchange for extension of life. Some of the promises are not made to God, but to someone on the hospital staff. . . .

Promises are never kept; patients say, "If I could live just long enough for my children to go through high school," and then they add college, and then they add,

"I just want a son-in-law, and then would like to have a grandchild," and it goes on and on.

If, in the denial stage, they say "No, not me," then in the anger stage they say, "Why me," and in the bargaining stage they say, "Yes me, but." When they drop the "but" it is, "Yes me." Then the patient becomes very depressed.

There are two kinds of depression and it is important to understand the two different kinds. The first type is a reactive depression in which the patient cries when he talks about it, and mourns the loss which he has experienced. Later on he becomes quiet and depressed. . . .

If I were to lose one beloved person, I would be allowed to mourn and everyone here would respect that as being socially acceptable. But who has the courage to face not only the loss of one person, but the loss of everybody he has ever loved? It is a thousand times more sad, and takes much more courage to face. What we should be trying to do is to tell our patients that it takes a man to cry and that we mean it completely and willfully. We should help them express their grief, which, in fact, is a preparatory grief. It is not mourning and grieving over things lost; rather, it is a grieving and mourning over impending loss. The patient is beginning to separate himself from the people that he has to leave in the near future. This is what we call preparatory grief; the patients will ask once more to see the relatives, then the children, and at the very end, only one beloved person, who is usually husband or wife and, in the case of children, naturally, the parents. This is what we call the stage of decathexis: when the patient begins to separate; when he begins to feel no longer like talking; when he has finished all his unfinished business; when he just wants the companionship of a person who is comfortable, who can sit and hold his hand. It is much more important than words in this final stage. If the physician can help the patient express his rage and his depression and assist him sincerely through the stage of bargaining, then most patients will be able to reach the stage of acceptance. It is not resignation—there is a big difference. Resignation, I think, is a bit like giving up. It is almost a defeat. A stage of acceptance is almost beyond any affect. It is the patient who has said, "My time comes very close now and it is all right."

A woman who was always hoping for a miracle drug that would cure her suddenly looked with an almost beaming face and said, "You know, Dr. Ross, a miracle has happened." I said, "What miracle?" and she replied, "The miracle that I am ready to go now and it is not any longer frightening." This is the stage of acceptance. It is not happy; the time is rarely ever right. People almost always want to live, but they can be ready for death and they are not petrified any more. They have been able to finish their business. . . .

Certain generalizations based on interviewing more than 400 dying patients in the past four years can be stated. All patients know when they are terminally ill, whether they have been told or not. Patients usually state that they would like to be told if it is serious, but not without hope.

Most, but not all, patients pass through five stages (denial, anger, bargaining, depression, and acceptance) between their awareness of serious illness. The knowledgeable physician, particularly one who is himself comfortable in facing the dying patient, can help these patients pass through one or all of these stages by appropriate verbal and nonverbal support—particularly the support engendered by the patient's realization that his physician will stay with him until the end.

Although the Grand Rounds were for physicians, you as a nurse must be aware

TABLE 6–4. LEADING CAUSES OF DEATH: UNITED STATES, 1973, 1975, 1978

Cause of Death	1973	1975	1978
NATURAL CAUSES			
Cardiovascular-renal Disease			
Diseases of the Heart			
and Hypertension			
Ischemic Heart Disease and Other			
Myocardial Insufficiencies	32.9%	32.3%	31.7%
Hypertensive Heart Disease			
and Hypertension	1.8	1.3	1.2
Other Diseases of the Heart	4.1	4.6	5.4
Total Diseases of the Heart	38.8	38.2	38.3
Cerebrovascular Disease	7.1	6.7	6.1
Arteriosclerosis and Other			
Diseases of Arteries, Arterioles			
and Capillaries	3.4	3.3	2.9
Other	1.6	1.6	1.5
Total Cardiovascular-renal	50.9	49.8	48.8
Cancer	20.1	21.4	22.4
Pneumonia and Influenza	2.9	2.8	2.7
Diabetes	1.0	1.0	.9
Other Diseases			
Bronchitis and Other			
Respiratory Diseases	2.9	2.9	3.1
Cirrhosis	1.4	1.3	1.2
Other*	11.9	12.0	12.4
Total Other Diseases	16.2	16.2	16.7
Total Natural Causes	91.1	91.2	91.5
EXTERNAL CAUSES			
Motor Vehicle Accidents	3.5	3.0	3.3
Other Accidents	3.1	3.1	2.7
Suicide	1.6	1.8	1.7
Homicide	.7	.9	.8
Total External Causes	8.9	8.8	8.5
Total All Causes	100.0%	100.0%	100.0%

Source: American Council of Life Insurance, *1979 Life Insurance Fact Book*, p. 95 (compiled).

of your role, which is very similar to that of the physician in this instance. Please refer to Dr. Ross's books for additional readings on this most important topic.

Expressing their grief often functions as a safety valve for the family. Let them cry. It is a normal, natural, and healthy way to express grief. Grief is expressed in different ways by different people. Your supportive role—your dignity and calmness—will leave a lasting impression.

The late Pope Pius XII said in 1957 that "human life continues for as long as its vital functions, distinguished from the simple life of the organs, manifest themselves spontaneously without the help of artificial processes." Since that time, clergy of all faiths, physicians, lawyers, civic leaders, and legislators have been meeting to discuss this problem of modern medicine; hopefully, they will find a solution with guidelines for what is to be considered "life" and "living," as differentiated from "existing," which is now medically feasible.

When is a person clinically dead? What are our responsibilities in prolonging and protecting life and relieving suffering? What are the rights of the patient to die? Should patients be kept alive by technical means even though they are not aware of their surroundings? These are only a few of the many questions you may encounter as science improves the artificial means of supporting and maintaining life. In our society many families prefer that death occur in the hospital, provided there is dignity and peace.

Death may be preferred to the artificial extension of life in the old and severely diseased person or to those who merely exist. However, the right to live and the right to die should rest with the patient, if rational, or with the family, if not. The doctor is the agent of the patient (and family) and therefore must consider their feelings when deciding to use or not use extraordinary measures to maintain life.

If the patient and family have discussed "the right to die" with the physician, the doctor then interprets the patient's wishes to the nursing team, writing orders accordingly. If your patient has expressed specific wishes to you, be sure you bring them to your team leader's attention so that they are discussed further with the patient's physician. You should also alert the physician and advise the patient to be sure to bring these wishes to the doctor's attention as prescription of patient care. The health care team carries out the physician's orders as authorized and cannot alter them. (See Chapter 7, Euthanasia.)

A physician usually pronounces a patient dead and signs the death certificate prior to the removal of the body by the mortician. In most institutions it is also the physician's responsibility to notify the family. If the death was caused by accident, suicide, or some illegal act, or if the patient was not under medical care and died within 24 hours after admission to a health care facility, the death must be reported to the medical examiner (coroner), who will rule whether an autopsy is desired. In order to perform an autopsy, the physician must receive permission from the next of kin and obtain a signed permit. Just as you were considerate in meeting the patient's needs, your responsibility now must extend to the family of the deceased. You must respect their wishes, and be aware that they need your guidance and sympathy. Sometimes it is difficult for the family to grasp the fact that their loved one died without asking for them; or that they were unable to be present when death occurred; or perhaps that they had no opportunity to ask forgiveness for some specific personal matter. You should try to find privacy for them and assist in providing whatever information or assistance is necessary. Unless your employer's regulations state differently, the personal belongings and valuables of the deceased should be handled carefully and released only on signature to the next of kin.

VISITORS

A patient's visitors may radically influence the course of recovery, for better or worse. Because of your responsibility to the patient, you should cultivate the friendship of family and friends and include them in your patient-care plans. You will need their cooperation on many occasions, and so the better you understand one another, the more benefit will accrue to the patient.

Relations with the patient's friends, family, and others who may visit will call for tact on your part. Because you know more than the visitors about what is best for the patient, you will have to be firm at times, but always pleasant and understanding as well. For instance, if a visitor arrives in a highly disturbed frame of mind, you might gently persuade postponement of the visit rather than upset the patient. No matter how unreasonable a visitor may be, never fail to be kind and considerate if only for the sake of your own reputation and that of the institution as well.

Visitors should be made comfortable, and if they must wait in lobbies or other areas, be sure that someone notifies them immediately when the patient is ready to receive them. If they must wait outside the patient's room while you give nursing care, be sure you tell them where to wait. Never expose the patient in the presence of visitors, and do not discuss illness with them in any detail. Ideally, the number of visitors a patient is allowed should be prescribed by the physician and should depend on the patient's condition. However, this is not always possible; therefore, decide for yourself if there are too many visitors at one time, if the frequency of visits is exhausting to the patient, or if there are certain individuals whose presence is not beneficial for the patient.

Be friendly and tolerant toward patients' visitors, but at the same time make sure that visitor regulations are not violated. If one patient's visitors interfere with another patient's welfare in a semiprivate or ward unit, be sure that you consider all the patients in that room, and if you cannot solve the "visitor problem," refer it to the attention of the person in charge of the unit.

Questions

A. Select the correct answer and either write the letter in the space provided, or circle the corresponding number.

1. "I baptize thee in the name of (Catholic version)
    A. The Father and of the Holy Spirit."
    B. The Holy Spirit and the Son of God."
    C. The Son of God, the Holy Father, and Holy Spirit." _____
    D. The Father, and of the Son, and of the Holy Spirit." Amen.
    E. The Father, and of the Son, and of the Holy Spirit."

2. A patient observing the kosher diet could drink milk and eat
    A. ham
    B. peaches
    C. rice
    D. eggs
    E. clams
    F. tomatoes
    G. chicken
    H. cheese

    1. C, D, F, G, H
    2. A, B, D, F
    3. B, D, F, G
    4. B, C, D, F, H
    5. B, D, H
    6. B, D, G, H

3. The supreme head of the Roman Catholic Church is known as a
   A. Bishop
   B. Pope
   C. Cardinal
   D. Mohel
   E. Father

   _____

4. In meeting the needs of the patient, the nurse must understand his
   A. religion
   B. illness
   C. visitors
   D. fears
   E. ambition

   1. B only
   2. All except C
   3. All except E
   4. All of these

5. Protestants include
   A. Methodists
   B. Quakers
   C. Friends
   D. Jehovah's Witnesses
   E. Eastern Orthodox
   F. Episcopalians

   1. A, C, E
   2. B, C, F
   3. A, F
   4. E

6. The Sabbath that begins at sunset on Friday and extends until Saturday night is observed by
   A. Jehovah's Witnesses
   B. Seventh-Day Adventists
   C. Christian Scientists
   D. Jews
   E. Quakers
   F. Eastern Orthodox

   1. A, B, D, F
   2. D
   3. B, D, F
   4. B, D

7. A Catholic patient who may be dying should receive
   A. Mass
   B. Holy Sacrament
   C. Penance
   D. Sacrament of the anointing of the sick
   E. Eucharist

   _____

8. The number one external cause of death is
   A. cardiovascular/renal disease
   B. suicide, homicide
   C. motor vehicle accidents
   D. malignant neoplasms

   _____

9. Infant baptism, in cases of death, is most important to the
   A. Catholic
   B. Orthodox Jew
   C. Seventh-Day Adventist
   D. Baptist

   1. A
   2. A, B
   3. A, C
   4. A, D

10. Nursing care plans should include
    A. diagnosis
    B. religion
    C. doctor's orders
    D. nursing orders

    1. All of these
    2. All except B
    3. All except C
    4. All except D

B. Complete the following statements.
    1. Vegetarians are usually (state religious faith) _____
    2. If a Catholic baby is dying, the nurse (if a Catholic priest is not available) should administer the sacrament of _____
    3. To receive Communion a Catholic must abstain from food for (indicate time) _____
    4. The Jewish spiritual leader is called _____
    5. Bar Mitzvah is celebrated following a boy's _____ birthday.
    6. The Day of Atonement is known also as _____
    7. A Catholic patient who may be dying should receive _____
    8. The "Rights of Patients" was published in 1972 by _____
    9. When a Christian Scientist is admitted to a hospital, a _____ should be called.
    10. A patient's death certificate must be signed by _____

C. True or False. Write *T* or *F* in answer space.
    _____ 1. Rehabilitation applies only to geriatric patients.
    _____ 2. Ethnic and empathic are identical.
    _____ 3. Rosh Hashanah is the most important Jewish holiday.
    _____ 4. Seventh-Day Adventists refuse blood transfusions.
    _____ 5. Communion and penance are sacraments.
    _____ 6. Quakers, Lutherans, and Presbyterians are classified as Protestants.
    _____ 7. The Jews are a race.
    _____ 8. "The Patient's View of the Patient's Role" was published by the National League for Nursing.
    _____ 9. Children less than three years of age will verbalize their fears.
    _____ 10. A nurse may sign an autopsy permit for the family.

D. Match the best associated expression from Column *B* with Column *A* and insert the letter in the space provided.

A	*B*
_____ 1. Seventh-Day Adventist	A. refuse blood transfusions
_____ 2. Jews	B. anointing
_____ 3. "Death and Dying"	C. NLN and AHA
_____ 4. sacrament of the sick	D. Dr. Elisabeth Kübler-Ross
_____ 5. teaching self-care	E. penance and confession
_____ 6. Jehovah's Witnesses	F. Yom Kippur
_____ 7. "Rights of Patients"	G. empathy
_____ 8. TLC	H. racial grouping
_____ 9. social behavior of people	I. usually vegetarians
_____ 10. nursing care plans	J. NLN and ANA
	K. rehabilitation technic
	L. saying the right thing at the right time
	M. sympathy
	N. nursing history
	O. culture
	P. communion

E. Identify the five stages between awareness of a serious illness and death that Dr. Elisabeth Kübler-Ross has pinpointed and explain the nurse's role in each.

Answers (2 points each)

A. Multiple Choice
1. E
2. 4
3. B
4. 4
5. 3
6. 4
7. D
8. C
9. 1
10. 1

B. Completion
1. Seventh-Day Adventists
2. Baptism
3. one hour
4. rabbi
5. 13th
6. Yom Kippur
7. sacrament of the anointing of the sick
8. AHA
9. Christian Science practitioner
10. a physician

C. True or False
1. F
2. F
3. F
4. F
5. T
6. F
7. F
8. F
9. F
10. F

D. Matching
1. I
2. F
3. D
4. B
5. K
6. A
7. C
8. L
9. O
10. N

E. 1. denial
2. anger
3. bargaining
4. depression
5. acceptance

Use of appropriate verbal and nonverbal support technics. (Plus 10 points for your explanation.)

7

Ethical and Legal Responsibilities

Codes of Ethics (NFLPN and NAPNES) • Legal Role of State Boards of Nursing • Contracts • Laws and Torts • Crimes • Organ Transplants • Wills • The Patient's Chart • Questions and Answers

Objectives

Upon the completion of this chapter, you should be able to

1. understand the principles that govern a nurse's conduct,
2. compare the NFLPN and NAPNES Code of Ethics for the licensed practical/vocational nurse (LP/VN),
3. explain the legal role of the state boards of nursing,
4. identify the licensure requirements for your state,
5. list at least five reasons for disciplinary actions by state boards of nursing,
6. differentiate between negligence and malpractice,
7. analyze informed consent and its important implications,
8. define assault and battery, civil law, defamation, euthanasia, false imprisonment, and tort,
9. understand your role in handling controlled drugs properly,
10. discuss your role when the patient wishes to make a will,
11. review why the patient's chart is considered a legal document.

This chapter deals with broad principles that govern the nurse's professional conduct. These principles are really your primary responsibilities and are considered from two standpoints: *legal* and *ethical*. Like any other profession, nursing is a specialized service rendered for the benefit of the public. Because of the nature of this relationship, certain laws have been passed that serve to protect both the nurse and the public that you serve. Knowledge of these laws, or what are called the legal aspects of nursing, is obligatory. The laws governing nursing can be considered to be the minimum responsibilities that the public demands that you fulfill, with failure to abide by them incurring a penalty.

A much broader concept of the nurse's responsibilities is the ethical one. "Ethical" comes from the Greek (*ethikos*) and means knowledge of the right and the wrong of human conduct. A nurse's legal obligations are only a part of the much more extensive code of ethics that has been established by the nursing profession. Consider it this way: if you were to ignore all ethical obligations except your legal ones, theoretically you would not be a public menace, but this is about all that could be said for you. By contrast, when you live by a nurse's code of ethics, you are not only fulfilling your legal obligations automatically but also you are conforming to the much higher standards that the nursing profession has set for its members.

CODES OF ETHICS

A code of ethics (the word "code," incidentally, comes from the Latin *codex*, a kind of writing tablet) is a list of the rules of good conduct. They are principles to live by. You should understand the difference between ethics and civil laws. Laws are rules made by a society for the purpose of preserving order and promoting the safety of that society's members. Because laws apply to everybody, they leave little up to the individual. For instance, laws cannot compel you to develop an exemplary character, but they can prohibit you from committing certain acts, such as crimes, that are against the public interest and therefore undesirable.

Conversely, a code of ethics is drawn up by an individual group (such as a profession), and the members of the group are expected to voluntarily live up to this ethical code. Unlike civil laws, ethical rules are more than a means of keeping people from doing wrong. They reflect the highest ideals of the group—aspirations so lofty that perhaps not every member is expected to live up to them in both letter and spirit.

National Federation of Licensed Practical Nurses (NFLPN) Code

By and large, ethics are practical rules, appealing to common sense, and are followed easily. The following Code of Ethics was adopted in 1961 (revised in 1969 and 1979) by the NFLPN as a principle of conduct by which and through which its members, all licensed practical nurses, should govern their private lives and nursing careers. This code is an excellent guide for students and graduates as well and "provides a motivation for establishing and elevating professional standards. Each licensed practical/vocationsl nurse, upon entering the profession, inherits the responsibility to adhere to the standards of ethical practice and conduct set forth in this code." Pertinent discussions are included to demonstrate more clearly the ethical implications.

1. "Know the scope of maximum utilization of the LP/VN and functions within this scope." Refer to the "Nursing Practice Standards for the Licensed Practical/Vocational Nurse," and be familiar with the Nurse Practice Acts of your state and the policies of your employer. As a student you too, are liable for your own negligence if injury results to the patient. The patient has the right to expect the competent performance of nursing care, by a student or licensed nurse. Therefore, "When in doubt find out"; have your instructor supervise you, and do not assume responsibilities for which you have not been prepared. This will be discussed further under "Negligence and Malpractice." You have a responsibility to evaluate properly your concern for the patient in relation to your own responsibilities. Perhaps you will be faced with decisions pertaining to your family and home obligations, preferences for tours of duty and work areas, or your acceptance of assignments. You are justified in making an individual decision in each case and, if necessary, discussing these problems with your immediate superior. It is impossible to adhere to a double ethical standard, one for your working life and the other for your private life. One invariably influences the other. Therefore, think of your code of ethics as something that is more than a guide for your career. Make it a part of you.

You must also refuse to participate in any unethical procedure. Examples of unethical procedures would be deliberate misuse of narcotics, barbiturates, and other dangerous drugs; charting procedures and observations that have not been performed; or giving medications you have not poured and measured. You should always report such incidents to the charge nurse or supervisor and refuse to be part of them. You have the responsibility to report to the appropriate authority incompetence or unethical conduct in others. Reporting should always be factual and objective.

2. "Recognize and appreciate cultural background and spiritual needs, respecting the religious beliefs of individual patients." Your obligations in this instance have already been covered in Chapters 4 and 6. Some trying situations can be caused by the particular religious beliefs of a patient. For example, at least one religious sect prohibits the giving of blood transfusions to its members. See The Patient's Religion in Chapter 6. Other sects may prohibit the administration of certain medications. Remember, forbidden treatment cannot be forced on such people without the consent of the patient or a legal guardian. However, most religious leaders will place the physician's orders above the doctrines of their religion.

3. "Safeguard the confidential information acquired from any source about the patient." Such information is not public, and you have an ethical and legal obligation to keep it to yourself. In "shop talk" sessions with your colleagues, or at home with your friends, you may be tempted to divulge a few tidbits of information about your patients, especially if these fragments have any sensational value. Understandably, the temptation is hard to resist, because it gives one a feeling of power to be the custodian of secrets, particularly about important people. But do not violate the position of trust in which your vocation has placed you. In Legal Aspects

(which follows) you will find additional reasons for not talking about your patients.

4. "Refuse to give endorsement to the sale and promotion of commercial products or services." Very often nurses are asked to endorse or sponsor certain commercial products, especially pharmaceuticals. They may be asked to participate directly or indirectly in an advertising and promotional sales campaign. It is against all nursing interests to participate in such endeavors, and nurses are forbidden to do so. Although you may be associated with a research program pertaining to a product or take part in some other commercial undertaking that may contribute to advances in health or medicine, you may not lend your name or vocational status to help its promotion. Whenever nurses advertise their services, they must do so in a dignified manner approved by the nursing profession.

5. "Uphold the highest standards in personal appearance, language, dress, and demeanor." Your responsibilities in this area have been fully discussed in Chapter 4. You are one of the image-makers for nursing and represent your fellow colleagues in the employment setting as well as in the community life you lead. Practice high personal standards in appearance, language, dress, and demeanor and you will indeed reflect nursing in an acceptable manner.

6. "Accept responsibility of membership in NFLPN and participate in its efforts to maintain the established standards of nursing practice and employment policies conducive to quality patient care."

The NFLPN is the official spokesmen for LP/VNs on the national level and has committees and representatives who work with other national organizations such as the American Nurse's Association, National League for Nursing, American Hospital Association, American Nursing Home Association, and others to implement the "Nursing Practice Standards for the Licensed Practical/Vocational Nurse." However, on state and local levels they need your active involvement. See Chapter 8 (Nursing Organizations) for further discussion.

Work with and through NFLPN in establishing and maintaining employment policies conducive to quality patient care. Since employment policies and practices vary from community to community and employer to employer, it is really on the local level where the action is! By being actively involved with the local division of NFLPN you will be represented.

Become an "involved" nurse in your community. The problems of comprehensive health care planning, air and water pollution, migrants, the ghetto, the aged, the mentally ill, drug addiction, alcoholism, communicable disease control, school health programs, fluoridation of water, and many other areas of concern are important to you. You cannot isolate yourself from your responsibilities as a citizen living in a community. Your role as a nurse and a health teacher increases your obligations to your community. Join various organizations and be aware of the problems in your community. Volunteer your services and become involved in fighting social ills. Many civic groups and health organizations look for nurse representation and will welcome you.

National Assocation for Practical Nurse Education and Service (NAPNES) Code

In 1971, NAPNES adopted the following Code of Ethics for the LP/VN. It states that the LP/VN should

1. Consider as a basic obligation the conservation of life and the prevention of disease.
2. Promote and protect the physical, mental, emotional, and spiritual health of the patient and his family.
3. Fulfill all duties faithfully and efficiently.
4. Function within established legal guidelines.
5. Accept personal responsibility (for his acts) and seek to merit the respect and confidence of all members of the health team.
6. Hold in confidence all matters coming to his knowledge, in the practice of his profession, and in no way and at no time violate this confidence.
7. Give conscientious service and charge just remuneration.
8. Learn and respect the religious and cultural beliefs of his patient and of all people.
9. Meet his obligation to the patient by keeping abreast of current trends in health care through reading and continuing education.
10. As a citizen of the United States of America, uphold the laws of the land and seek to promote legislation which shall meet the health needs of its people.

Throughout this book, principles, proper conduct, and ethical relationships have been stressed and clarified. Unfortunately, the biggest factor in any ethical code is the problem of enforcement. Very often nurses hope that somehow, somewhere, the "other nurse" (the one you are not very proud of) will change. Very often you may be wrong and overestimate the insight of such nurses into their behavior and their willingness to improve. You must assume the responsibility for helping to enlighten them and must try to show them right from wrong. This is not easy; it takes tact and courage. In the long run, though, if you do not act, your own standards and conduct may deteriorate also.

A new approach to understanding ethical decision making, *situation ethics*, or the new morality, has evolved. According to this concept, the rights and wrongs of behavior must be decided by the individual himself. Every individual has the responsibility and freedom to make the "right" decision, depending upon the circumstances involved. This is a person-centered rather than principle-centered approach. Although you may become involved in situation ethics through your personal beliefs, be cautious in its application in your daily life at the hospital and in patient-care contacts. Analyze the situation, asking yourself what would happen "if everyone did what I want to do or did," "if everyone took home a hospital sheet," "if everyone charted procedures that were not done," "if no one washed their hands in the nursery," "if no one replaced equipment," and so on. It may sound simple to the proponents of situation ethics to say everyone must decide for one's self what is right for the individual, but are you not a member of society with additional responsibilities?

LEGAL ROLE OF STATE BOARDS OF NURSING

All professions, including nursing, are subject to legal control, since they operate in the public interest. Each state has its own laws pertaining to nursing, called Nurse Practice Acts, and responsibility for the administration of these laws is granted to an official agency, usually known as the Board of Nursing, the Board of Nurse Examiners, or Nurse Registration. The Board may function under one of several state departments or be appointed directly by the governor of the state. It usually consists of experienced registered nurses, and in many states it includes LPNs and consumers. The Board may be authorized to employ an educational director and other personnel as necessary for the performance of its duties, which include the preparation of prescribed curricula and standards for schools of nursing and the survey of such schools for accreditation purposes ("accreditation" meaning that the school is state-approved). The Board also examines, licenses, and renews licenses of qualified applicants and conducts hearings on charges calling for discipline of a licensee, which may include revocation or suspension of license. The Board has the power to issue subpoenas (that is, it has the power to call a person to a hearing) and administer oaths to persons giving testimony at hearings. It is responsible for the prosecution of anyone violating the Nurse Practice Acts. State Boards of Nursing are actually the nurses' greatest protection, because through state licensure the nurse assumes legal status and meets legal requirements. See the Appendix for the addresses of the State Boards of Nursing and write for a copy of "The Law Governing the Practice of Nursing and Nursing Education" in your state.

In June 1978 the National Council on State Boards of Nursing was formed. It is now composed of 53 State Boards. The primary objective of the Council is to strengthen and coordinate the credentialing of nurses on a national scale. They control the State Board Test Pool licensing examinations for both professional and practical nurses. The National Council of State Boards of Nursing, Inc. is located at 303 East Ohio St., Chicago, Illinois 60611.

Licensure

In order to protect the public, any person practicing or offering to practice nursing for hire in all states must be licensed as either a registered nurse (RN) or a LP/VN. Possession of a license usually means that the nurse has passed a state examination that has required a demonstration of minimal safe practice. Professional and technical nurses licensed to practice hold the legal title of registered nurse. A practical nurse who is licensed has the title licensed practical nurse. In

California and Texas practical nurses with licenses are titled licensed vocational nurse. Legal titles are conferred only on those individuals who have met the requirements; they cannot be borrowed or assumed. An unqualified person who does so can be prosecuted.

The entire United States and the outlying areas of Guam, Puerto Rico, and the Virgin Islands have passed laws permitting the licensure of practical nurses. In some states licensing of the practical nurse is mandatory; that is, you must have a license before you are allowed to practice. In other states licensing of practical nurses is permissive, meaning that you can practice without a license if you wish (but, of course, cannot then use the title LPN or LVN or represent yourself as licensed). The advantage of mandatory licensing is that it offers greater protection to the public by weeding out unqualified practitioners, thereby raising the standards of the vocation. Actually, a mandatory law protects the practice of nursing, but a permissive law protects only the title.

If you are aware of persons who are practicing nursing or calling themselves nurses, without being licensed, you have an important responsibility: that of notifying the Board of Nursing in your state. In some state statutes it is considered "an offense against the State if you do not report unlicensed persons that are practicing nursing in any hospital, clinic, office, nursing home, etc., or as a private duty nurse." This offense is usually punishable by fine or imprisonment. You, are therefore, urged to report this crime.

Mandatory licensure is becoming common in many states; in these states it has become compulsory for the nurse to obtain the legal document that permits offering one's services to the public before charging fees. In 42 jurisdictions (states and territories) the Nursing Practice Act for practical nurses is part of the same law that provides licensure for professional nurses.

During 1975, the licenses renewed for practical nurses totaled more than 470,770. However, this figure does not reflect the actual total number in force, since nine states currently have a two-year renewal period whereas others require an annual renewal. Some 50,000 licenses were issued to practical nurses receiving their first United States license in 1975. The vast majority of these were to persons who had just completed their training. There were over 49,500 candidates for the licensing examination and 89% of these passed successfully. In 1975, 13,470 licenses were issued to practical nurses on the basis of interstate endorsement (that is, the formal recognition of their qualifications from one state by another state).

Qualifications for Licensure

The State Board of Nursing, as we saw, sets the definitions for the practice of nursing and the qualifications and fees required of the applicants for licensure (Table 7-1).

Although each state has its own qualifications for licensure, uniformity in these laws is slowly being achieved. Although the minimum age for licensure varies from 17 to 18 years, in most states the candidate for licensure must have attained the age of 18 years.

TABLE 7-1. STATE AND TERRITORIAL BOARD LISTING FOR MINIMUM AGE, EXPIRATION DATE AND LICENSURE FEES, 1976*

State or Territory	Minimum Age	Expiration Date	Examination Fee	Endorsement Fee	Renewal Fee
Alabama	—	September 30	$30	$30	$ 4
Alaska	18	June 30[1]	30	30	15[1]
Arizona	—	December 31	35	35	6
Arkansas	—	April 30[1]	25	25	10[1]
California	17	Birthdate[1]	15	15	15[1]
Colorado	—	June 30[1]	30	30	10[1]
Connecticut	—	December 31[1]	25	25	5
Delaware	—	December 31[1]	30	30	10[1]
District of Columbia	18	June 30	30	30	10
Florida	—	March 31	40	20	6
Georgia	18	Birthdate[1]	30	30	10[1]
Guam	—	June 30	5	5	2
Hawaii	—	June 30	[2]	[2]	[2]
Idaho	—	June 30	40	40	10
Illinois	18	May 1	15	15	10
Indiana	—	December 31[1]	25	20	10[1]
Iowa	—	June 30	30	25	6
Kansas	—	Birthdate[1]	25	25	12[1]
Kentucky	18	October 31	25	15	4
Louisiana	—	January 31	15	17	5
Maine	—	June 30	30	30	10
Maryland	—	January 31[1]	15	15	2[1]
Massachusetts	—	Birthdate[1]	30	50	6[1]
Michigan	18	March 31	20	20	5
Minnesota	—	December 31	25	25	5
Mississippi	—	December 31[1]	35	35	8[1]
Missouri	18	June 30	20	20	5
Montana	—	December 31	35	35	10
Nebraska	—	December 31	35	35	5
Nevada	18	February 28 or 29[1]	27.50	20	10[1]
New Hampshire	—	Birthdate[1]	25	25	6[1]
New Jersey	18	December 31[1]	25	15	10[1]
New Mexico	—	Birthdate[1]	30	30	10[1]
New York	17	August 31[1]	60	40	10[1]
North Carolina	—	December 31[1]	25	30	8[1]
North Dakota	—	December 31	25	25	4
Ohio	18	August 31	20	20	3
Oklahoma	—	June 30	15	15	8
Oregon	—	March 31[1]	35	25	15[1]
Pennsylvania	—	June 30[1]	5	5	2[1]
Puerto Rico	—	[2]	[2]	[2]	[2]
Rhode Island	—	March 31	25	25	5
South Carolina	18	December 31	30	30	7.50
South Dakota	—	Birthdate[1]	25	25	15[1]
Tennessee	—	December 31[1]	30	30	8[1]
Texas	18	August 31	25	25	3
Utah	—	December 31	25	25	7.50
Vermont	18	April 30[1]	25	25	10[1]
Virgin Islands	18	June 30	5	—	1
Virginia	—	December 31	25	25	4
Washington	18	Birthdate	25	25	8

TABLE 7-1. STATE AND TERRITORIAL BOARD LISTING FOR MINIMUM AGE, EXPIRATION DATE AND LICENSURE FEES, 1976*—Continued

State or Territory	Minimum Age	Expiration Date	Examination Fee	Endorsement Fee	Renewal Fee
West Virginia	—	June 30	32	25	7.50
Wisconsin	18	June 30	40	25	10
Wyoming	—	June 30	40	40	6

* Compiled from 1976–1977 *Facts About Nursing*, ANA. (State Boards of Nursing, 1977)
[1] Biennial renewal.
[2] Not listed.

If you meet the age requirement, your application then must prove you to be capable of safely performing the duties of a practical nurse according to the usual State Board definition: the performance of nursing acts in the care of the ill, the injured, or the infirm, under the direction of a licensed physician, a licensed dentist, or a registered nurse, provided, however, that all such acts do not require the specialized skill, judgment, and knowledge of an RN. In order to demonstrate your knowledge and capability in this respect, you must take and pass the State Board of Nursing examination for practical nurses. Licensure examinations are generally given two times annually and include a written test and sometimes a practice section to test the skills of the applicant. It is usually an all-day examination, with the administration and the conduct of the examination completely in the hands of the State Board of Nursing. In most cases, the application, properly notarized and filled out, must be sent in a month or two before the examinations are offered, and the State Board office then sends you an admittance card.

Ordinarily, candidates for licensure are eligible to take the State Board examination only if they have met the educational qualifications, namely, to have completed a one-year course of study in an accredited school of practical nursing. In some states 18 months of study in an accredited school of nursing for the preparation of RNs, with satisfactory bedside nursing experience, are considered to be the equivalent of the approved course of study required in schools of practical nursing. In addition, most states require two years (the range is one to four years) of high school (or its equivalent), good physical and mental health, good character, as well as the other entrance qualifications previously discussed. Once the candidate has passed the examination and met the other qualifications, a license is issued. The fee for the examination ranges from $5 to $60, with most states charging $25 (see Table 7-1).

The State Board Test Pool Examination is prepared by the National League for Nursing and is used in all states, which individually set the standards for passing and failing grades. You will be given an identification number and your school has a specific code number that is used on the special answer sheets. The test is usually in two parts, one booklet to be used in the morning and another in the afternoon. Four suggested answers are usually given for each test question; after reading the question and answers carefully, you must choose the *best* answer and record it in the prescribed manner (with a special pencil) on the answer sheet. As with all examinations, it is very important to follow the examination instructions carefully.

In most states it was possible for practical nurses to be licensed without examination if they had been practicing capably before licensing laws went into effect. Usually, a group of people (RNs, physicians, patients, and others) endorsed these nurses, who then obtained their licenses by meeting certain requirements and by paying the set fee. In most states, however, this method of licensing (called the *waiver method*) is no longer in effect.

Interstate Licensure (Endorsement)

Endorsement, more correctly referred to as interstate licensure, is the formal recognition by one state of the qualifications of a nurse from another state. For instance, once a person has been licensed to practice as a practical nurse, one may be eligible for licensure in another state without examination, provided that in the opinion of the State Board of Nursing the applicant's qualifications are satisfactory and the requirements of that state are met; therefore, nurses who may have obtained their licenses by the waiver method may not be eligible for licensure in another state if that particular state does not accept the waiver method. Also, since each state has its own standards and passing grade on the examination, an applicant who has barely passed the State Board examination in one state may not necessarily be considered to have a passing grade in another. Standards in practical nurse education have varied from state to state, and even the curricula in the state-approved schools will not necessarily be acceptable from state to state. Because determination of the passing grade and acceptance of clinical experience, classroom hours, and other educational requirements is the prerogative of each state and territory, eligibility for licensure by reciprocity is not always available to the practical nurse. If you decide to move to another state, it is important that you check with its State Board of Nursing before you accept a position there. Some states may ask that you take their State Board of Nursing examination in order to become eligible if you do not meet their standards. In most states you must be eligible for licensure within 30 to 90 days after beginning your new position if you expect to practice as a licensed nurse.

Renewal

Your license must be renewed periodically. Failure to renew, as provided for in the licensure law, automatically may suspend your license; a satisfactory explanation for this failure must accompany the fee that the Board will charge before reinstatement is granted. An inactive or nonresident nurse licensed in the state may request to be placed on an inactive list, usually without cost. At the time that you wish to recommence the practice of nursing, you may pay the regular renewal fee and be reinstated actively. Any person who practices as a nurse during the time in which the license has lapsed or has been suspended would be an illegal practitioner and would be violating the Nurse Practice Acts.

Continuing education is required for relicensure in several states. Other states are currently making decisions as to whether continuing education should be a mandate for relicensure. Continuing education has been defined as planned learning experience beyond a basic education program. These experiences are designated to promote the development of knowledge, skills, and attitudes for the achievement of nursing practice, thus improving health care to the public. A continuing education unit, or CEU, is the equivalent of 10 contact hours. A contact hour equals a minimum of 50 minutes and a maximum of 60 minutes of organized learning experience.

Each state, through its rules and regulations, will decide what the State Board of Nursing feels is recognized continuing education. Continuing education must be approved and/or accredited by designated agencies in order to be recognized for the relicensure requirements.

There is no uniform date on which the license expires; each state or territory sets its own date. Most of them use the fiscal year, some having biannual rather than annual renewal. Renewal dates and other information pertaining to licensure laws can be obtained from the State Board of Nursing. In the Appendix is a list of the addresses of Boards of Nursing (see Table 7-1, as well).

Disciplinary Action

The State Board of Nursing has grounds for disciplinary action if the holder of a license is immoral or unethical in conduct; if the licensee is a habitual intemperant or addicted to the use of narcotics or other habit-forming drugs; and if the person circulates untrue and misleading advertising, is unfit or incompetent, or willfully violates any Nurse Practice laws. A hearing is usually called, at which time the Board reviews the charges and the findings, and if its verdict is guilty, it institutes proper disciplinary action. If a nurse is in prison, or adjudged incompetent, and in some instances if convicted of a felony, the Board may deny or refuse to renew the license without a hearing. Remember that the State Board of Nursing protects the public and the patients as well as the nurses themselves; therefore, you must be aware of these regulations and abide by them.

Institutional Licensure

Institutional licensure applies to institutionally based health care employees who would be regulated by the employer, institution, or agency, within certain bounds established by state institutional licensing boards. The accountability, responsibility, and liability of the employee would then belong to the institution, rather than to the individual licensee.

CONTRACTS

A contract is an agreement between two or more people for a "consideration" (a legal term meaning some recompense such as a fee). A contract is legally binding on both parties. If you do not uphold your end of the agreement, you have committed a "breach of contract" and can be sued for damages by the other person.

In order for a contract to be legal, there must be a mutually understood offer and acceptance. Some contracts are very formal; the terms are elaborated in a document that you read and then sign, formally giving your acceptance. However, most contracts are much more casual; the offer and the acceptance can be "implied" or "silent." If you go to a newsstand, pick up a newspaper, and leave the proper change before the vendor, who pockets it, both of you have made a contract even though not a word was spoken.

Doctor Brown discusses the conditions of employment with Mrs. Smith; Mrs. Smith approves and tells the doctor that she will report for work next day. The doctor says that he will expect her. She arrives for work at the appointed time. Here again, both parties have entered into a contract even though nothing was actually said about a contract. The contract is "implied," because there is no doubt as to the intentions of both the doctor and the nurse.

Private duty nurses should make as definite as possible contractual terms with their patients. Phrases such as "usual wage and hours," "regular salary and time off," or "reasonable payment and working hours" are so vague as to be meaningless. Spell out the terms precisely, so that there is no doubt on the part of either you or your patient.

An offer may be withdrawn before it is accepted. For example, Mrs. Greene offers Miss Dixon (the nurse) a position but changes her mind before Miss Dixon has accepted the offer. This is her privilege, and she incurs no penalty. Even if Miss Dixon had accepted, and there were a contract, the contract could be dissolved by mutual agreement.

A nurse who foresees certain circumstances making it impossible to carry out these responsibilities in a contract must discuss them at the time of employment and reserve the right to stop work or to adjust the schedule, if necessary. These reservations might be stated, for example, by nurses who have dependents whom they must care for.

Everyone has both a legal and a moral obligation to abide by the terms of a contract. But sometimes some event beyond our control, such as an "act of God" (say, a hurricane or a blizzard), may prevent one from carrying out the terms of a contract, in spite of the best intentions. Most states would allow you to be excused from your obligations in such an eventuality. You should be familiar with your own state's opinion of such situations.

If one person does not perform *all* the obligations as required by the contract, one commits a breach of contract (unless the performance has been excused on a legal ground). A patient who has suffered injury through a nurse's negligence may sue on the basis of the contract, claiming a breach, since care was not rendered with ordinary skill or judgment. In many instances nurses have sued successfully for damages for breach of contract, collecting unpaid salaries or reimbursements for patient expenses, and holding the employer to other obligations that had been agreed upon.

LAWS AND TORTS

Civil laws deal with legal rights and duties between individuals. A civil suit usually pays money for the damages incurred. Criminal law is for offenses against the public and those crimes and criminals that are detrimental to society. The crime is prosecuted by the state. If the person is found guilty, the punishment may be fines and/or imprisonment.

A tort is a wrongful act committed by one person against another. You might think immediately of the word "crime," but there is a difference. A crime can be a tort—that is, committed against another person—but it also is by nature an act against the whole of society. A crime, then, is a more serious act than a tort. Remember that you are responsible for any tort or crime that you may commit, even if you had no intention of doing wrong. As the law sees it, "Ignorance is no excuse."

Negligence and Malpractice

A common legal problem in nursing, and one often difficult to interpret, is that of negligence.

Negligence is defined as the failure to do what a person of ordinary judgment or prudence would do, or doing what a reasonable person would not do. It may be intentional or unintentional.

Malpractice is a particular type of negligent conduct. The term "malpractice" refers to the negligent acts of persons who have had specialized professional education and training. In the performance of nursing duties, every nurse is required to exercise reasonable care so that no harm or injury comes to a patient. The actual furnishing of nursing care to the patient constitutes a nurse/patient relationship and involves the legal responsibility of giving care in a reasonable, competent manner. This includes both acts of omission and commission. Any professional misconduct—what you do or do not do—can lead to a malpractice suit if injury to the patient results. The nurse rather than the employer is always responsible for his or her own acts; therefore, you are responsible for your own negligence and must know the consequences of your actions.

The fundamental rule of personal liability—that is, every person is liable for one's own tortious conduct—applies here. However, under the doctrine *respondeat superior*, the employer may become responsible for the legal consequences of the employee's actions within the scope of employment. Therefore, your employer could be held legally responsible for your conduct in the course of your employment. The employer has the right and responsibility to control, direct, and supervise you. Even though *respondeat superior* may apply here, the negligent employee is always liable for personal conduct and may be sued alone or jointly with the employer.

A nurse who in some manner causes injury to a patient can be sued by that patient. If the nurse is careless in the performance of duties to the extent that human like is jeopardized, the act of negligence may then be considered as "gross negligence," which may be viewed as a crime rather than a tort. The nurse's act of negligence may result in a liability suit.

Many practical nurse organizations are sponsoring liability insurance plans through the state associations or through other groups, and this may be worth looking into, since people are becoming more and more lawsuit-conscious every day.

Typical acts of malpractice for which nurses have been sued include the following:

> Leaving side rails down, so that patients fall out of bed.
>
> Burning the patient from hot-water bottles, enemas, heating pads, inhalators, douches, sitz baths, or overheated solutions.
>
> Giving a wrong medication, incorrect dosage, or administering a drug by faulty technic.
>
> Leaving a thermometer in the rectum of an unconscious patient.
>
> Using apparatus that is obviously defective.
>
> Misuse of a patient's personal belongings—for example, breaking or losing dentures.
>
> Failure to count sponges accurately during an operation, so that one or more are left inside the patient.
>
> Abandoning a patient in a situation in which the nurse's presence is constantly needed; for example, if you go to lunch and leave your critically ill unconscious patient without first notifying the head nurse (or another nurse) to observe the patient.

Always remember that since you are responsible for your own actions, it is your right and duty to refuse to obey an order under certain circumstances. A nurse may refuse to carry out a physician's order whenever this order is contrary to hospital regulations, medical ethics, standing orders, good health care practice, or if the welfare of the patient is endangered, and the nurse's common sense or judgment indicates that it is wrong. This will depend entirely on the education, training, and experience of the nurse as well as the licensure interpretations. The nurse has the choice of carrying out the physician's orders as written or refusing to do so. Under no circumstances may you alter an order or substitute something else that you feel would be more effective for the patient.

Most employers will not expect nurses to perform acts for which they are not qualified; but if you do, and you accept these responsibilities, *you will be liable for your acts.* If you practice professional nursing because your employer expects you to, then I recommend very strongly that you resign, or else have your employer adjust your duties, since you are gambling with the loss of your license, your reputation, and your future. Do not assume duties for which you are not trained. Have all your nursing skills shown to you, be supervised in them, and then practice them safely.

If the orders of physicians seem incomplete to you, do not hesitate to call this to their attention. Be sure that you have the amount of the drug, the method of administration, the frequency with which it is to be given, as well as all other necessary information before you attempt to give a medication. Remember that you are responsible for your acts, and guesswork must be left out. There is no "usual dosage, frequency, or method of administration"; when you give the medication, the order must be complete. Do not give medications that someone has poured or prepared for you, even if it is your charge or head nurse. It is your right to refuse an order of this nature, just as it is your responsibility to obtain clarification from the physician on orders that are not clear to you. You must know the limits of your responsibilities and not carry out orders that are not clearly written out.

Sometimes you may be assured by the charge nurse or the physician that you are protected if you do what they direct you to do, even if it is not within the limits of practical nursing. This is not so. If a patient should be injured because of your carelessness or incompetence, you are also personally liable. It is wiser to say that you do not know how to do the procedure, or that this procedure does not come within the scope of your work, than to take the risk of injuring the patient. Very often you may not be sued directly for your actions but may be named as codefendant (that is, accused) together with a physician or a hospital on the basis of joint negligence, if your actions are not legal. Remember that you are protecting yourself, the reputation of the practical nurse and, most important of all, the patient. *If in doubt, find out* is perhaps the best slogan for you to remember in trying to understand the legal aspects of nursing.

In emergencies you may be permitted by the law to perform certain functions that ordinarily would be outside the scope of your duties. Certain first-aid procedures, for example, qualify as medical practice. However, a nurse must know when an emergency is an emergency, and use good judgment and common sense.

Remember that in assuming duties of the RN or the physician, you are exposing yourself to severe penalties, including the loss of your license. Therefore, it is imperative that you keep calm, cool, and collected, and do only those things that are essential for the safety of the patient, knowing the circumstances that surround the emergency. It may be better to wait a few minutes for the arrival of a physician or an ambulance with qualified personnel than to assume the practice of medicine.

Another way in which a nurse inadvertently may practice medicine is to volunteer to treat the physical injuries and the ailments of friends and neighbors. If someone seeks medical help or advice from you, the best policy is to recommend seeing a physician as soon as possible. You must convince your acquaintances that it is for their best interests that you decline to offer direct medical aid, and you must teach them the habit of seeking help only from a qualified person.

You should also caution the well-meaning person who prescribes personal medications for someone else with the same or similar symptoms, and, above all, do not dispense medications that you have in your home medicine closet for those "minor ailments" that you think you can cure.

Good Samaritan Statutes

Many states have enacted so-called Good Samaritan Statutes (laws) to encourage medical aid at the scene of an accident by limiting the legal liability that might arise. Some statutes apply only to physicians, whereas others may include nurses and other persons. In some states, the laws are effective only if the services are gratuitous, performed in "good faith" without proper equipment, and are restricted to injuries resulting from emergency medical aid. In most states, it is expected and implied that the person rendering aid act "as any reasonable prudent person would act under similar circumstances.'' The law usually requires a higher standard of medical aid by the nurse, the physician, the member of a rescue squad, and others trained in first aid than by the average member of the general public.

Informed Consent—Patient's Consent

The fundamental principles of our legal system is that all persons have the right to make major decisions involving their bodies. Therefore, the patient who is of sound mind has the right to make personal decisions about what becomes of the body and what should be done to the body. No one has the right to compel the patient to accept treatment that is not wanted. The doctrine of informed consent, therefore, may be defined as the duty to warn and explain to the patient all the hazards that are possible in the procedure, any complications that could be developed, and the expected and unexpected results that may result under these usual and normal circumstances. If the treatment or therapy is new and/or experimental or unusual, it is even more important to warn the patient that all the effects of the treatment are not as yet completely known.

In summary, the patient has the right to know what is involved and must be able to understand the risk of the proposed procedure. If the patient does not understand this or does not give consent, the procedure cannot be carried out.

Although the consent form that the patient (or parent, for a minor) signs for certain hospital procedures is designed primarily to protect the hospital or the physician, it is important to you, as well. You could be held liable if you obtained the consent signature for a procedure *after* the patient had been medicated. If a patient is not mentally or physically competent, or, if, while serving as a witness to the signature, it is your responsibility to describe the procedure to be performed and you fail to do so, you could also be held liable. If a patient refuses to sign a consent form, it becomes your responsibility to notify the team leader or physician accordingly and to protect the patient from the performance of an unauthorized procedure. If a true emergency condition exists in which the patient's life is jeopardized, or if there is a possibility of losing one or more limbs, a consent signature may be obtained from the next of kin. However, the physician must first have the agreement of another physician in the same specialty that if the procedure is not performed as an emergency *at the time*, the patient might die or, if such is the case, lose one or more limbs. The person who is a minor (younger than 18 years of age) must be married, or financially independent, or emancipated from one's parents to sign the consent form; since the age of majority is 21 years in some states, be sure you are familiar with your own state's requirements prior to asking any patient to sign a consent form.

Assault and Battery

An assault is a threat or an attempt to contact the body of another person without the privilege of doing so and without consent. A battery is the *act* of making this unauthorized contact. Almost invariably, an assault is a threat to use force, and a battery is the actual employment of force or merely touching someone, in each instance against the will of another. Therefore, never under any circumstances threaten a patient, because you can be sued for it. No treatment can be performed without the consent of the patient or someone qualified to speak for the patient (such as a parent or legal guardian in the case of a minor or an adult patient who is mentally incompetent). Unauthorized medical or nursing treatment can bring a charge of assault and battery.

There are exceptions to this rule: for instance, in emergencies (provided, of course, that a genuine emergency existed); and also in some cases involving mental patients, in which any threat or force used by the nurse was clearly for the purpose of self-defense.

Child Abuse—The Battered Child

In all states, the Virgin Islands, and the District of Columbia, hospitals are now legally responsible for reporting suspected cases of child abuse to the designated law enforcement or health and welfare agencies. Legal impunity is assured those who make the report and you, as a nurse, are in a key position to observe the defenseless victims of parental assault. Whether the child is seen in the emergency room, the pediatric unit, or the pediatrician's office, welts, scars, bruises, long bone fractures, cranial trauma, malnutrition, and starvation may indicate child abuse. In many of these cases, further investigation is warranted.

Duty of Care

Reasonable care, standard of care, and duty of care are terms defined as the care that can be measured against that which is given by other reasonable prudent nurses under similar circumstances. It includes all those acts that were performed or omitted that a nurse would have or would not have done. All nurses have the legal duty to exercise independent judgements to protect the patient from harm and to give reasonable care that is their "duty of care."

False Imprisonment

In general, false imprisonment means the unwarranted restriction of the freedom of another. Under this heading would be included not only the unlawful detention of a patient but also the misuse of restraints by hospital personnel. A patient cannot be restrained unnecessarily.

The nurse has the right to use some type of restraint without a physician's order if the patient is to be protected from self-injury. Bed rails, sheets, or other restraining devices to hold patients in wheelchairs, beds, or on stretchers may be used as precautionary measures. It is considered negligence when the nurse has the knowledge that these means may be used to protect the patient but does not use them. Crib and side rails should be up and in place on all children's beds and should be checked during and after visiting hours when well-meaning parents and visitors sometimes forget to replace them. The use of side rails on patients older than 65 years of age, on unconscious and postoperative cases, as well as others who may be under the influence of sedatives, has become routine in many hospitals, and this may be done without a doctor's order. When a patient's movements are restrained, caution must be used to prevent the patient or family from getting the idea that this confinement is unnecessary. Explain that you are doing this for the patient's safety. Since the advent of tranquilizers, mechanical restraints are applied very rarely, but if they are, they must be checked constantly. The detention of a patient for failure to pay the bill or for some other reason is another form of false imprisonment and therefore is unlawful.

Invasion of Privacy

Every patient has the right to privacy, and a nurse may not make unauthorized disclosures about the patient, who must give permission to have this information released. If the patient is unconscious, the nearest of kin may grant this permission.

In police and accident cases the only facts that may be released without the patient's consent (according to Press and Police Code Rules, which vary in each community) include the patient's name, address, sex, marital status, approximate age, occupation, employer, and the name and the address of the nearest relative.

The condition of the patient may be stated as good, fair, serious, critical, or dead on arrival. Do not describe the injuries, or how the accident was caused, and do not imply that the patient may have been intoxicated or poisoned, had attempted suicide, was addicted, or had received specific injuries. Merely state that the patient received injuries, and if they were serious, this may be included. The name of the attending physician may not be released unless permission is granted to do so. Most hospitals have regulations about the disposition of information on accidents, this usually is not within the province of the nurse.

Photographs may not be taken, unless the patient can give you this permission in writing. Photographing unconscious patients, or those with severe injuries, is not permitted. If the patient is a child, it is necessary to obtain permission for photographs from the parents or guardians.

Perhaps one of the most frequent invasions of the patient's right to privacy is the "shop talk" that goes on inside and outside of the hospital or even the doctor's office. Quite often nurses may discuss diagnoses, important patients, or types of surgery to be performed. Sometimes this type of discussion may lead to gossip and later perhaps to lawsuits for defamation of character (see the next section of this chapter). A nurse may safely discuss a patient's condition with another nurse on duty on the same case; as long as the discussion centers around medical treatment and nursing care, there is no invasion of privacy. However, if additional information is exchanged that involves the patient's private and personal life, it may constitute an invasion of the right of privacy.

There are, however, occasions when a nurse has a legal obligation or duty to disclose information. The reporting of certain communicable diseases, child abuse, criminal abortions, gunshot wounds, attempted suicides, drug abuse, and other matters are required by law. These requirements vary from state to state, and it is important for you to be familiar with the health regulations and laws pertaining to the reporting of specific situations brought to the attention of the hospital, physician, or nurse.

Defamation

A nurse should be very careful in personal remarks about patients, physicians, coworkers, hospital supervisors, and others encountered in daily work. By making derogatory remarks the nurse may be guilty of defamation, a wrongful act meaning to injure the reputation of another person. If the defamation is oral, it is called slander; if written, it is known as libel. In either case the intent is to expose the person to contempt, ridicule, or hatred and thereby endanger the person's reputation.

For a statement to be considered as slander or libel, in effect there must be another person present who either hears or sees it, in addition to the person involved. A disparaging statement by a nurse to a physician about himself or herself is not considered slanderous unless this same statement is made about the physician to another person; however, if this statement is made to the physician in the presence of another person, it would also be slanderous. It is important to note that nurses must not be careless in this respect and should remember to think before they either say or write anything that may be a defamation of another person.

CRIMES

As previously stated, crime (a criminal act) is any offense that is perpetrated against the public interest. If you commit a tort, the injured person is the one who takes action against you. However, if you commit a crime, it is the state that seeks to punish you.

There are two categories of crimes: misdemeanors and felonies. Misdemeanor means "misbehavior," and includes the less serious forms of crime. Felonies are more serious crimes, carrying penalties ranging from imprisonment in the state penitentiary to death.

Keep in mind that many of the torts already discussed can be considered criminal acts. As we saw, the tort of negligence can be so serious as to be called "gross negligence," a criminal offense (for instance, when the nurse leaves a critically ill patient without being relieved, an act that no nurse has the right to do). Assault and battery can also be a crime under certain circumstances.

Remember that it is quite possible to commit a crime without having any evil intent. For example, if the state has a mandatory licensure law, the practice of nursing in that state by one who is unlicensed is a willfull violation of the law of that state, and the nurse is committing a misdemeanor even though the unlawful practice may be due to ignorance and not to actual intent. Some acts are considered crimes only because the laws of a particular state or other jurisdiction make them so; for example, to drive a car at 55 miles per hour may be a crime in one state but not in another. Conversely, offenses such as robbery and murder are considered crimes everywhere. Apropos of this point, if a nurse must render care to a criminal or a lawbreaker, this must be reported to the nearest police station or sheriff's office as soon as possible. The fact that you rendered care under threat of injury, or even death, will not be held against you as long as you report your acts to the proper authorities at the very first opportunity.

Abortions

In January, 1973, the United States Supreme Court ruled that individual states could no longer deny women the right to abortions during the early months of pregnancy. This was based on the Supreme Court's conclusion that the fetus is not a person in any constitutional sense and thus is not entitled to protections normally accorded to human life. This decision, coupled with similar ones passed previously in certain states, has made therapeutic abortions legally available to most women in the United States. It is more difficult to obtain a legal abortion in some states than in others, and here as in the past, illegal abortions continue to exist. Anyone engaged in the practice of illegal abortions is criminally liable. In many instances, state medical societies and legislators have instituted a "conscience clause" in abortion legislation; these clauses usually maintain that no person or hospital can be required to take part in an abortion. Some states also prohibit the extension of public welfare or benefits to abortion patients. (See The Abortion Patient, Chapter 6.)

If you are called to take care of a critically ill patient who has had a criminal abortion, you should stay with the patient until legal medical aid is obtained; meanwhile you should give this patient your best, as you would any other, and refrain from making moral judgments. It could also happen that you will be asked to give emergency care to someone suffering complications after a legal abortion. Under normal circumstances your conscience will determine your participation in such care, but if you choose to take part, remember that tenderness and compassion are essential.

Euthanasia (Mercy Killing)

One of the fundamental responsibilities of the nurse and physician is to do everything in their power to preserve and prolong life, even when the medical situation is not accurately known. Euthanasia is the practice of painlessly putting to death persons who have incurable, painful, or distressing handicaps or diseases. The term comes from the Greek word meaning *easy death*, and is commonly referred to as *mercy killing*. Euthanasia is illegal in the United States and other civilized countries, although there are almost faultless arguments justifying it. Euthanasia is opposed by most religious groups and, even though requested by the patient, could be called suicide or murder. Euthanasia should not be confused with *agathanasia*, the right of the patient to make a "death with dignity." (See Chapter 6, Death.)

Unlawful Death

To cause the death of another person unlawfully is called an act of homicide. Practically the only acts of homicide excusable by the law are in cases of preventing the commission of some atrocious crime or in defending oneself or one's close relatives. Otherwise, to take a human life is a crime. If a person kills with deliberate intent and what the law calls "malice aforethought," the crime is murder. To commit a mercy killing, no matter how justifiable it may seem under certain circumstances, is still murder. In all states an illegal abortion is considered a felony; and if death results from a felony, the crime is murder. Therefore, anyone who participates in an illegal abortion resulting in the death of the woman is guilty of murder.

If a person kills another without malice aforethought, the crime is called manslaughter. Manslaughter may be voluntary or involuntary. One person may kill another in the heat of passion, without premeditation, when self-control is temporarily lost. In such a case the crime would probably be classed as voluntary manslaughter rather than murder, since the law recognizes this trait of human nature. Involuntary manslaughter is the killing of a person without malice aforethought and as the result of an offense no greater than a misdemeanor. For instance, if the death of the patient results from negligence (ordinary or gross) on the part of the physician or the nurse, the charge may be involuntary manslaughter. Similarly, anyone engaging in the unlawful practice of medicine or nursing (such unlawful practice being a misdemeanor) who causes the death of a patient will have committed involuntary manslaughter.

Narcotics and Other Drugs

The Drug Abuse Prevention and Control Act of 1970 updated the Harrison Narcotic Act, in effect since 1914. It is a federal law passed primarily for the purpose of regulating the manufacturing, dispensing, selling, and prescribing of narcotic drugs. These drugs are defined to mean opium and coca and all their preparations, natural and synthetic derivatives, and salts. Some of the most commonly known drugs in this group are morphine sulfate, codeine, papaverine, pantopium hydrochloride, and apomorphine hydrochloride. This law makes the possession of narcotics a crime. Many states have passed legislation restricting the sale of hypnotic drugs of the barbituric acid family. These laws are patterned after the federal drug act and prohibit the possession or the sale of derivatives of barbituric acid except under proper licenses, and they may not be dispensed except on prescription. Some of the most commonly known drugs in this group are pentobarbital, amobarbital, phenobarbital, and barbital. Find out whether the laws of your own state have legal restrictions on this category of drugs.

The Drug Abuse Prevention and Control Act of 1970 does provide that a nurse may have legal possession of narcotics (or barbiturates) for treatment as a patient, if prescribed by a physician holding a narcotics license for administration to patients, provided that they are returned to the physician when the nurse leaves the case, or when the patient no longer needs them. In addition, a nurse may give narcotics if they are supplied in an institution that has a narcotics license, provided that the dispensing of them is carefully recorded on legal records indicating the patient's name, the physician, the name of the drug, the dosage, and the time given, as well as the nurse's signature. These records are checked, and a narcotic count is done three times a day by two people (usually one from the off-going and one from the on-coming tour) to ensure accuracy. Discrepancies, wastes, errors, and breakage of ampules must be explained and signed for by the person responsible and must be countersigned by another nurse if the total amount of the drug has been wasted. When it becomes necessary to discard a partial dose, an account for the portion not given must also be recorded and signed for by a witness. When narcotics or barbiturates become unfit for use because of breakage, contamination of solution, or broken tablets, they must not be destroyed but are returned to the pharmacy or other sources from which they were obtained. Narcotics must be safeguarded, and most hospitals require that they be kept under a double lock at all times. If the key is lost, the inner lock must be replaced.

The Joint Commission on Accreditation of Hospitals has also issued regulations pertaining to the administration of dangerous drugs. For the protection of patients, an automatic stop order has been set for narcotics and anticoagulants at 48 hours or two days, whereas hypnotics and antibiotics may be given for five days without obtaining a renewal order from the physician in charge of the patient. This should point out to you the serious responsibilities involved in the administration of these medications and the importance of clear and concise orders before these drugs are given to patients. (Automatic stop and renewal orders may vary from hospital to hospital.)

Nurse Practice Acts in several states now authorize nurse practitioners both to prescribe and dispense certain drugs. As these acts become more common, nurses will undoubtedly assume increased responsibilities in the handling of drugs.

ORGAN TRANSPLANTS

As transplants of kidneys or other vital organs from one human being to another become more and more common, their ethical and legal implications must be considered. First of all, there must be assurance that the potential donor, if given the most intensive and best medical care available, cannot possibly recover from the disease or injury. One must remember that the donor's life is just as important as the recipient's. The recovery of a heart or other organ transplant patient may be as uncertain as the ultimate fate of the donor. The general opinion of most experts in the field is that artificial organs would be preferable to human organ transplants. Anytime you are involved in the care of a potential transplant donor or recipient, make sure you are familiar with all the applicable laws in your state and institution.

WILLS

A nurse may be asked by a patient to help make a will, which is a legal declaration of a person's wishes as to the disposition of property after death. Because a nurse is untrained in legal matters, you should never volunteer to help the patient directly in this matter. Instead, you should assist the patient in securing the services of an attorney, either by referring the patient to the list of lawyers in the classified telephone directory or by getting in touch with the Legal Aid Society.

If a patient does make a will, the nurse may be asked to serve as a witness. All witnesses (some states require two, others, three) must be present simultaneously and sign in the presence of the person making the will. For the will to be valid, the patient must be of sound mind (that is, have full knowledge of what is happening) and should not be under the influence of any person or drug.

When the will is made, the nurse should record this fact on the chart and also be sure that the chart is accurate and up to date on the patient's condition at this time. If the will is contested (that is, if a dispute over its validity arises), the chart will be important.

When death is imminent, many patients, in addition to making wills, very often bestow personal presents on certain individuals. These gifts are legally valid if the patient has full control over these properties, and the gift is accepted by the receiver. Here again, just as in a will, the patient must be free of influence or deceit on the part of anyone else, and must understand the actions taken and be responsible for them. If the nurse is asked to be a witness to such acts or even to be a recipient of a gift, it would be advisable to record the patient's condition on the chart at the time that the presents were given. A witness should be at least 18 years of age.

THE PATIENT'S CHART

The patient's chart is considered to be a legal document. The patient is safeguarded through the chart, and in turn it may also protect the doctor, the nurse, or the hospital in the event of unjust accusation or lawsuits. The chart provides a written account of the patient's hospitalization. Therefore, medications, treatments, and nursing care as well as physician's reports, laboratory procedures and results, and all other pertinent information should be recorded accurately and as soon as possible, so that there will be an accurate, up-to-the-minute log of the entire health history and physical condition from admission to discharge.

The arrangement of the sheets on the chart will vary somewhat in different hospitals; however, all recorded information must be legible, complete, and informative. Words must be spelled correctly, and only standard acceptable abbreviations may be used. Each nursing service will have its own standards of what should be recorded on the nurses' notes, graph sheets, and other nursing forms, and it will be your duty to be familiar with the charting procedure practiced in the particular hospital in which you are studying or practicing. It must be remembered that only important and pertinent observations should be recorded and signed, and above all, that the date, the time, and the patient's name must appear on every chart page on which a notation is made.

Questions

A. Selected the correct answer and circle the number that answers the question best.

1. The Drug Abuse Prevention and Control Act regulates (A) morphine, (B) codeine, (C) papaverine, (D) anticoagulants.
   1. All of these
   2. All except B
   3. All except C
   4. All except D

2. Nurse practice acts are (A) administered by the State Board of Nursing, (B) enforced by ANA and NFLPN, (C) protection for the nurse, (D) permissive in most states.
   1. All of these
   2. All except B
   3. All except C
   4. All except D

3. Malpractice suits may include (A) burns from hot-water bags, (B) falling out of bed when the side rail is down, (C) giving wrong medication, (D) improper use of patient's personal belongings.
   1. All of these
   2. All except B
   3. All except C
   4. All except D

4. A derogatory remark is considered (A) defamation, (B) slander, (C) libel, (D) "malice aforethought."
   1. A, B
   2. A, C
   3. B, C
   4. B, D

5. The State Board of Nursing may refuse to renew a nurse's license if that nurse is proved to be (A) incompetent, (B) intemperate, (C) addicted, (D) in prison.
   1. All of these
   2. All except B
   3. All except C
   4. All except D

6. A will could be valid if (a) the patient is of sound mind, (B) the patient is under the influence of medication, (C) it is written in pencil, (D) it is witnessed by two people.
   1. All of these
   2. All except B
   3. All except C
   4. All except D

7. As a nurse you may have legal possession of narcotics if (A) you have them on prescription for a patient you are taking care of, (B) a patient has given them to you when you left the case, (C) a doctor has prescribed them for you, (D) a doctor gave them to you at completion of a private duty case.
   1. All of these
   2. A, B, C
   3. A, C, D
   4. A, C

8. Licensure for practical nurses is (A) usually obtained by passing State Board examination, (B) permissive in most states, (C) enacted in all states, (D) mandatory in some states.
   1. All of these
   2. All except B
   3. All except C
   4. All except D

9. The graduate practical nurse should write the licensure examination (A) anytime within one year after graduation, (B) the first time it is offered after graduation, (C) according to the rules of NFLPN, (D) under the regulations of the Board of Nursing.
   1. A, C
   2. B, C
   3. A, D
   4. B, D

10. The NFLPN Code of Ethics (A) is enforced by NFLPN, (B)   1. All of these
    is regulated by State Boards of Nursing, (C) serves as a guide   2. All except B
    to the LPN as a citizen and in relationships with the employer,   3. All except D
    the patient, and co-workers, (D) is renewed annually.   4. C

B. Complete the following statements.
    1. To cover the claims as well as the legal counsel nurses might need, they should
       carry _____
    2. A will should be signed by at least _____ witnesses.
    3. In order for a will to be valid, the patient must be _____
    4. To cause an unlawful death is called _____
    5. An oral defamation is called _____
    6. An unwarranted restriction of freedom is called _____
    7. Failing to count sponges accurately during surgery may result in a _____
    8. A wrongful act of one person against another is called _____
    9. Interstate licensure for licensed nursing personnel is done by _____
    10. The Drug Abuse Prevention and Control Act controls narcotics and in some states
        also _____

C. True or False. Write *T* or *F* in answer space.
____   1. The patient's chart is considered to be a legal document.
____   2. The Drug Abuse Prevention and Control Act requires that narcotics be counted
           four times a day in all hospitals.
____   3. Felonies are more serious crimes and carry imprisonment penalties.
____   4. Battery is the act of making unauthorized body contact.
____   5. A nurse may alter a physician's order if it is known that a mistake was made in
           writing it.
____   6. A wrongful act by one person against another is called "malice aforethought."
____   7. Graduate practical nurses are eligible for licensure by endorsement.
____   8. All State Boards of Nursing have the same licensure fees.
____   9. Endorsement may be called waiver licensure.
____   10. JCAH has recommended automatic stop dates for dangerous drugs.

D. Match the best associated expression from Column *B* with Column *A* and insert the
   letter in the space provided.

                        A   *B*
____   1. interstate licensure   A. cocoa
____   2. Drug Abuse Prevention and Control Act   B. euthanasia
____   3. mercy killing   C. slander
____   4. written defamation   D. codeine
____   5. "gross negligence"   E. tort
                                                          F. combiotic
                                                          G. endorsement
                                                          H. libel
                                                          I. crime
                                                          J. waiver

Answers

A. Multiple Choice (4 points each)

1. 4
2. 2
3. 1
4. 1
5. 1
6. 2
7. 4
8. 1
9. 4
10. 4

C. True or False (2 points each)

1. T
2. F
3. T
4. T
5. F
6. F
7. F
8. F
9. F
10. T

B. Completion (3 points each)

1. liability insurance
2. two or three
3. of sound mind (competent)
4. homicide
5. slander
6. false imprisonment
7. malpractice suit
8. a tort
9. endorsement
10. barbiturates

D. Matching (2 points each)

1. G
2. D
3. B
4. H
5. I

8

Organizations

Nursing Organizations • Health and Welfare Organizations • Department of Health and Human Services • Department of Education • Other Public Health Agencies • Voluntary and Private Health Agencies • United Fund • Questions and Answers

Objectives
Upon completion of this chapter, you should be able to
1. understand the importance of joining nursing organizations and what the responsibilities of a member are,
2. compare the aims and membership of the ANA, NAPNES, NFLPN and NLN,
3. describe the structure and objectives of the Department of Education and the Department of Health and Human Services,
4. identify the components of the Department of Health and Human Services,
5. explain the purposes of the Social Security Administration,
6. summarize the roles of at least 15 national voluntary or private health organizations,
7. review the role of the World Health Organization,
8. elaborate the responsibilities of a state health department,
9. summarize the role and responsibilities of the United Fund.

NURSING ORGANIZATIONS

Organizations are important to further the interests of any group. The fundamental principle of "united we stand, divided we fall" is most appropriate when you begin to think about your obligations to your school and your vocation. You

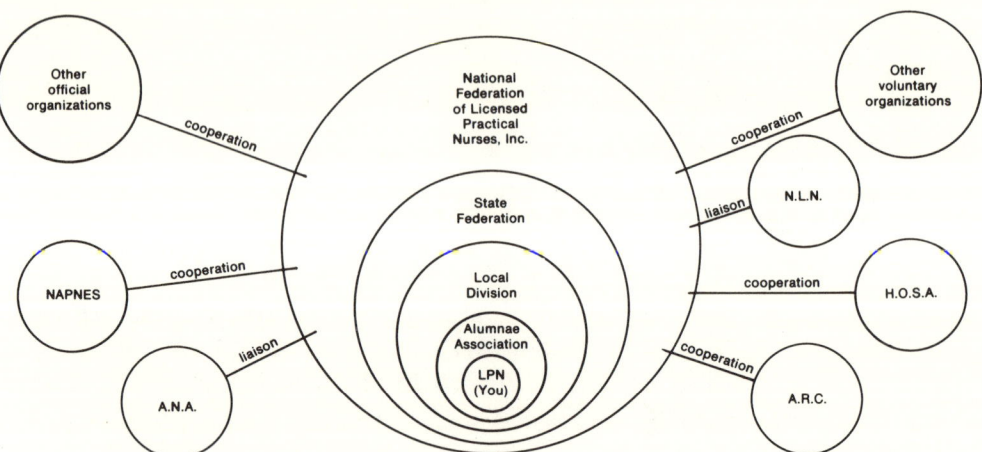

FIGURE 8-1. *The practical nurse and the sphere of organizational activities.*

cannot expect national and state organizations to do the job alone. It is your responsibility as a nurse to join those organizations that will assist you in becoming a better practitioner and will advance the interests of nursing and nurses. Annual dues are necessary in order to support various causes and functions; but it is not enough merely to pay dues. It is even more important to become an active member who participates in the programs offered. You must realize that the progress of any organization depends on the support and the cooperation of individual members. At the same time, it is only through these organizations that you will be able to retain your vocational security and to share in the benefits and the success that group effort has achieved. "One for all, and all for one," the slogan of the Three Musketeers, is certainly a good reason to join and to take an active interest in your alumnae association, the district or state Licensed Practical Nurse association, or any other organization interested in practical nursing. Outlined here are several for your consideration. Learn about them, attend their meetings if you can, or write for descriptive literature so you can make your choice (Figure 8–1).

Alumnae Associations

Good public relations begins with you and your classmates, who must maintain the standards of your school and elevate them whenever possible. A public relations program can be put into effect by the efforts of students and alumnae. If your school has not founded a student or alumnae association, you should discuss this with members of the faculty and attempt to organize such a group. Most schools of practical nursing have some type of student government that, through its elected officers, forms the Student Council. This Council should work very closely with the Alumnae Association and the faculty in representing the interests of students and graduates, assisting in recruitment, and explaining the meaning of the practical nurse program and the role of the practical nurse to the community. This is accomplished by sending speakers to other organizations and sponsoring an "open house," whereby interested persons can visit the school and discuss practical nursing with students and graduates.

Every organization has bylaws, which state its objectives and duties, as well as the means for carrying them out. These must be written for your group also, and their complexity will depend on the size of the group and on your immediate as well as long-term goals. One way of generating interest and achieving success in your organization is to have a definite stated purpose. Such objectives could be to establish a scholarship and loan fund, to provide programs that will keep alumnae members up to date in nursing skills, or to join as a group the local division of your state association of licensed practical nurses, so that you can have an active voice in its activities.

Health Occupations Students of America

Health Occupations Students of America (HOSA), a national vocational organization, was founded in 1976 for students enrolled in health occupation education. Local and state chapters provide programs and activities to help students develop their physical, mental, and social well being. Members strengthen their leadership and citizenship abilities through interaction with professional, business, and other student organizations. They also learn to appreciate their ability to help people who need health care or to help people achieve a better understanding of health-related issues. HOSA stresses the need for individuals to develop good decision-making skills that can help them reach full learning potential. As a practical nursing student, this organization gives you an excellent opportunity to meet other students in health careers and to become involved in improving health conditions in the community.

The national organization can be contacted through the New Jersey Department of Education, Division of Vocational Education, 225 West State Street, Trenton, New Jersey 08625. Your State Department of Education, Vocational Technical Education (Occupational Education) also has information pertaining to the state and local chapters. The National HOSA motto is: "The Hands of Youth Mold the Health of Tomorrow."

National League for Nursing*

The National League for Nursing (NLN) is a membership organization whose purpose is to improve nursing, and thereby all health services, through a coalition of community leaders, nurses, allied professionals, nursing service agencies, and schools of nursing. NLN advocates community planning for nursing as a primary component of comprehensive health care, the development of nursing personnel, and high standards of nursing service and education.

It is located at 10 Columbus Circle, New York, New York 10019, with branch offices in San Francisco and Atlanta. In 1952, after 10 years of studying existing

---

* Based on information submitted by Sister Mary Walsh, R.N., Director, Department of Practical Nursing.

nursing organizations, three national organizations and four committees voted to combine their programs and resources to become the NLN. They were the National League of Nursing Education, established in 1893; the National Organization for Public Health Nursing (1912); the Association of Collegiate Schools of Nursing (1933); the Joint Committee on Practical Nurses and Auxiliary Workers in Nursing (1945); the Joint Committee on Careers in Nursing (1948); the National Committee for the Improvement of Nursing Services (1949); and the National Accrediting Service (1949).

NLN membership includes more than 15,000 individual members and 1,800 agency members. *Individual members* are citizens concerned with nursing and health care in all parts of the country—registered and practical nurses, educators, doctors, social scientists, therapists, hospital administrators, board members of health services, and other interested persons. *Agency members* are nursing services and nursing schools. Organized into six national councils, each relating to a specific type of service or education program, they are the Councils of Associate Degree Programs, Baccalaureate and Higher Degree Programs, Diploma Programs, Home Health Agencies and Community Health Services (sponsor also of an Assembly of Home Health Agencies), Hospital and Related Institutional Nursing Services, and Practical Nursing Programs.

Forty-five constituent leagues for nursing implement national programs at the community level. These leagues are organized on city, state, or area bases. Many have local action groups to stimulate community interest in and cooperative planning for nursing and comprehensive health services. A national Assembly of Constituent Leagues for Nursing and five regional assemblies make possible the coordination of planning and action among the constituent groups. Programs are carried out through the constituencies and by direct national assistance to nursing services of hospitals, public health agencies, extended care facilities, and nursing homes and to nursing education programs, including associate, bachelor's, master's, and doctoral degree programs in colleges and universities, diploma programs in hospital schools, and practical nursing programs. The NLN also aids community groups and individuals needing information, guidance, or a means of channeling efforts to improve or expand community health services. Following are the major services of the NLN:

- NLN offers consultation services to its constituencies and other community groups, nursing services, and education programs on a wide range of interests—among them establishing new community health services and education programs, evaluating existing programs, improving administrative practices, and developing staff, faculty, and community leadership personnel.

- NLN nationally accredits all types of nursing education programs. More than 1,000 education programs now hold NLN accreditation. Accreditation of community public health nursing services is conducted by NLN in cooperation with the American Public Health Association. Seventy-three of these services are now fully accredited. NLN also develops self-evaluation criteria for hospitals and other institutional nursing services.

- NLN conducts one of the largest professional testing services in the country. It constructs and processes licensing examinations for registered and practical nurses, administers NLN preadmission tests for nursing school applicants, and provides achievement and qualifying tests for nursing students, practical nurses, and aides. Over 1 million tests are processed each year.

- NLN annually conducts surveys and publishes statistics on nursing school admissions, enrollments, and graduations. It studies costs, salaries, policies, and practices of public health nursing agencies. Some NLN special studies related to nursing education, service, and community action have been on the career patterns of nurses, financial aid available to nursing students, and community planning for health services.

- NLN is a central source of information on trends in nursing, personnel needs, community nursing services, schools of nursing, and governmental programs affecting nursing services and education. It publishes a wide variety of materials, including guides and manuals, reference matter, case histories, statistics, and newsletters. NLN is cosponsor with the American Nurses' Association, professional organization of registered nurses, of a national nursing careers program and the magazine, *Nursing Research*. "Nursing and Health Care" replaced "NLN News" in 1980. All League members automatically receive this journal as a membership benefit.

- NLN holds biennial national conventions and national, regional, and local meetings, workshops, and conferences for continuing education of nursing and other health care personnel and the exchange and dissemination of new ideas, information, and technics.

NLN Philosophy on Practical Nursing

The following statement, approved by the National League for Nursing's Board of Directors on February 1, 1971, reaffirms the philosophy formulated and approved by the Board in 1958.

GENERAL BELIEFS

The National League for Nursing recognizes that there are basic health needs common to people of all ages and in all settings. Within this broad scope, there are certain needs that the practical, or vocational, nurse meets in assisting the patient to return to and maintain optimum health.

Practical nursing is an integral part of all nursing. Therefore, the service rendered by the practical nurse and the educational programs for the preparation of this practitioner can be developed properly only when viewed as an interrelated, coordinated part of all nursing service and nursing education. The National League for Nursing, through its organizational structure, provides for such coordination.

NLN supports practical nursing service and practical nursing education in fulfillment of its purpose of improving nursing service. NLN will continue this support in order to help meet the increasing health needs of the people. The major aspects of NLN's program for practical nursing pertain to recruitment of suitable candidates into practical nursing, to education and utilization of the licensed practical nurse, and to interorganizational relationships.

RECRUITMENT

The team relationship of practical nurses to professional nurses is an important concept to be interpreted in all recruitment materials.

Prospective students should be informed of all opportunities in nursing education, so that each may select the program appropriate to his or her abilities, interests, and goals. To meet the challenge of recruiting adequate nurse manpower, those who counsel potential candidates should understand the present and developing trends in nursing education.

EDUCATION

Educational programs in practical nursing should be designed according to sound educational principles. They should incorporate selected learning experiences appropriate to the role of the practical nurse on the health team.

The faculty of a practical nursing education program must be responsible for developing and implementing a course of studies having a realistic articulation of foundation knowledges and clinical learning experiences. The student's learning experiences should form a meaningful sequence that spans the entire program. Inherent in a soundly planned curriculum is the necessity to evaluate outcomes according to stated goals.

Practical nursing students may be prepared in the same clinical facilities as professional nursing students, but each group should have its own faculty in order to ensure proper implementation of the respective programs.

Teachers in practical nursing schools need preparation for the broad scope of nursing to which practical nursing must relate. In addition, they need preparation for teaching. NLN bears responsibility for helping teachers in practical nursing schools implement their programs through such means as curriculum conferences and workshops.

IMPROVEMENT ON THE JOB

Licensed practical nurses come to the employing agency with varying backgrounds. NLN therefore expects that employing agencies will make provision, through planned programs of inservice education, for meeting the needs of the licensed practical nurse as they relate to on-the-job improvement.

CONTINUING FORMAL EDUCATION

Those individuals who wish to change career goals should have the opportunity to do so. Opportunity should be provided to validate previous education and experience and to apply earned credits to the achievement of additional educational objectives.

NLN Council of Practical Nursing Programs

The Council of Practical Nursing Programs, founded in 1957, is primarily concerned with the continuous improvement and development of educational programs in practical nursing. There are about 150 agency members who have a voice and vote in the affairs of the NLN's activities. The Board of Review for Practical Nursing Programs (seven regular and seven alternating members) is appointed by the executive committee. The Board of Review is responsible for the evaluation of NLN accreditation of programs in practical nursing education. Other functions of the Council are to

a. Collaborate with other membership groups to promote and achieve the objectives of the NLN.

b. Promote general professional understanding and active participation in the support of sound practical nursing education.

c. Develop and approve statements of characteristics that programs in practical nursing should have in order to make their appropriate contributions to society.

d. Develop and approve criteria for the evaluation of educational programs in practical nursing.

e. Develop and approve the policies and procedures of accreditation of practical nursing programs.

f. Cooperate with the American Nurses' Association, the National Association for Practical Nurse Education and Service, the National Federation of Licensed Practical Nurses, and other national organizations, federal agencies, and such international agencies as are appropriate in matters related to nursing education.

g. Recommend to the NLN Board of Directors the adoption of appropriate programs and policies.

h. Conduct meetings of special interest to members.

i. Establish committees as needed to implement any Council function or activity.

j. Promote appropriate studies and research and encourage experimentation in practical nursing programs.

k. Develop and publish materials pertinent to practical nursing education.

l. Issue statements in the name of the Council provided they are in accord with the overall policies of the NLN.

Through the NLN's Council of Practical Nursing Programs, agency members work together to raise overall standards and to improve the preparation of practical nurses within the programs. New outlooks and new goals for practical nursing result from the interchange of ideas, imagination, and knowledge at council meetings.

The Council of Practical Nursing Programs also recognizes the need for the continuing education of licensed practical nurses, and urges them to broaden their education by taking courses in educational institutions. Such courses are available to anyone who meets admission requirements.

National Association for Practical Nurse Education and Service, Inc.*

The National Association for Practical Nurse Education and Service, Inc. (NAPNES) established in 1941, is the oldest organization totally committed to practical nursing and the only one of its kind that is concerned both with schools of practical nursing and the welfare and continuing education of licensed practical nurses. Its central office is located at 122 East 42nd Street, New York, New York, 10017.

The main goals of NAPNES are (1) to promote an understanding of practical nursing, (2) to further the development of basic practical nursing education, (3) and to promote opportunities for LP/VNs in continuing education to keep abreast of current trends in the health care delivery system.

Two of NAPNES' activities contribute to the attainment of all these objectives: publication of the monthly magazine, the *Journal of Practical Nursing,* and the annual convention, a continuing educational activity, which brings together LP/VNs, RNs, hospital and nursing home administrators, physicians, and others concerned with practical nursing.

In addition, NAPNES is committed to

1. Promoting an understanding of practical nursing by:
   a. Preparing and disseminating the *Declaration of Functions of the Licensed Practical/Vocational Nurse.*
   b. Publicizing the important contribution of LP/VNs in national magazines and over the radio and television.
   c. Representing the interests of practical nursing on committees and in other groups concerned with health and education.
   d. Disseminating information about practical nursing to prospective students and career counselors.
   e. Serving as a clearning house for information about practical nursing.

2. Furthering the development of basic practical nursing education by:
   a. Providing assistance and guidance to today's practical nursing schools.
   b. Developing and promoting the use of sound standards for practical nursing education.
   c. Maintaining a national accreditation service recognized by the United States Commissioner of Education and the Council on Post-Secondary Accreditation for basic and postgraduate programs in practical/vocational nursing education.
   d. Maintaining a consultation service for institutions conducting or contemplating the establishment of practical nursing programs.
   e. Sponsoring national and regional workshops and seminars for practical nursing educators.
   f. Preparing materials that are useful to faculties in schools of practical nursing.

* Based on information submitted by Mrs. Lucille L. Etheridge, RN, Executive Director.

g. Encouraging research directed toward the development of more effective educational practices.

h. Providing scholarships for practical nursing students.

3. Promoting opportunities for licensed practical nurses to continue their education by:

a. Preparing course outlines for use in continuing education programs and issuing certificates to those who complete these courses and pass a national examination.

b. Sponsoring workshops and seminars.

c. Encouraging the development and accreditation of specialized (postgraduate) programs.

d. Encouraging the development of methods whereby LP/VNs who wish to become registered nurses can do so without being retaught material and skills they have already mastered.

4. Promoting the welfare of licensed practical nurses. All of the activities that have been mentioned benefit LP/VNs. In addition, NAPNES does the following:

a. Provides consultation and assistance to state licensed practical/-vocational nurse associations on matters relating to their organization and programs.

b. Publishes information about the legal aspects of nursing practice.

c. Keeps LP/VNs informed about legislation and other developments that affect their welfare.

d. Sponsors low-cost group insurance programs for NAPNES members (including students).

It is obvious that this broad program requires the participation of people with varying backgrounds—LP/VNs, practical nursing educators, people who employ or supervise LP/VNs, practical nursing students, and members of the public. For this reason, membership in NAPNES is open to anyone who is concerned with the advancement of practical nursing. Agency membership is available to institutions and groups.

LP/VNs constitute the largest group of members, and practical nursing students, the second largest. Members in these categories contribute to the NAPNES program not only at the national level but also through participation in the activities of NAPNES constituent state and district vocational nurse associations. An LP/VN member of a constituent association is automatically a "per capita" member of NAPNES, but many such members choose to become individual or life members through the payment of additional dues. All other members join as individual, life, or student members, who receive subscriptions to the *Journal of Practical Nursing* as a privilege of membership. The student dues are equivalent to the cost of a subscription to the journal.

The voting body, which consists of the constituent state associations, determines the broad policies of the association. Responsibility for the general management of the association rests with the Board of Directors, the majority of whose members are LP/VNs. Many of the activities of the association are assigned to standing committees, which sometimes delegate tasks to work committees whose members are especially prepared for the assignments. In addition, provision is made in the bylaws for the formation of councils whose members have special interests in common.

National Federation of Licensed Practical Nurses, Inc.*

The National Federation of Licensed Practical Nurses, Inc. (NFLPN) is a national membership organization for all licensed practical and vocational nurses. Membership is also open to students, who may participate in some of the local and state activities, such as the student-of-the-year and essay-writing contests.

There are two types of membership for licensed practical and vocational nurses: (1) joining NFLPN through a constituent state association and (2) joining NFLPN as members-at-large. The latter are members who live in a state that licenses practical nurses but whose state is not a constituent member of NFLPN. In 1972, the NFLPN had 39 constituent state or territorial associations and individual members from 13 states.

Each member participates in developing the policies and program of NFLPN through the House of Delegates. The House of Delegates consists of elected representatives of each constituent state association, whose responsibility is to conduct the business of the association during the convention. The NFLPN Executive Board is elected by the House of Delegates to conduct the business of the association between conventions. A national headquarters with an administrative staff is maintained at 250 West 57th Street, New York, New York, 10019. NFLPN was founded in May, 1949, and publishes a monthly publication, *The Journal of Nursing Care,* which is mailed to all members and is available to nonmembers by subscription.

The goals of the NFLPN are as follows:

- To preserve and foster the ideal of comprehensive care for the ill and the aged.
- To associate together all licensed practical nurses and groups of licensed practical nurses or persons with equivalent titles.
- To secure recognition and effective use of the skills of licensed practical nurses.
- To promote the welfare and interests of licensed practical nurses.
- To improve standards of practice in practical nursing.
- To speak for licensed practical nurses and interpret their aims and objectives to other groups and the public.
- To cooperate with other groups concerned with better patient care.
- To serve as a clearing house for information on practical nursing.

* Based on information submitted by Mr. Charles W. Hull, Jr., Managing Director.

- To further the continued improvement in the education of licensed practical nurses.
- To organize leadership training programs for licensed practical nurses.
- To promote the effective functioning of constituent state and local associations.

In order to accomplish its many objectives, NFLPN has formed various interorganizational committees and an Interorganization Council composed of official representatives of the major medical and nursing associations. For example, the Economic and General Welfare Committee is responsible for planning and implementing the Collective Action Program. Various consultants on labor and government relations assist NFLPN in implementing its short- and long-range goals. One major thrust has been in the area of continuing education, as illustrated by the following "Criteria for Continuing Education of the LPN/LVN."

Continuing Education includes those organized educational experiences which are planned to help practical nurses achieve more productive and satisfying fulfillment of their roles as health workers. Improved patient care is the primary goal of all continuing education of the LPN/LVN.

I. To Remove a Waiver
1. A program in each state providing opportunity for removal of the waiver administered by an educational institution with the approval of the state board of nurse examiners and the cooperation of LPN associations.
2. Consideration and evaluation of the competence gained by work experience and continued learning of the LPN in meeting requirements of the program.
3. Provision of counseling services as an integral part of the program.
4. No limitations on age for admission to the program.
5. Provision of financial assistance when required.

II. To Improve Practice
1. Varied opportunities for continuing education geographically and financially accessible to all LPNs.
2. Wide dissemination of information about learning opportunities in the area.
3. Cooperative efforts of educational institutions, division, state and national nursing and health organizations, and health care agencies in development of programs.
4. Motivation of LPN/LVNs towards continuing education.

III. To Change a Career Goal
1. Admission to higher education institutions available to all LPN/LVNs for systematic study.
2. Guidance in planning a change in career goal provided by educational institutions.

3. Consideration and evaluation of the competence and knowledge gained through work and life experience in meeting the requirements of the program.

4. Provision of financial assistance where required.

Among the resolutions passed in 1978 by the NFLPN's House of Delegates, the following were included:

"Whereas, the technologically sophisticated health care industry of the future will require sound credentials for nursing practice, and

Whereas, Present credentialing and licensure mechanism for statutory law in the United States have tended to strengthen identification of a nursing practice level which the general public and nursing commonly identify as practical/vocational nursing, and for which the title "licensed Practical/vocational nurse" is both specific and appropriate, and

Whereas, There is a continuing need to identify and define the expanding scope of the practice of practical nursing, therefore be it

RESOLVED, That an entry level into nursing pactice be the licensed practical/vocational nurse."

And,

"Whereas, The National League for Nursing is a recognized agency for the accreditation of all educational programs in nursing, therefore be it

RESOLVED, That the National Federation of Licensed Practical Nurses supports the continuance of national accreditation services by the National League for Nursing for all educational programs in nursing."

The education and research arm of NFLPN is the National Licensed Practical Nurses Educational Foundation, which was formed in 1962 for educational and charitable purposes. The Foundation administers NFLPN's achievement point program in continuing education. This program, launched in 1968, was the first in the United States to set a standard of awarding recognition for continuing education in nursing. Certificates of achievement are awarded to NFLPN members and student affiliates who have participated in organized, validated educational events, including conferences, workshops, meetings, and courses. Points are determined by the number of hours of participation. The Foundation also administers an annual scholarship program that provides financial assistance for a select number of deserving practical nursing students throughout the United States.

The National Licensed Practical Nurses Educational Foundation, in 1970, under a contract from the United States Department of Health, Education, and Welfare developed two textbooks to prepare qualified licensed practical nurses for charge nurse positions in nursing homes and extended health care facilities. "Practical Nursing in the Nineteen Seventies—A Position Paper," a very thought-provoking publication was released in 1972, and included these 12 recommendations:

The Field of Licensed Practical Nursing Should:

1. Take a stand now professionally to lead and to act for its own ranks.

2. In spite of past episodes and concomitant deep feelings, seek to achieve a high degree of unity between existing LPN organizations and/or associations in order to consolidate strengths and to present a unified, professional front. To that end *immediately,* joint cooperative committees should be inaugurated to deal with the several essential issues set forward in this paper.

3. Inaugurate a national program beamed to every licensed practical nurse to aid her in building a healthy self-concept. This should be both an "internal" public relations and educational program.

4. Take steps as a unified group to stimulate accrediting and licensing bodies to evaluate their posture and procedures for the purpose of bringing them into line with the realities of health care needs and field practices.

5. Move instantly toward having greater LPN representation on all accrediting and licensing boards and bodies.

6. Stimulate programs to prepare, gain acceptance of, and use selected LPNs for filling full-time faculty posts.

7. Prepare now the methods and techniques for involving more of their "publics" in gaining recognition and support.

8. Redefine its own occupation in terms of extant facts and not rely primarily on the definitions of non-LPN bodies. Concurrently with this, the LPN occupation should start with renewed earnestness a national thrust:
   a) to improve the access to quality training curricula based on sound theory and "field realities";
   b) to improve and professionally monitor sanctions for graduation, licensure, and practice;
   c) to develop continuing education activities for maintaining and improving competency.

9. Seek to have the LPN receive full credit for demonstrated competence upon entering an RN program.

10. Alert the public, especially employers, to fuller utilization of LPNs because of (a) their geographic stability, (b) their ability and (c) their amenability to definitive additional education for specialized functions and responsibilities.

11. Take a more mature, professional stand in stating the LPN case in a positive and forthright manner to off-set any tendency to be an overly dependent or subservient occupation.

12. Urge through concerted action all appropriate bodies to use measures of competence as the final criteria for licensure, certification, registration and in employment assignments.

These recommendations show clearly that the NFLPN, and practical nursing as a whole, are entering a new era. It is a time of unlimited challenge and increased responsibility. You, as a future LPN, must be fully aware of its possibilities.

American Red Cross Nursing Services

The purpose of the American Red Cross Nursing Services (ARCNS) is to maintain a nationwide program that extends the normal nursing and health resources of the community. Emergency services and instructional programs formerly given only by and for the RN have been expanded and now include the LPN, who is usually supervised and assigned by a member of Nursing Services. The national office is located in Washington, D.C. Nursing Services was organized nationally in 1909. Although the local programs vary in each community, the general scope of activity includes disaster nursing, training of volunteer nurse aides, and instruction in the care of the sick and the injured and in mother and baby care. Special needs in health education are met by adaptations in the nursing and health programs of the local county chapters. ARCNS projects may include educational programs on sickle cell anemia, family planning, drug abuse, and venereal disease; special services in nutrition for the elderly; free clinics; and health education programs for teenagers. A new program, which the Public Health Service and the American Nursing Home Association requested from the ARCNS, is training in home nursing for aides employed in nursing homes.

An official Red Cross pin for LPN volunteers was approved in 1968 and may be earned by LP/VNs. Practical nurses are important members of the Red Cross nursing team, which includes RNs, volunteer nurses' aides, and lay people who have completed the required courses. Disaster training courses are conducted in the adaptation of nursing skills to meet patient needs under disaster conditions. LPNs as well as RNs attend these courses. In addition, student nurses may participate in many of the same programs.

For further information contact your local American Red Cross chapter or write to the National Director, American Red Cross Nursing Services, Washington, D.C. 20026.

American Nurses' Association

The national organization and official voice for all professional RNs is the American Nurses' Association (ANA), founded in 1896, and located at 2420 Pershing Road, Kansas City, Missouri 64106. The ANA is to the RN what the NFLPN is to the LPN. In 1980 the association had 53 state or territorial constituents with over 800 district nurses' associations. Each of the state or territory constituents has local district associations that carry out various programs for improving the standards of nursing practice and for promoting the general welfare of professional nurses. The membership of this organization is kept informed of pertinent issues through the official newspaper, *The American Nurse* and the periodical, the *American Journal of Nursing*.

ANA's policies and programs are established by the membership through representation in a House of Delegates, which is the highest authority in the Association. The Board of Directors transacts the general business of the Association between biannual conventions. The Board is also responsible for establishing policies governing the affairs of the Association and for implementing measures for the Association's growth and development. This is done through the Congress for Nursing Practice and through standing and special committees and task forces. In 1973, the American Academy of Nursing was founded and elects fellows (F.A.A.N.) annually.

TABLE 8–1. MEMBERSHIP ORGANIZATIONS FOR NURSES (Summary)

Name	Year Founded	Membership Open to	Magazine of Organization	Comments
ANA	1896	RNs only	*Am. Journal of Nursing*	State & local districts
NAPNES	1941	Anyone interested	*The Journal of Practical Nursing*	State & local units
NFLPN	1949	LPNs, LVNs, and student PNs	*The Journal of Nursing Care*	State & local divisions
NLN	1952	Anyone interested	*Nursing and Health Care*	State & local divisions

The ANA, like the nursing organizations previously discussed, works closely with other health and welfare agencies.

Your Membership Responsibilities

Once you have joined the organization(s) of your choice (Table 8–1), you will be able to help in the advancement of practical nursing through your financial support, personal interest, and participation in meetings and conventions. You must realize that it takes many types of people to make up an organization, and that each one has a part in deciding on the policies, the functions, and the responsibilities. Through active membership participation you will have an opportunity to share in planning and shaping the thinking of the association; you will be working toward the acceptance, the understanding, and the advancement of practical nursing and practical nurse education.

An organization can only be as effective as the officers who are authorized to plan and direct its activities. The officers should be elected by a written and confidential vote in the form of a ballot and should be chosen (nominated) from the general membership for their leadership qualifications and not because they are the most popular. A strong president or chairperson is needed to pull together various factions and administer the work of the organization; the other officers must be capable of carrying out their duties and guiding the membership properly. Qualifications for officers should include their willingness to serve the organization, to fulfill the responsibilities of the office, and to attend all meetings (unless ill). Also, they should be familair with the needs of the group as a whole and yet be able to give attention to the requirements of individual members. Leaders should be able to understand individual differences in human beings; they should also be acquainted with the technics of human relations. Good leadership will make each member feel vitally needed, an important asset to the group.

The general membership of any organization has certain individual responsibilities. They must support the officers they have elected and they must be able to understand the aims of the organization. In addition, their loyalty, cooperation, and participation at routine meetings and as members of various committees is necessary to the organization's success. Each member should try to attend as many meetings as possible, be on time, and participate actively in an orderly fashion. (If you work on the afternoon tour and cannot attend all meetings, you might join a telephone committee or some other committee that does not necessarily have to meet during evening hours.) Express your opinions while attending the meetings and not afterward. If you have any criticisms, make them constructive, and think first, "Could I do as well or better?" and, "Would I take on this responsibility?". You certainly need not agree with or approve of every policy or procedure, but you should wait until the appropriate time and then voice your opinion objectively. Once the majority has made a decision, you should abide by it whether you agree or not, because your cooperation is vital to the welfare of the organization.

Every organization must have its constitution and bylaws that state clearly the rights and the responsibilities of the members and the officers. Once these have been accepted, they must be abided by until they are changed or amended.

Parliamentary Procedure

Parliamentary procedure or law has been generally accepted as the rule for conducting meetings, preserving order, and transacting the business of the association in an organized manner, thereby promoting cooperation and harmony. Usually the *Robert's Rules of Orde* or a simplified version of it will serve as the guide in parliamentary procedure, and the order of business should follow a set pattern or agenda.

Officers of the organization should include the president, the vice-president(s), secretary (recording, corresponding, or executive), the treasurer and sometimes a parliamentarian who rules on correct procedures. The size and the scope of the organization will determine the number of officers as well as the standing and special committees. Standing committees are formed for a definite period of time and usually function for the length of time that the officers hold power. Special committees, as the name implies, are formed for a specific task; when this is accomplished, the committee is dissolved. All duties of officers and standing committees should be defined clearly and included in the constitution and the bylaws of the organization.

HEALTH AND WELFARE ORGANIZATIONS

During the past century a growing sense of responsibility toward others has been a primary factor in the establishment of health and welfare agencies in the community. Local citizens have always assisted a neighbor in distress, whether the plight was the result of illness, fire, flood, or some other cause, and community agencies are a modern expression of this spirit. By the early 1900s many agencies were founded by special interest groups and by charitable citizens. Some of these were backed by religious organizations; others were supported through taxation and were under government auspices. Regardless of their support and special interest, they were all dedicated to service and to improving the health and the welfare of the needy.

In 1830 there were about 1 billion people living on the earth. In 1930 there were 2 billion; and according to United Nations' figures, the world contained an estimated 4.32 billion persons on January 1, 1980. It is estimated that the world' population will reach 7 billion by the year 2000 if current trends continue. It is also estimated that the United States alone will have approximately 250 million people by 1985 and 310 million by the year 2000. Some authorities estimate that about half of all our citizens will be living in three huge metropolitan complexes: San Francisco–Los Angeles–San Diego; Milwaukee–Chicago–Detroit–Cleveland; and Boston–New York–Philadelphia–Baltimore–Washington–Norfolk. It is also anticipated that the population of people older than 65 years will reach a total of 25 million by that time. Hence, we must rapidly expand our health services to meet the predicted demands. Under the terms of Medicare, persons older than 65 years of age will have the ability to pay for most of their health services. No one can yet predict with certainty the eventual impact of Medicare and National Health Insurance on health care facilities.

Although there is no known limit to the number of persons the earth can support, overpopulation has already become a reality. We have reached a point at which the major agricultural producers, such as the United States, simply cannot produce enough food for the world's masses. Internationally, scientists are busily engaged in extensive research on food production, air and water pollution, energy consumption, and other areas affecting general health and welfare.

It is easy to see that with the improvement of communications and transportation, and exploration into outer space, the world becomes smaller and smaller, and, as a result, the role of health and welfare agencies becomes even more important. In a sense such agencies must ask the biblical question: "Am I my brother's keeper?"

Most health and welfare agencies have a stated function and usually develop and administer their programs around education, service, and research. They are generally in accord with the broad concept of the World Health Organization (see later in this chapter) that the field of public health represents the art and the science of preventing disease, prolonging life, and promoting physical and mental efficiency through organized community effort. The various health and welfare agencies plan such an effort on a cooperative basis as shown in Figure 8–2.

Official or public agencies are supported through public funds from the Government (taxes) and are administered by appointees of the Federal, state, or local government. Many are staffed with Civil Service employees. One of the most important and influential federal agencies was the Department of Health, Education, and Welfare (HEW), which in October 1979 was divided into the Department of Health and Human Services and the Department of Education. The regional offices of these departments are shown in Table 8–2.

DEPARTMENT OF EDUCATION

The Department of Education (DE) is a cabinet level department that establishes policy and administers and coordinates most federal assistance to education. The

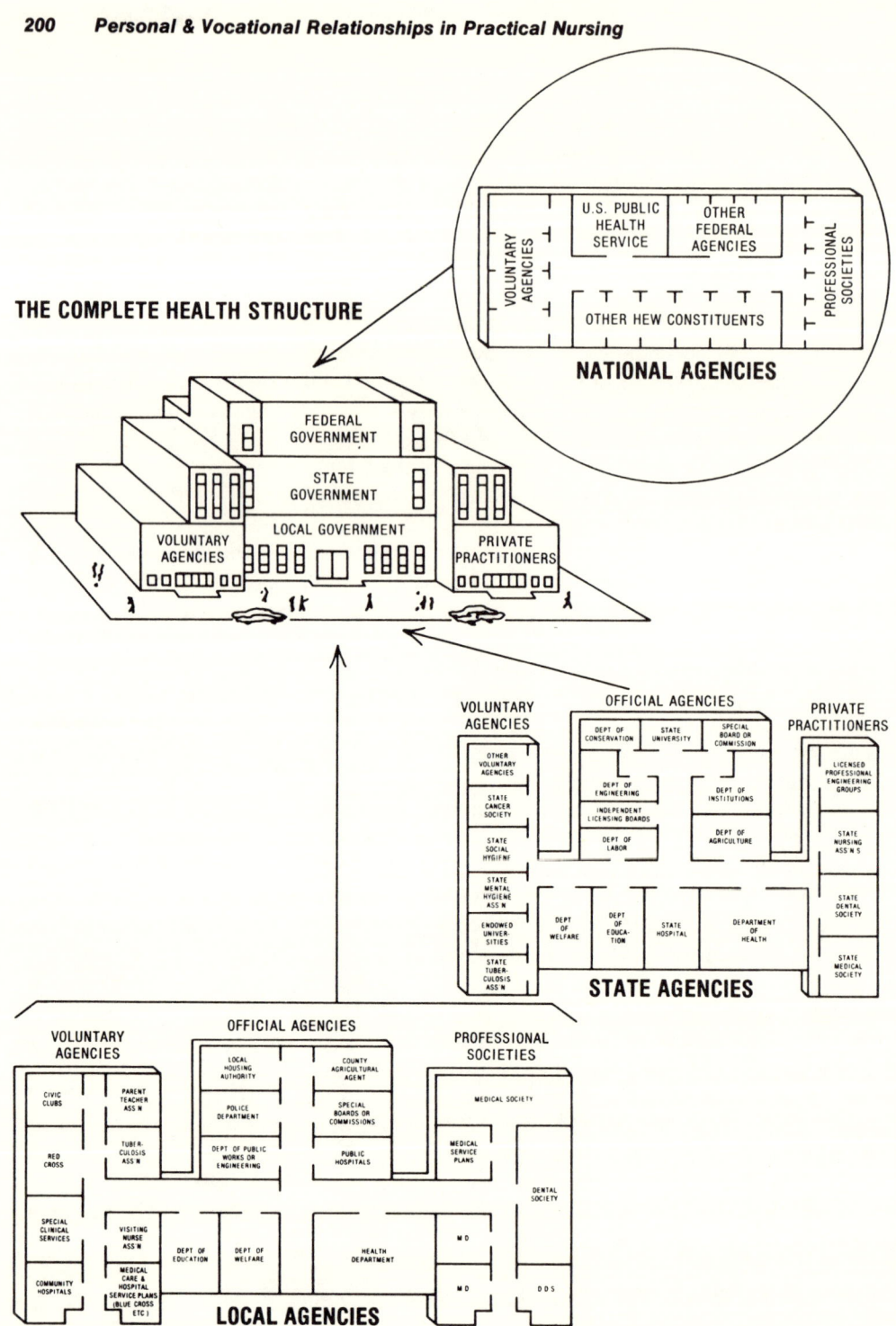

FIGURE 8-2. *The complete health structure—working together for improved public health. (U.S. Department of Health, Education, and Welfare)*

TABLE 8–2. STATES AND TERRITORIES INCLUDED IN EACH OF THE TEN REGIONS, AND THE LOCATION OF THE REGIONAL OFFICES

I. **Conn., Me., Mass., N.H., R.I., Vt.**

    John F. Kennedy Federal Bldg., Boston, Mass. 02203 617-223-6831

II. **N.Y., N.J., P.R., V.I.**

    26 Federal Plaza, New York, N.Y. 10007 212-264-4600

III. **Del., D.C., Md., Pa., Va., W.Va.**

    3535 Market St., Philadelphia, Pa. 19101 215-596-6492

IV. **Ala., Fla., Ga., Ky., Miss., N.C., S.C., Tenn.**

    50 7th St. NE., Atlanta, Ga. 30323 404-221-2442

V. **Ill., Ind., Minn., Mich., Ohio, Wis.**

    300 S. Wacker Dr., Chicago, Ill. 60606 312-353-5160

VI. **Ark., La., N.M., Okla., Texas**

    1200 Main Tower Bldg., Dallas, Tex. 75202 214-655-3301

VII. **La., Kans., Mo., Nebr.**

    601 E. 12th St., Kansas City, Mo. 64106 816-374-3436

VIII. **Colo., Mont., N.D., S.D., Ut., Wyo.**

    1961 Stout St., Denver, Colo. 80202 303-837-3373

IX. **Ariz., Calif., Hawaii, Nev., Guam, Am. Samoa**

    50 Fulton St., San Francisco, Calif. 94102 415-556-6746

X. **Alas., Idaho, Ore., Wash.**

    1321 2d Ave., Seattle, Wash. 98101 206-442-0420

Department was created by legislation proposed by President Carter and was approved by Congress in September, 1979. The Secretary of Education advises the President on plans, policies, and programs of the Federal government and is responsible for the four federally aided corporations: The American Printing House for the Blind, Gallaudet College, Howard University, and the National Technical Institute for the Deaf. The total functions of the Department are shown in Figure 8–3.

The Under Secretary and many other assistant secretaries are responsible for the administration and enforcement of laws related to education of private and public students in this country and overseas for dependents of the Department of Defense. The educational needs of preschool children through adults are considered in the various components of the Department. Ten regional offices serve as centers for dissemination of information and provide technical assistance to state and local agencies.

DEPARTMENT OF HEALTH AND HUMAN SERVICES

The Department of Health and Human Services (HHS), a cabinet level Department, was formerly the Department of Health, Education, and Welfare. The Secretary of HHS advises the President on programs of the Federal government concerning health, welfare, and income security plans and policies. It is the Department "most concerned with people and most involved with the nation's human concerns. In one way or another—whether it is mailing out social security checks or making health services more widely available—HHS touches the lives of more Americans than any other Federal agency. It is literally a department of people serving people, from newborn infants to our most elderly citizens."* The complete structure is shown in Figure 8–4.

The *Office for Civil Rights* is responsible for the administration and enforcement of the policies prohibiting discrimination with regard to race, color, national origin, sex, age, or handicap in programs receiving Federal financial assistance.

Office of Human Development Services

The HDS administers a broad range of programs designed to deal with the problems of specific populations, including the elderly, children of low-income families, persons with mental or physical handicaps, runaway youth, and native Americans. The major components include:

1. Administration on Aging (AOA), which is responsible for identifying the needs, concerns, and interests of older persons and for carrying out the programs of the older Americans Act.

2. Administration for Children, Youth, and Families (ACYF), which consists of the Office of Services for Children and Youth, the Office of

---

* U.S. Government Manual, 1980–81, p. 293.

Department of Education

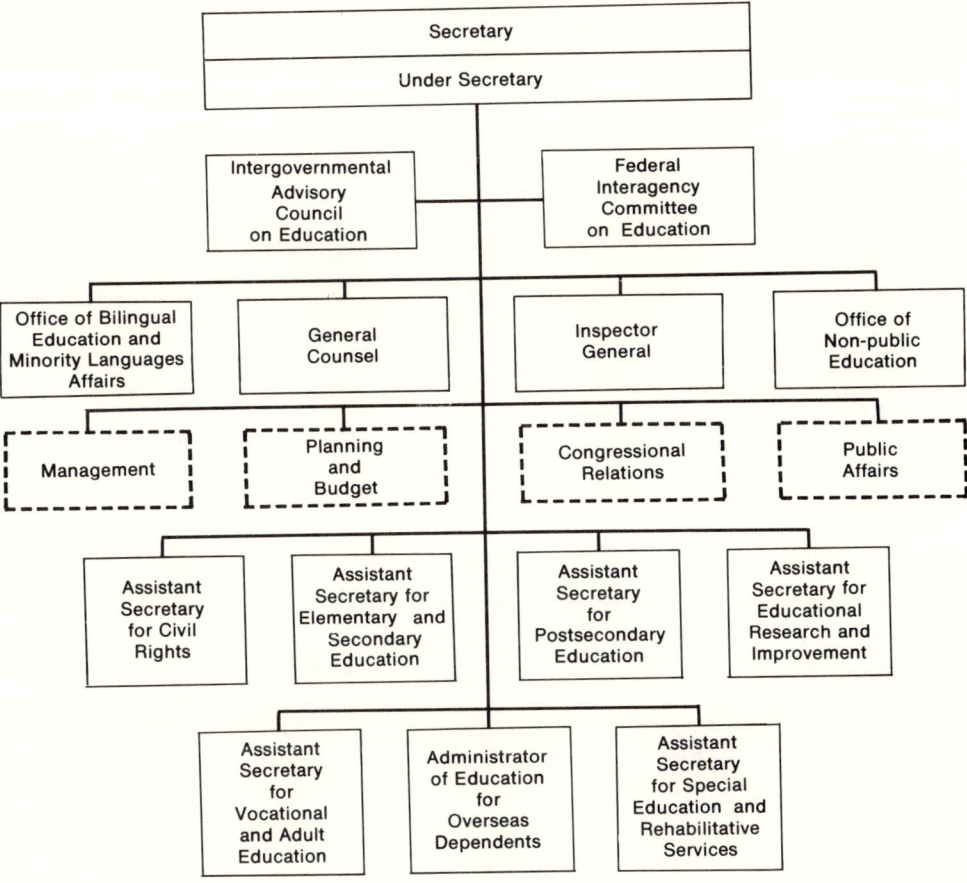

FIGURE 8-3. *Organization of the U.S. Department of Education. (U.S. Government Manual, 1980–81, p. 266)*

Developmental Services, the Office for Families, and the Office on Domestic Violence. These offices operate federally funded programs such as Head Start, the National Center on Child Abuse and Neglect, and Child Welfare Services Program. Each coordinates the intradepartmental activities in the field of runaway youth.

3. Administration for Native Americans (ANA), which is concerned with the special needs of American Indians, Alaskan natives, and native Hawaiians.

Department of Health and Human Services

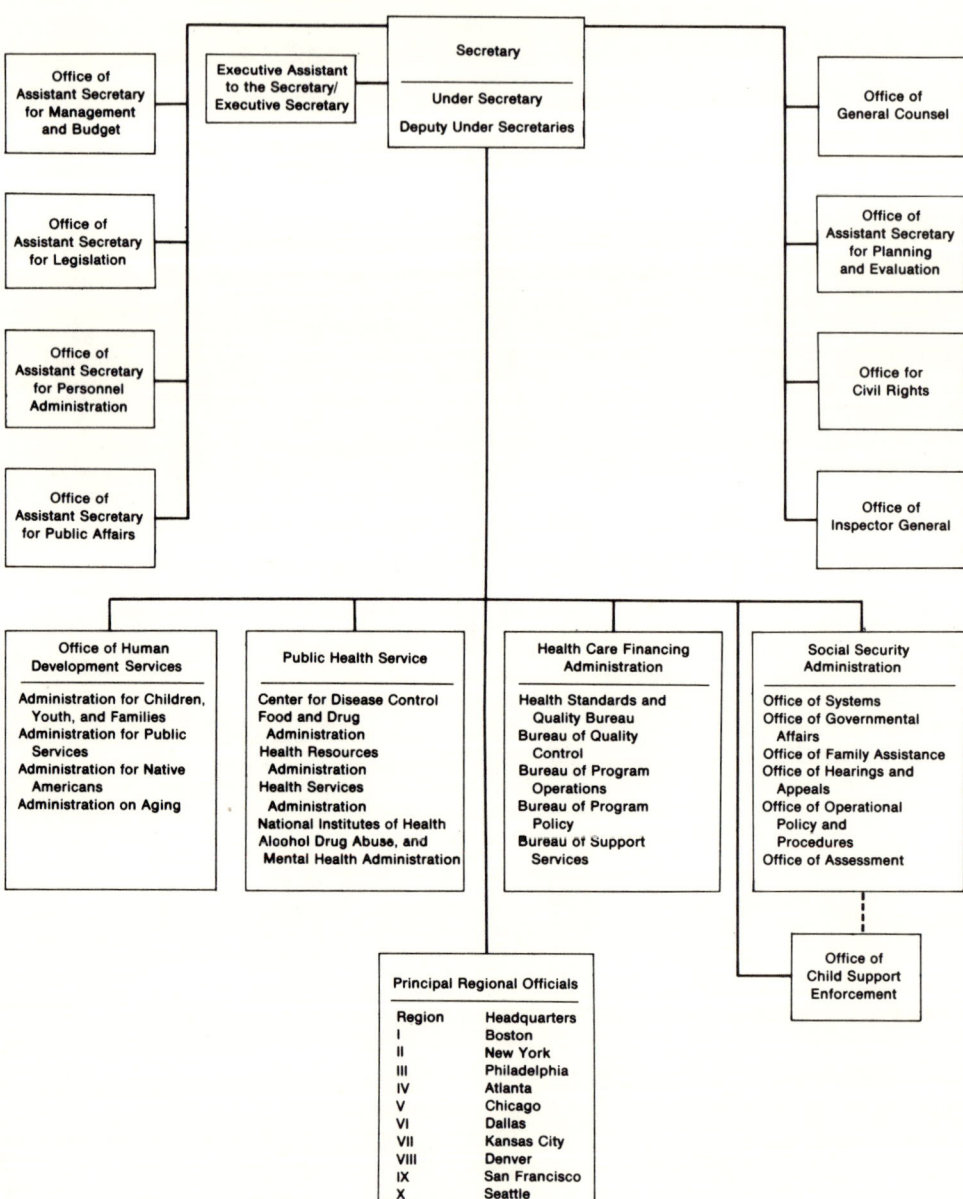

FIGURE 8–4. *Organization of the U.S. Department of Health and Human Services. (U.S. Government Manual, 1980–81, p. 294)*

4. Administration for Public Services (APS), which provides leadership for social services programs authorized under the Social Security Act and coordinates the HHS programs designed to improve employment potential and job opportunities for Americans who are unemployed, underemployed, or in need of training.

Health Care Financing Administration

The HCFA was created in 1977 to oversee the Medicare and Medicaid programs and related Federal medical care quality control staffs. The Medicare program provides basic health benefits to recipients of Social Security and is funded through the Social Security Trust Fund. The Medicaid program provides grants to States to offer health services to those who cannot afford adequate medical care. An HCFA quality assurance program was established to carry out the quality assurance provisions of the Medicare and Medicaid programs. This responsibility includes the implementation of the Professional Standards Review Organization (PSRO) program and the End Stage Renal Disease (ESRD) program. It also includes the monitoring of health and safety standards for providers of health care services. The Long Term Care program is another aspect of the quality assurance effort and includes the aged and chronically ill in nursing homes.

Office of Child Support Enforcement

The OCSE was established in 1975 to provide leadership in the planning, development, management, and coordination in the efforts to require States to enforce support obligations owed by absent parents of their children, establishing paternity when necessary, and obtaining child support. Although a separate organization, the Commissioner of Social Security Administration serves as Director of OCSE.

Social Security Administration (SSA)

In 1935 the Social Security system was established by the U.S. Government. The basic program has changed through the years, just as the needs of the people have changed. This program is the national system of health, old age, survivors, and disability insurance that now covers practically all persons who work for a living. Social insurance against other risks is provided through worker's compensation and unemployment insurance, administered by each state. Complementing these social insurance programs is a program of federal grants to the states to help them provide financial assistance, medical care, and other services for needy people. Closely related are vocational rehabilitation services and public health and welfare services, particularly those for mothers and children, which also come under Social Security. Nine out of ten workers are earning protection under social security. Following is a brief description of Social Security.

The basic idea of social security is a simple one: During working years, employees, their employers, and self-employed people pay social security contributions. This money is used only to pay benefits to the nearly 35 million people getting benefits and to pay administrative costs of the program. Then, when today's workers' earnings stop or are reduced because of retirement, death, or disability, benefits will be paid to them from contributions by people in covered employment and self-employment at that time. These benefits are intended to replace part of the earnings the family has lost.

Part of the contributions made goes for hospital insurance under Medicare so workers and their dependents will have help in paying their hospital bills when they become eligible for Medicare. The medical insurance part of Medicare is financed by premiums paid by the people who have enrolled for this protection and amounts contributed by the Federal Government.*

Nearly one out of every seven persons in this country receives monthly Social Security checks. About 23.4 million people 65 and over, or nearly all of the nation's aged population, have health insurance under Medicare. Another 2.8 million disabled people under 65 also have Medicare. Since 1973, Medicare coverage has been available to people under 65 who have been entitled to disability checks for 2 or more consecutive years and for people with permanent kidney failure who need dialysis or kidney transplants. Legislation affecting Social Security benefits is enacted frequently. There are over 1300 local Social Security offices in communities throughout the United States. Since changes in retirement, survivors, and health insurances occur very rapidly, contact the office nearest you for the latest free materials available.

Account Number Cards

If your work is covered by the Social Security Act, you must have a social security number. This account number, which is shown on your social security card, is used to keep a record of your earnings. You should use the same account number all your life. There are more than 100 million individual accounts in the social security records, and some of them may be under names exactly like yours. Your social security account number keeps your record from being confused with the social security record of anyone else. Both your name and account number are needed to make sure that you get full credit for your earnings. If you are employed, show your card to each employer so that your name and account number will be used exactly as they appear on the card when reporting your wages. If you are self-employed, copy your name and account number on the form you use to report your net earnings for social security credit.

Your social security office will help you get a social security card or a duplicate card to replace one that has been lost. If there is no social security office in your town, ask at the post office for an application blank. If your name has been changed, ask your social security office for a new card showing the same account number with your new name.

---

* Department of Health, Education, and Welfare: *Your Social Security,* p. 5 (DHEW Publication (SSA) 79-10035, June 1979).

Each employer is required by law to give you receipts for the social security taxes deducted from your pay. This must be done at the end of each year and also when you stop working. These receipts (Form W-2) will help you check on your social security account, because they show not only the amount deducted from your pay but also the wages paid you. You may check the official social security record of wages and self-employment income credited to you by writing to the Social Security Administration, Baltimore, Maryland 21235, and asking for a statement of your account. You can get an addressed post card form at your social security office for use in requesting this information. This information cannot be given out without a signed request from you.

Remember, your statement of earnings shows the amount of earnings reported for you. It does not show the amount of taxes you or your employer paid. Benefits under the retirement, Medicare, and disability insurance programs are based on earnings from work covered by the law, not on the amount of taxes paid, and these earnings are shown on the statement which is sent to you on request.

Public Health Service (PHS)

The Public Health Service had its origins in an act passed in July 16, 1798 authorizing marine hospitals for the care of American merchant seamen. Subsequent legislation has broadened its scope and, under the direction of the Assistant Secretary for Health, is charged with the responsibility of protecting and improving the health and environment of the people of the nation. It is also responsible for collaborating with governments of other countries and with international organizations involved in world health activities.

The programs of the Public Health Service are related closely to those of the other agencies of the Department of Health and Human Services, and to many state official and voluntary agencies as well. Research programs are conducted in laboratory, clinical, engineering, statistical, epidemiologic, and administrative fields and are centered on various health problems. Financial grants are given to states for general and specific health services and for the construction of health centers, medical facilities and hospitals. Grants are available also to professional personnel for advanced study in certain specialized fields. These research grants augment the nation's medical research and educational efforts. The Public Health Service also provides medical and hospital care for eligible groups, such as American Merchant Marine and United States Coast Guard personnel; American Indian tribes; civilian employees of the Government; and others whom the Congress of the United States may deem to be eligible. It also administers Saint Elizabeth Hospital, the largest federally operated hospital for the mentally ill.

There are six major agencies in the public health service: the National Institutes of Health; Food and Drug Administration; Center for Disease Control; Alcohol, Drug Abuse, and Mental Health Administration; Health Resources Administration; and Health Services Administration. Each of these agencies has its own particular area of concern. You may write for further information to the following: Office of Public Affairs, Public Health Service, Room 17-22, 5600 Fishers Lane, Rockville, Maryland 20852 for specific information pertaining to the six public health agencies. You may wish to contact them individually as follows: National Institutes for Health, Division of Public Information, Building #1, Room 307, Bethesda, Maryland 20014; Food and Drug Administration HFI-10, 5600 Fishers Lane, Rockville, Md. 20852; Center for Disease Control, Atlanta Georgia 30333; Health Resources Administration, Room 10A-31, 5600 Fishers Lane, Rockville, Md. 20852; Health Services Administration, Room 14A-55, 5600 Fishers Lane, Rockville, Md. 20852; Alcohol, Drug Abuse, and Mental Health Administration (ADAMH), Room 16-95, 5600 Fishers Lane, Rockville, Md. 20852.

Center for Disease Control

The Center for Disease Control (CDC) was established within the Public Health Service to provide leadership and direction in the prevention and control of diseases and other preventable conditions. It is comprised of eight major operating components: National Institute for Occupational Safety and Health, Bureau of Epidemiology, Bureau of Health Education, Bureau of Laboratories, Bureau of Smallpox Eradication, Bureau of State Services, Bureau of Training, and Bureau of Tropical Diseases. The Center also provides consultation to other nations in the control of preventable diseases.

Food and Drug Administration

Although the FDA, first established in 1906, has functioned under different organizational titles, its main purpose has been to protect the health of the Nation against impure and unsafe foods, drugs, cosmetics, and other potential hazards. The Bureau of Biologics administers regulations of biological products shipped in interstate and foreign commerce, inspects facilities, approves licenses of manufacturers, tests products, and conducts research. The Bureau of Drugs develops policy pertaining to the labelling of all drugs, evaluates new drugs, develops standards for the safety and effectiveness of the over-the-counter drugs, monitors the quality of medications, directs the antibiotic and insulin certification programs, and disseminates toxicity and treatment information. The Bureau of Foods conducts research and develops standards on the composition, quality, nutrition, safety of foods, food additives, colors, and cosmetics; reviews and develops regulations for food standards to permit the use of color and food additives; and maintains a nutritional data bank. The Bureau of Radiological Health carries out programs designed to reduce hazardous exposure of individuals to ionizing and nonionizing radiation. The Bureau of Veterinary Medicine conducts programs relating to the safety and efficacy of veterinary preparations and other medical matters. The Bureau of Medical Services is charged with the responsibility of developing policy regarding the safety, efficacy, and labeling of medical devices. The National Center for Toxicological Research conducts research programs to study the biological effects of potentially toxic chemical substances found in our environment to determine the health effects resulting from long-term exposure to chemical toxicants.

Health Resources Administration (HRA)

The HRA identifies health care resource problems and administers programs to improve the health care systems, as well as the health status of Americans. Major components include:

1. The Bureau of Health Manpower which provides national leadership in coordinating the development and utilization of the Nation's health care personnel.
2. The Bureau of Health Facilities Financing, Compliance, and Convention develops policies for Federal programs pertaining to the modernization, utilization, continuation, and closure of non-federal health facilities.
3. The Bureau of Health Planning administers the program of federal, state, and areawide health planning and health care delivery systems development.

Health Services Administration (HSA)

The mission of the HSA is to provide professional leadership in the delivery of health services. Through the Bureau of Community Health Services, the implementation of Maternal and Child Welfare, Community Health Centers, Migrant Health, Family Planning, and the National Service Camps occurred, a primary health care program supported the initiation of several hundred ambulatory health care centers in urban and rural areas. The *Indian Health Service* operates a comprehensive health program for eligible American Indians and Alaska natives. The *Bureau of Medical Services* provides complete health care services to designated Federal beneficiaries and includes the medical care programs of the Federal Bureau of Prisons and the U.S. Coast Guard, and Public Health Services hospitals and clinics.

The National Institutes of Health

The mission of the NIH is to improve the health of American people by conducting and supporting research into the causes, prevention, and cure of disease; supporting research training and the development of research services; and making use of modern methods to communicate biological medical information. NIH is comprised of the following: the National Cancer Institute; National Heart, Lung, and Blood Institute; National Institute of Antibiotics, Metabolism, and Digestive Diseases; National Institute of Allergy and Infectious Diseases; National Institute of Child Health and Human Development; National Institute of Dental Research; National Institutes of Environmental Health Sciences; National Institute of General Medical Sciences; National Institute of Neurological and Communicative Disorders and Stroke; National Eye Institute; National Institute on Aging; Clinical Center; Fogarty International Center; Division of Computer Research and Technology; Division of Research Resources, Division of Research Services; and the Division of Research Grants.

Alcohol, Drug Abuse, and Mental Health Administration

The mission of the ADAMHA is a federal effort to provide leadership to reduce and eliminate health problems caused by alcohol and drug abuse, and to improve the mental health of people. Major components include:

1. The National Institute on Alcohol Abuse and Alcoholism (NIAAA), which is responsible for the prevention, control, and treatment of alcohol abuse and alcoholism and the rehabilitation of affected individuals.

2. The National Institute on Drug Abuse (NIDA) which is involved with the prevention, control, and treatment of narcotic addiction, drug abuse, and the rehabilitation of affected people.

3. The National Institute of Mental Health (NIMH), which operates Saint Elizabeth's Hospital and provides leadership in the promotion of mental health, the prevention and treatment of mental illness, and the rehabilitation of affected people.

It is through these agencies that the Public Health Service meets its main responsibility, that of promoting and assuring the highest level of health attainable for every individual and family in the United States. PHS also collaborates with governments of other countries and with international organizations in world health activities.

OTHER PUBLIC HEALTH AGENCIES

State Health Department

The State Department of Health is supported by funds from the state treasury. The governor of the state appoints the various officials who are responsible for the development and the functioning of local health departments. When a local office (county, township, or municipality) is not prepared to deal with health problems in the community, the State Department may send workers to assist the local health officers, or it may take control of the entire program by administering it from the state level. The Commissioner of Health for the state will usually appoint directors for the various departments, and these will vary from state to state. The licensing of undertakers, embalmers, and manufacturers and wholesalers of narcotics and other important drugs, as well as licensing of hospitals, nursing homes and other agencies, may also fall under this administrative office. Health education materials, including a film library, pamphlets, books, and folders on various health subjects, are usually available free of charge from the Health Education or Information Division. Other divisions may include Vital Statistics, Communicable Disease Control, Public Health Nursing, Maternal and Child Health, Laboratories and Research, Sanitation, Nutrition, Dental Health, Tuberculosis, Sexually Transmitted Disease, and Mental Health.

Local Health Department

The local or official community health organization may have the same divisions or sections as those on the state level. However, its functions and administration vary with each county, township, or city, since the funds available, as well as the type of men and women appointed as officers and employees, will affect the efficiency of the organization. The quantity and the quality of health service given by this agency also will depend on the advisory board, the mayor, the councilmen or councilwomen, and in some instances, county managers and commissioners. The general activities and responsibilities are usually (1) reporting of communicable diseases, which encompasses the entire field of epidemiology; (2) keeping accurate vital statistics such as reports on the population, birth rate, mortality, or death rate (including infants, stillborns, and mothers), morbidity or disease rates, and divorce and marriage rates; (3) public health nursing and health education; (4) environmental sanitation, including milk, water, rodent and insect control; and (5) maternal and child health services, including school, dental, nutritional, and mental health aspects.

World Health Organization

The World Health Organization (WHO) is a specialized agency of the United Nations and is the one directing and coordinating authority on international health. It is a cooperative organization that works on a worldwide basis to raise health standards by such measures as correlating information on epidemiology, statistics, and drug standardization. It disseminates health information in various languages through pamphlets, films, and demonstrations. The main function of the organization is to assist countries in strengthening their own health services by providing advisory services through public health experts in disease control. These consultants are available through regional offices in Africa, the United States, Southeast Asia, Europe, the Western Pacific, and the Eastern Mediterranean. International sanitary regulations that afford protection against the international spread of disease by sea, land, or air traffic have been established and are enforced by the WHO. Also, it has sponsored international health legislation that provides for the uniform registration of diseases and deaths in all countries, in order to achieve an adequate appraisal of health problems and better planning of health campaigns. Another important function of the WHO is the standardization of all important drugs. An international description of drugs giving standards of purity, potency, and testing procedures is published, ensuring that drugs used or ordered by physicians anywhere in the world are of proper quality and are uniform in strength.

The control of communicable diseases has been singled out for a worldwide plan of attack by this organization, in order to lessen the toll in human lives, suffering, and economic loss due to such infectious diseases as malaria, tuberculosis, venereal infections, leprosy, anthrax, typhus, diphtheria, and many others. Other areas of its work include the fields of maternal and child health, social and occupational health, rehabilitation, public health education and administration, mental health, nutrition, and sanitation. To summarize the work of the WHO, it is perhaps best to state the following excerpts taken from its constitution.

> The following principles are basic to the happiness, harmonious relations and security of all peoples:
>
> Health is a state of complete physical, mental and social well-being and not merely the absence of disease or infirmity.
>
> The enjoyment of the highest attainable standard of health is one of the fundamental rights of every human being without distinction of race, religion, political belief, economic or social condition.
>
> The health of all peoples is fundamental to the attainment of peace and security, and is dependent upon the fullest cooperation of individuals and States.
>
> The achievement of any State in the promotion and protection of health is of value to all.
>
> Unequal development in different countries in the promotion of health and control of disease, especially communicable disease, is a common danger.
>
> Healthy development of the child is of basic importance; the ability to live harmoniously in a changing total environment is essential to such development.
>
> The extension to all peoples of the benefits of medical, psychological and related knowledge is essential to the fullest attainment of health. Informed opinion and active cooperation on the part of the public are of the utmost importance in the improvement of the health of the people.

VOLUNTARY AND PRIVATE HEALTH AGENCIES

Private or voluntary agencies receive their support from such sources as the United Fund, donations, gifts, endowments, patients, membership fees, and sometimes from public funds allocated to these agencies for rendering a specific service that is recognized as a public responsibility. An example of this would be the payment to a voluntary hospital, by official agencies, for treating public charges or indigents as patients.

These private organizations are usually administered by a Board of Directors who volunteer their services because of their interest in the organization and their belief in its necessity. A salaried executive secretary or director is usually in charge of the paid staff and is responsible for the administration of the agency and for carrying out the wishes of the Board members. Many private agencies have volunteers who offer their services and provide many hours of important service free of charge.

The professional groups of health and welfare workers have formed organizations such as the American Public Health Association, the American Medical Association, the American Dietetic Association, the National Association of Social Workers, the American Association for Health, Physical Education and Recreation, the American Pharmaceutical Association, the American Society of Clinical Pathologists, the American Hospital Association, and many others, which, through committees or councils, arrange for national and international meetings and conventions.

The list of agencies whose memberships and activities are national in scope is very long. Many national organizations have provisions in their bylaws or charters that prevent them from combining their fund-raising activities with other agencies; therefore, many of the national organizations are not participating members of the local United Fund or Community Chest agencies. All national agencies, particularly those interested in the control of a particular disease, such as the American Lung Association, the American Heart Association, and the American Cancer Society, have united in an effort to bring about some sort of coordination among national health organizations. In 1921 the National Health Council was incorporated to study the functions and the relationships of these groups.

Since it is difficult to administer organizational activities on a national level, most voluntary agencies operate on state and local levels. In some instances the national or state organization grew from a small local unit that was founded by a few citizens interested in a specific health problem. Most agencies, though different in their functions and interests, play an important role in the total health program of the community, the state, and the nation. The agencies that are being discussed here have been selected for their variety of functions and are most important to you in meeting your responsibilities as a citizen and as a nurse. Refer to this list if you are able to use their facilities and materials in your patient care and community activities. Help in their fund raising, health education, and volunteer services. Acquaint yourself with the local units by reading their annual report, visiting their offices, and seeing how your contribution is being spent. If there is no local office, and you cannot find a particular agency either by contacting the health or the welfare councils, you can write to the National Health Council, 1740 Broadway, New York, New York 10019, for the location of the state or national office.

> *Alcoholics Anonymous* (AA) helps the alcoholic only if one wishes to be helped. There are over 16,000 active AA groups in the world. The fellowship is made up of more than 400,000 members who have recovered from alcoholism, and in sharing their recovery they help others overcome the same problem.

> The *American Cancer Society* educates the public, keeps doctors and professional people informed, and supports facilities for the detection, diagnosis, and treatment of cancer. It improves medical and social services for patients and conducts a broad research program.

> The *American Diabetes Association* educates the public and professional workers in the nature and the treatment of this disease and encourages the formation of subsidiary groups. It improves standards of treatment, promotes medical research, and distributes accurate information to the public as well as to patients.

> The *American Heart Association* supports research in the cardiovascular diseases, the leading cause of death in the United States. It provides educational programs for professionals, patients, and the general public, and it sets standards to maintain and promote better medical care for patients.

The *American Lung Association*, formerly the *National Tuberculosis and Respiratory Disease Association*, provides professional and public educational materials for anyone interested in respiratory and lung diseases. It also participates in rehabilitation programs for patients and funds vast research programs. (Christmas Seals help support this organization.)

The *American Red Cross* conducts war and disaster relief programs; collects blood; offers educational programs in first aid, accident prevention, and water safety; and helps to promote social welfare. It sponsors activities in schools and colleges and conducts volunteer programs that include the Gray Ladies, Braille readers, nurses' aides, motor corps, and canteen services. For further information, see the section on Nursing Organizations.

The *Arthritis and Rheumatism Foundation* carries out research programs in the causes of these diseases and develops methods of prevention, diagnosis, and treatment. It promotes educational programs, supports local treatment facilities, and assists in the training of physicians and other health care personnel.

The *Association for the Aid of Crippled Children (and Adults)* offers instructional materials for orthopedic physicians, nurses, physical therapists, and others. It conducts scientific conferences and research programs and prepares various educational tools for patients and professional workers in this field. (Easter Seals help support this organization.)

The *Muscular Dystrophy Association of America, Inc.*, conducts research programs for the discovery of the cause and the cure of this progressively crippling disease that afflicts more than 250,000 Americans. It assists individuals in the purchase and repair of necessary appliances and equipment and renders patient services in physical therapy, counseling, education, recreation, and transportation.

The *National Association for Mental Health* carries out a nationwide program of clinical research, works for better preventive and treatment facilities for the mentally ill, and promotes mental health through public and professional educational programs. It informs the public about how to avoid serious mental breakdown.

The *National Association of the Physically Handicapped* promotes rehabilitation and employment for the handicapped. It sponsors recreation programs, including competitive sports, for the physically disadvantaged and furthers the social, economic, and physical welfare of this client group.

The *National Consumers' League* is a very important consumer pressure group interested in consumer protection by attending federal hearings, monitoring advertising, advising consumers on their legal rights and directing consumers to appropriate state and federal agencies for grievance actions. It also prepares educational materials and lists of various inspections that have been held on health care providers (nursing homes, for instance).

The *National Coordinating Council on Drug Abuse* seeks to coordinate the educational and informational efforts of groups in the area of drug abuse. It evaluates educational programs, encourages research, and establishes interdisciplinary committees to respond to area needs. The council offers an excellent drug information service that provides publications and audiovisual aids.

The *National Cystic Fibrosis Research Foundation* has more than 116 cystic fibrosis research, care, and teaching centers located throughout the United States. It is also developing local diagnostic and treatment clinics that reach the public through films, literature, symposia, and other means of communication.

The *National Foundation* (originally the National Foundation for Infantile Paralysis) extended its facilities, which formerly dealt with polio research, prevention, and aid, to include other virus diseases, arthritis, birth defects, and central nervous system disorders. It now offers educational programs, research projects, and patient aid in these areas.

The *National Health Council* helps member agencies to work together more effectively and helps to identify, publicize, and promote efforts toward the solution of national health problems. It also encourages better state and local health services, whether governmental or voluntary. The Council sponsors a National Health Forum and publishes the *Forum Report, A Guide for Community Health Planning, Health Careers Guidebook,* and other aids for local health councils. There are almost 200 member agencies, and a national health library is maintained at the central office at 1740 Broadway, New York, New York 10019, where information regarding health and welfare agencies may be obtained.

The *National Hemophilia Foundation* is dedicated to finding a cure for hemophilia. It also works toward the management and control of the disease so that the hemophiliac can live a normal, full, and productive life. In addition, it supports research and special clinics for emergency care and for diagnostic, dental, orthopedic, and other special care.

The *National Interagency Council on Smoking and Health* is composed of governmental and private groups fighting cigarette smoking. It cooperates closely with state and local agencies in antismoking campaigns.

The *National Multiple Sclerosis Society* is dedicated to finding the cause of this disease, and seeing that effective treatment may be developed. It offers a research program that fosters medical and scientific advances in the cure and prevention of the disease and provides educational material for professional people and the general public.

The *National Rehabilitation Association* promotes practical ways for the complete rehabilitation of all physically and mentally handicapped persons. It also strives to improve the standards of care rendered by professional and other interested groups.

The *National Safety Council* works diligently to reduce the number and the severity of all kinds of accidents (from automobiles, home and industrial hazards, fires, poisonings, and so forth) by gathering and distributing information about the causes of accidents and the means of preventing them. It provides literature and posters and sponsors institutes and safety programs for industry, high school seniors, and other interested groups. Accidents are the fourth largest cause of death in the United States.

The *National Society for Crippled Children and Adults* provides treatment, rehabilitation, education, employment, and recreation for crippled persons. It owns and operates facilities that provide these services and conducts many public education and research programs.

The *National Society for the Prevention of Blindness* awards grants for research to determine causes of blindness and to develop better diagnostic procedures. It provides industry with safety programs, promotes legislation, and cooperates with federal, state, and local agencies in sight-conservation programs. It also offers special educational facilities for those with partial vision, gives vision screening tests, and publishes teaching materials.

Planned Parenthood (Federation of America, Inc.) and *World Population*, in their various centers, conduct research and deal with the issues of marriage, education, child spacing, population control, and infertility. Their literature and other materials are available to physicians, nurses, religious leaders, social workers, civic leaders, and others who are interested in the total well-being of family life.

The *Salvation Army* offers emergency relief, food, shelter, guidance, and counseling for families and individuals. It aids local or migrant homeless men and women, acts as an employment bureau for them, and offers them recreational and religious programs with group work activities to assist in rehabilitation.

The *United Cerebral Palsy Association* operates diagnostic and treatment clinics for the cerebral palsied; offers therapeutic treatment, speech therapy, manipulations, and training for the palsied; and carries on an educational program for those who are interested.

The *United Health Foundation* coordinates the research and health education activities of the members of local and state health foundations and organizations, as well as United Fund agencies.

The *United Ostomy Association* is a federation of state and local groups composed of persons who have lost the normal function of their bowel or bladder, necessitating colostomy, ileostomy, ileal bladder, or ureterostomy surgery. These groups offer aid in rehabilitation through mutual assistance, moral support, and exchange of practical information on the management of stomas.

The *Visiting Nurse Association* provides home nursing under medical care to the acutely ill, chronic invalids, mothers with newborn babies, convalescents, and others who cannot leave their homes for treatment. It teaches members of the family to care for the ill and guides the patient in regaining and keeping his health. (It is a local agency only.)

UNITED FUND

In the early 1900s less than 2% of the population of our large cities gave financial support to local charitable institutions. As individual organizations attempted to raise money, well-meaning volunteers approached prominent businessmen, politicians, and professional people asking them to lend their names and prestige and influence to fund-raising campaigns. Citizens were no longer approached by one agency for their contributions but by many, and the number of charitable organizations grew and grew. Fund-raising efforts were often duplicated. The individual costs of soliciting funds ran from 10 to 30% of the money collected. The names that were lent to fund-raising appeals began to be used over and over by different organizations. Out of this situation grew the need for joint fund raising, with an allocation of funds on a basis of community need and the particular purpose of the organization. By the end of World War I in 1918, more than 300 cities had organized war chests, and later the names Community Chest and Red Feather Agency were coined.

During the 1950s the name United Fund replaced the Red Feather symbol as well as its name in many communities. The general function of the United Fund (or the Community Chest) is to raise funds each year by *one* community-wide appeal for all the affiliated voluntary social, welfare, and health agencies. These funds are then distributed in accordance with a mutually agreed upon budgeting procedure. The results of this joint effort of fund raising were lower administrative costs and better social, welfare, and health programs, established through the cooperation and the coordination of existing programs. Duplication of effort was prevented through the study of agency activities, and there was improvement in the standards of work and research, as well as better community understanding and citizen support. This cooperative plan of combining the various community agencies and their fund raising activities into one general drive has been accepted by many organizations; however, there are still many very worthwhile charitable organizations that for one reason or another, have not become members of the combined effort. These are supported through the efforts of interested citizens.

Questions

A. Select the correct answer and circle the number that answers the question best.

1. A voluntary agency usually (A) is supported primarily by taxes, (B) is supported by donations, (C) is supported by patient charges, (D) has civil service employees.

   1. All of these
   2. All except B
   3. A, D
   4. B, C

2. An official local agency (A) may be supported by federal funds, (B) is supported by local taxes, (C) never charges patients, (D) usually has civil service employees.

1. All of these
2. All except C
3. A, B
4. B

3. Official agencies include (A) American Lung Association, (B) American Mental Health Society, (C) Public Health Service (D) Department of Health and Human Services, (E) State Health Department.

1. All except B
2. All except A
3. C, D, E
4. D, E

4. Official agencies include (A) Red Cross, (B) Salvation Army, (C) St. Elizabeth Hospital, (D) National Institute of Health, (E) State Health Department.

1. All except B
2. All except C
3. C, D, E
4. D, E
5. A, D, E

5. The Department of Health and Human Services includes (A) Howard University, (B) Food and Drug Administration, (C) WHO, (D) National Health Council, (E) United Ostomy Association.

1. All except E
2. All except C, E
3. A, B, C
4. A, B

6. The field of Vital Statistics includes (A) birth and death, (B) divorce and marriage, (C) accident and fire prevention, (D) morbidity, (E) census, (F) mental health.

1. All of these
2. A, B, D, E
3. A, B, C, F
4. A, C, E

7. The NLN (A) publishes the *Journal of Nursing,* (B) publishes *Nursing and Health Care* (C) is interested in RN education only, (D) founded a Practical Nurse Council in 1950, (E) organized the Council of Practical Nursing Programs in 1957.

1. All except D
2. All except D, E
3. B, C
4. B, E
5. B, D

8. A practical nurse may belong to (A) NAPNES, (B) NFLPN, (C) NLN, (D) ARC, (E) ANA.

1. All of these
2. A, B, C
3. All except E
4. A, C
5. A, B

9. NAPNES (A) publishes the *Journal of Practical Nursing,* (B) accredits schools, (C) sponsors summer schools, (D) prepares a list of approved schools, (E) was founded in 1941.

1. All except E
2. All except C
3. All except D
4. All of these

10. NFLPN (A) prepares a list of approved schools, (B) was founded in 1949, (C) has only PN members, (D) has state and local divisions, (E) will have RN members.

1. All except E
2. All except B, E
3. C, D
4. B, C, D

B. Place *O* for "official" or *V* for "voluntary" agency in the space provided.

____   1. United Fund
____   2. American Heart Association
____   3. State Health Department
____   4. Public Health Service
____   5. American Red Cross

_____ 6. American Lung Association
_____ 7. Visiting Nurse Association
_____ 8. National Health Council
_____ 9. World Health Organization
_____ 10. National Association for Mental Health

C. Match the best associated expression from Column *B* with Column *A* and insert the letter in the space provided.

A	*B*
_____ 1. WHO	A. three years
_____ 2. United Fund	B. study of epidemiology
_____ 3. American Lung Association	C. CP Control
_____ 4. State Health Department	D. Christmas Seals
_____ 5. Vital Statistics	E. PHS
_____ 6. National Formulary	F. Food and Drug Administration
_____ 7. Communicable disease control	G. United Nations
_____ 8. Department of Education	H. licensing of nursing homes
_____ 9. State Board of Nursing	I. licensure for nurses
_____ 10. Associate degree	J. technical nursing education program
	K. mortality rate
	L. four years
	M. Community Chest
	N. Vocational Nurse education
	O. cosmetic inspection

D. Select the *one* correct expression that will complete the sentence and place the letter in the answer space.

1. The broad aspects of training urgently needed health manpower or personnel were added to the responsibilities of (A) the Office of Education, (B) the Food and Drug Administration, (C) the Public Health Service, (D) Social Security. _____

2. Morbidity rate in the field of Vital Statistics applies to (A) deaths, (B) disease, (C) stillborns, (D) epidemiology. _____

3. Easter Seals are used to raise funds for the (A) Red Cross, (B) Cancer Society, (C) Crippled Children's Association, (D) Lung Association. _____

4. Research to eliminate the leading cause of death in the United States would be conducted by the (A) Lung Association, (B) Heart Association, (C) Cancer Society, (D) Mental Health Association. _____

5. The national vocational organization for students in health occupations is NHSA, (B) HASN, (C) NVSO, (D) HOSA. _____

6. *Journal of Nursing Care* is published by (A) NLN, (B) NFLPN, (C) NAPNES, (D) LPN, Inc. _____

7. Joint fund raising is carried out by (A) American Red Cross, (B) Health Foundation, (C) National Welfare Assembly, (D) United Fund. _____

8. The Council of Practical Nursing is under the (A) National Federation, (B) National League for Nursing, (C) Public Health Service, (D) National Association for Practical Nurse Education and Services. _____

9. Health Insurance or Medicare is under the (A) Public Health Service, (B) Office of Education, (C) Social Security Administration, (D) Social and Rehabilitation Service. _____

10. Pesticide tolerance tests are done routinely by (A) WHO, (B) PHS, (C) FDA, (D) OASDI.

Answers (2½·points each)

A. Multiple Choice	B. Classification	C. Matching	D. Selection
1. 4	1. V	1. G	1. C
2. 2	2. V	2. M	2. B
3. 3	3. O	3. D	3. C
4. 3	4. O	4. H	4. B
5. 4	5. V	5. K	5. D
6. 2	6. V	6. F	6. B
7. 4	7. V	7. B	7. D
8. 3	8. V	8. N or J	8. B
9. 4	9. O	9. I	9. C
10. 4	10. V	10. J	10. C

9

Career Opportunities and Responsibilities

Evaluating Yourself • Marriage and Your Career • Types of Positions • Evaluating Positions • Finding a Position • Resignations • Dismissals • Labor Laws • Collective Bargaining • Your Income and You • Federal Income Tax • Savings and Investments • Continuing Your Education • Self-Protection Rules • Questions and Answers

Objectives

Upon completion of this chapter you should be able to

1. identify the roles, responsibilities, and limitations of the practical nurse before graduation and after licensure,
2. compare the advantages and disadvantages in different types of career opportunities,
3. explain the importance of fringe benefits and what to look for,
4. write a resume,
5. apply for a position,
6. resign from a position,
7. understand the financial responsibilities and obligations of an employee,
8. discuss collective bargaining,
9. apply self-protection rules.

Because of the ever-changing responsibilities of the registered nurse (RN), as well as the expanded functions of practical nursing, today's practical nurse has become one of the most valuable members of the health team. Graduate practical nurses are in constant demand to work in hospitals, homes, physicians' offices, and industrial and community health agencies; the opportunities in the field of practical nursing are virtually unlimited.

The role of the practical nurse is two-fold. First, you may work under the supervision of an RN, or a licensed physician or a dentist, in those instances in which the patient's needs have been defined, and the treatments, medications, and general considerations of care do not require a more advanced scientific background. Second, you are able to assist RNs in rendering care in situations that require skills beyond those that you may have acquired. This role makes practical nursing a definite occupation within nursing; therefore, the practical nurse has an important responsibility to fulfill in practicing this career in an ethical and sound manner.

In the *Nursing Practice Standards for the Licensed Practical/Vocational Nurse* this caution appears: "Shall know the scope of nursing practice authorized by the Nurse Practice Act in the state wherein employed." Therefore, it is the responsibility of the practical nurse to know the State Board of Nursing's regulations pertaining to the practice of practical nursing. It is essential that you understand this role so that you may protect the title and the legal initials of LPN or LVN. The nurses using these titles are automatically expected to know the law of the state awarding the license, and it is presumed that they will practice within the limitations defined by it. (See Chapter 7, Ethical and Legal Responsibilities.)

EVALUATING YOURSELF

Before you choose a position in the nursing, medical, and allied health fields, you must be informed about the position and compare it with others, and, most important of all, you must judge yourself as an individual and decide whether or not you are suited for this type of position. Those of you who are graduating from approved programs, as well as those who have been practicing nursing for years, are asked to think seriously about your reasons for becoming a nurse. Have your motives changed during the past year? Do you still enjoy doing things for your patients? Do you understand their needs, and are you able to meet them? Are you able to analyze your feelings toward your patients, coworkers, superiors, and others? Are you able to meet the physical and the emotional demands imposed on you daily? Surely some of you know nurses who should not be nurses, and some of you have said, "Oh, I don't want to be like Mrs. Jones—she certainly doesn't do justice to nursing;" or, "Ken Smith is interested only in the paycheck and doesn't give two cents for nursing;" or, "Pam Davis is just putting in time till something better comes along." If you are not going to be an asset to the nursing profession, or if you yourself are dissatisfied with nursing and therefore cannot be happy in your work, certainly it would be advisable to leave nursing and find something else to do. You must be a happy, well-adjusted nurse to meet your responsibilities and to do justice to your patients. You must understand yourself, be emotionally mature, and know your nursing skills, as well as your legal and personal limitations.

If you drift from position to position and change jobs frequently, either by your employer's request or by your own choice, you will usually earn less money, miss promotional opportunities, and lose out on increments, sick time, holidays, vacations, and other benefits that are granted to employees on permanent status. In addition, you will probably derive little personal satisfaction and will find that you adjust poorly in the constant change of employee-employer situations. Therefore, by evaluating yourself along with the positions available to you, you should be able to choose the one that will afford you the most satisfaction. In self-appraisal you must be honest and consider the standard of living that you are accustomed to, and how much money it will take to maintain yourself and your dependents. Your instructors, supervisors, and others may be able to give you valuable suggestions as well as information. An intelligent approach in the selection of your future position is vital for job satisfaction. (See Self-Evaluation, Appendix C.)

MARRIAGE AND YOUR CAREER

For those of you who intend to be or already are married, combining your career with marriage may not be easy. For example, your mate may resent your outside interests, your income, the postponement of children, your working hours, and additional housekeeping responsibilities. It is, therefore, most important that you discuss all aspects fully with your prospective mate and reach an agreement, based on mutual knowledge and understanding, before you get married. Face the possibility of problems honestly and realistically and work them out together prior to the wedding. Build common interests and goals and share the activities you enjoy; discover each other and develop mutual leisure time activities so that your marriage will be built on a firm foundation.

Building a successful relationship that will stand the strains and stresses of modern living requires emotionally mature people who not only love and respect each other but also *know* each other well. Statistics prove that marriage is most successful if the backgrounds, likes and dislikes, and interests of the marriage partners are compatible, and if friends and parents approve of the marriage. All too often marriage may be an escape from home, school, or work responsibilities for one of the partners, or is entered into with the idea that a partner can be changed after marriage. There is almost one divorce in every three marriages, not including separations by mutual consent.

TYPES OF POSITIONS

The practical nurse may find job opportunities in private duty nursing; institutional nursing in general hospitals or in specific fields, such as obstetrics, pediatrics, surgery, general medicine, psychiatry, and other specialties; in nursing homes, physicians' and dentists' offices; in the Peace Corps and Armed Forces; in community health agencies, industry, and many other areas. Positions are usually classified according to the type of employer. Some of the many positions available are discussed here.

Private Duty Nursing

The private practitioner of nursing has an opportunity to care for patients in their homes, in an institution, or wherever the patient may desire to take the nurse. Private duty nurses are usually paid by the patient, even though they are directly responsible to the physician and the health care facilities' nursing administration for the performance of their duties. This field offers an excellent opportunity for the nurse to practice basic bedside nursing and teaching skills and have ample time to meet the comprehensive needs of patients including the physical, medical, emotional, nutritional, and rehabilitative aspects of nursing care. You will have an opportunity to get to know your patients and their families extremely well and to give them your undivided attention.

In private practice, whether in a facility or patients' homes, the condition of your patients and the physician's orders will determine your responsibilities. It is important that you keep the physician informed regarding your patient's condition to build confidence in you as a capable nurse by carrying out the instructions exactly, even though your patient may not like the procedures that the physician asks you to perform. Be sure that you bring to the physician's attention anything that needs clarification. Feel free to question orders and instructions if there is any doubt in your mind, and do not carry out orders if you think that there might be a mistake in the way they were written. The nurse is responsible for any action performed regardless of the orders. It is your responsibility to know the expected results of your ministrations before you carry them out (see Legal Aspects). When you are ordering or purchasing medications, ask the pharmacist to include descriptive literature regarding the medication if you are not familiar with it, so that you will know its mode of administration, usual dosage, and any side-reactions or dangerous symptoms that should be watched for.

Charting must be accurate and, if you are taking care of a patient in an institution, charts must be kept according to hospital policies. Charts are legal documents, and they must be kept and recorded accurately, even in the home. The condition of the patient, medications, treatments, and vital signs (such as temperature, pulse, respirations, blood pressure), nourishment taken, sleep and rest, processes of elimination, and fluid intake and output, are only some of the items that must be recorded. This chart in the home setting may become your possession, to be released to the physician upon request.

Although hospital private duty nursing does not require that you have your own personal equipment (other than scissors, pen, and a watch with a second hand), home nursing does. The nurse doing private duty in a home will find that inexpensive, disposable versions of equipment (emesis basins, bed pans, packaged dressings, enemas, syringes, and needles) as well as the ability to improvise are essential in helping to reduce the patient's expense. In addition, you are usually expected to own your own charting material, stethoscope, and blood pressure apparatus (sphygmomanometer). Remember, also, that in home nursing, though you are directly responsible to the physician, the medical and nursing team is not as readily available to assist you in an emergency as it is in the hospital. Narcotics and other medications left for you must be returned to the physician before you leave the patient.

Meal preparation, food purchasing, and many other housekeeping duties involved in home nursing will vary with the community in which you are practicing and the family that hires you. These obligations will depend, too, on the terms under which you were hired. The Registry rules usually state your responsibilities. It is imperative that you abide by them and be aware of the scope of the work outlined. The Licensed Practical Nurse Associations suggest salary scales, which are usually three fourths of the scale for the RN. In many states the current rate is $56 to 66 for eight hours of consecutive duty. If services are specifically requested on an hourly basis, and the total time does not exceed three hours per day, the first hour or fraction thereof is charged at $12, with each successive hour or fraction thereof at $10. In addition, the Official Registry usually has a Code of Ethics and Conduct for its members, and this office will enforce its standards in the local community or state in which you may be practicing.

In the health care facility, as in the home, you must remember that the private duty nurse always shows tact, respect, and understanding. You must realize that you are a guest and therefore must conform to the policies and the regulations of the institution or the customs of the home. Private duty nurses for institutional work are secured through the nursing office and must be familiar with the regulations of the institution. The private duty nurse is directly responsible to the head nurse of the area and must practice nursing skills in accordance with the rules and the regulations issued by the nursing office. Above all, you must be loyal to the institution in which you are currently working and must not discuss the advantages or the disadvantages of this institution with the patient or with other hospital employees.

The nursing office is responsible for all personnel doing nursing care. Therefore, if at any time the private duty nurse does not meet its health, social, ethical, or emotional standards, or if the quality of nursing is substandard, the nurse will be counseled by the supervisor; if this is not effective, he or she may be suspended by the Private Duty Nurse Committee representative or by the nursing office supervisor. If you are working in the home, you must prepare your own work schedules and patient-care routines so that you do not interfere with family routines.

The chief drawbacks in private duty nursing are the irregular hours and the economic uncertainty, since there are no guarantees as to the availability of work or, sometimes, even payment. To be reimbursed, the nurse should have the Registry statements for services rendered, or similar forms, which can be purchased in a stationery store. The statement usually is presented to the patient or family on a weekly basis, or at the termination of employment. In case of a patient's death, tact must be used with the patient's family; it is usually advisable to mail the statement to the patient's home, family, or attorney. Private duty nurses are covered by Social Security and must pay this as well as income tax; therefore, accurate records and a sound bookkeeping system should be maintained on a current and continuous basis, including names and addresses of patients, length of service, earnings, professional expenses, and any other necessary information. A sample is outlined in Table 9-1.

Institutional Work

The graduate practical nurse has many opportunities for demonstrating nursing skills in a hospital, and it is often here that the most personal satisfaction in practicing is to be found.

To the patient, the bedside nurse is usually the hospital's most important person. The nurse is with the patient for longer periods of time than the physician, and is more readily available. Your genuine interest in taking care of the sick will be as asset in this type of employment. Every day you will be busily engaged in patient care and will work as a teammate with RNs, doctors, social workers, dieticians, laboratory personnel, and others in caring for the sick, promoting health, and preventing further illness. Your scope of work will depend on the organization of nursing care and the definition of your duties, as well as on your training and work experiences. In most institutions, patient care is performed by RNs, practical nurses, nurse technicians, aides, orderlies, and attendants. Usually, the specific duties and responsibilities of all of these employees are described carefully in a job analysis; it is important for you to know what each person is expected to do, including yourself, so that your own role is defined clearly.

The nurse may participate in total patient care as a primary nurse or by being either a team member of (if qualified and the patient's condition warrants it) a team leader. You usually will receive your patient-care assignment from the charge nurse or team leader who is responsible for all the patients in the unit. You will then report back to the team leader or charge nurse the conditions of your patients, the results of treatments, and the completion of assignments. In addition to patient-care duties, it is expected that the nurse will see the unit as a whole and will show interest and understanding in assuming a place on the nursing team, assisting as needed. The nurse is expected by the employer to know all personnel policies and to be punctual, well-groomed, courteous, reliable, and ethical in all work relationships. In many institutions it is expected also that the LPN will become a member of the Licensed Practical Nurse Association, participate in any activities that may help vocational development, and attend all meetings and educational programs as assigned.

Nursing employees usually work a certain tour of duty or "shift." This may vary, but usually the day tour is from 7 AM to 3:30 PM; the afternoon or PM tour is from 3 PM to 11:30 PM; and the night tour is from 11 PM to 7:30 AM. In emergency staffing situations, and in order to safeguard patient care, some hospitals rotate their personnel or will expect them to work other hours or tours as indicated, including 10- and 12-hour tours. Days off usually are scheduled two weeks in advance, and special requests for particular days off must be submitted to the head nurse, usually the week preceding the posting of the time sheets or weekly schedule of nursing activities. Weekends and holidays are usually rotated, so that everyone has an equal opportunity for them.

There are many advantages in institutional work. Steady employment, with advantageous personnel policies, makes this position superior to many others and often compensates for some of the day-to-day problems and dissatisfactions. The practical nurse may choose a specialty area in a general hospital, or perhaps work in hospitals specifically intended for tuberculosis, pediatric, psychiatric, or other categories of patients. Your experience is varied, and the opportunities for learning are ample.

In hospital work the practical nurse will find many opportunities to extend the

TABLE 9-1. SAMPLE MONTHLY ACCOUNTING RECORD FOR PRIVATE DUTY PRACTICAL NURSE

Patient's Name	Address	Doctor	From-To	Payment	Comments
Zimmerman, Lois	1150 N. Meridian	Nathanson	5/1 to 5	$300	Chart to Dr. Went to St. Joseph's
Glockenspiel, Marion	Mount Zion	Green, L.	5/9 to 11	$180	Died
Andrews, Michael	St. Joseph's	Smith, B.	5/23 to 27	$200 Owe $100	Pd. 5/26
Johnson, Tina	4905 S. Benton	O'Leary	5/30 to 31	$120	Chart to Dr.

range of nursing skills. It is important to remember that State Boards of Nursing, as well as individual hospitals, will set their policies as to what you should or should not do, regardless of your preparation and experience. However, if your nursing skills are safely and well performed in those emergency situations for which the RN is not available, you will prove your abilities to others around you. You will then slowly but surely be able to carry out these responsibilities when the RN is present and available and thereby free the RN for other, more responsible duties. If you have been taught skilled procedures in your school program, or in a sound inservice program, do not hesitate to practice them, with supervision, so that your patients will receive safe care.

The LPN Charge Nurse

With the passage of Public Law 89-97, Title 18 (Medicare) and Title 19 (Medicaid), plus the changes in the accreditation standards for nursing homes, extended care, and related facilities, the use of the LPN as a charge nurse has become more and more acceptable. Both NAPNES and NFLPN have participated in the preparation of courses for LPNs who will assume these positions. These references are available from these organizations, and you may wish to write for them. Vocational schools, junior colleges, employers, and practical nursing organizations sponsor continuing education programs; you are urged to attend a course before you accept a position with the responsibilities of charge nurse.

Your main responsibilities revolve around the proper use of the nursing personnel assigned to you and the necessary supplies and equipment. Your patient care and personnel management will require many additional skills that you must develop. Satisfied patients and personnel reflect the leadership abilities that you, as charge nurse, must possess. Leadership skills are not inherited! They are developed by conscientious effort and sincere interest. Good human relationships are the foundation upon which you build your leadership potential. Qualities of good leadership include characteristics such as listening with an open mind, being emotionally mature, fairness, consistency, an outstanding character, exemplary performance, humanism, sensitivity, teaching ability, responsibility, and a problem-solving capacity (see job description, Appendix D, p. 267).

Office Nursing

The office of a physician or a dentist provides opportunities for the LPN who also has receptionist or secretarial talents. Usually, the office nurse is an efficient "jack of all trades." In addition to nursing duties, routine responsibilities in the office may include laboratory work; taking the patient's history; patient education; housekeeping of offices, waiting, and examining rooms; sterilizing equipment and instruments; requisitioning supplies and equipment; taking periodic inventories; and handling correspondence and office bookkeeping. The job of office nurse will vary with the specialty of the physician and the size of the practice. In offices in which several physicians share the premises, a receptionist or other personnel may be employed. Many physicians delegate routine treatments, changes of dressings, injections, and the collection of fees to their office nurse; therefore, you should be able to carry out such duties with ease and speed.

Your working conditions will vary with the physician, but be sure that you understand your responsibilities, working hours, and when and how your salary will be paid. Make sure that you will be working with a reputable physician before you accept this type of position. You can check with the county medical society as to whether or not this physician is licensed to practice.

Nursing and Convalescent Homes (Extended Care Facilities)

These institutions are becoming more common throughout the United States, since the general hospital usually will not care for chronic disease and geriatric patients except on an emergency basis or if they are acutely ill. The short-stay hospitals may transfer these patients to convalescent or nursing homes for further therapy as soon as the acute condition is taken care of. Good nursing and convalescent homes are badly needed throughout the country. These facilities are often supported by federal assistance, and with the increased cost of living, they are likely to be inadequately financed. Licensing of these homes has become the responsibility of the State Departments of Health and Welfare, and very often temporary approval is given even to substandard homes because patients could not be transferred elsewhere because of a lack of accommodations. While medical research is busily engaged in lengthening the life-span and improving treatment of the diseases of old age, the nurse plays a vital part in the care of geriatric patients. A nurse in this type of setting must be genuinely interested in older people and understand the mental, social, economic, rehabilitative, physical, and preventive aspects of their care. Reality orientation, occupational, recreational, and diversional therapy technics help to keep these people useful and contented.

Usually, one RN must be employed in a nursing or convalescent home to supervise routine care and to recognize symptoms that may lead to serious illness. A physician must be on call, and is responsible for standing orders or those that are written in advance and may be used as reference. Although the salaries and the working conditions in these homes do not always measure up to those of other institutional settings, the opportunities for advancement in nursing homes are much better, and as the standards of patient care improve, many practical nurses will find satisfaction in these facilities. The work atmosphere is usually more congenial and less formal, and here the older and more mature nurse may develop many friendships. Practical nurses who accept the challenge of providing quality care in these settings are true agents of change.

Occupational Health

There are many job opportunities for the practical nurse in industrial and commercial agencies as well as in labor unions and other organizations that have shown an increased interest in health programs for their members and employees. Health programs for employees are usually under the supervision and the administration of physicians and RNs; however, many of them employ qualified practical nurses as assistants. The industrial nurse must know what kind of work is performed by all employees, the skilled and unskilled laborers as well as the "white collar" workers. In order to plan safety and accident prevention programs, any industrial nurse must be aware of health and safety hazards and also the general relationship between management and employees. The nurse is usually very closely allied with both employees and employer and therefore must be able to understand the nature of the occupation, as well as the personal and health problems of the employees.

In some industries there are pre-employment as well as periodic physical examinations, various other health appraisal measures, and an active emergency and incidental care program. First aid care may be provided directly, and there may be screening tests for vision and hearing as well as regular diagnostic surveys for cancer, diabetes, tuberculosis, and other diseases. Job responsibilities of the industrial nurse will vary with each industry. The working conditions as well as the salaries will usually be better than those found in institutional nursing.

Psychiatric Nursing

Although psychiatric nursing experience is not a requirement for practical nurses, some schools are adding this specialty to their curriculum, since the role of the practical nurse in this type of care is becoming more and more important. Nonprofessional nursing personnel have been working in this specialty for a long time, and the RN complement is usually extremely low in relation to patient census. Practical nurses who are trained and qualified, and, even more important, who are tolerant, understanding, and able to derive personal satisfaction from rendering care to patients who have emotional disturbances, are encouraged to investigate the career opportunities in mental hospitals, psychiatric institutions, community mental health clinics, and mental health agencies. You will find that there is an extreme shortage of nurses in most institutions dealing with the mentally ill, and your inquiry will be welcomed. There are numerous opportunities for advancement after inservice programs and on-the-job training programs have qualified you. If you are mature (not necessarily in years alone) and able to carry out the job responsibilities, you will probably be able to advance to a leadership position in this type of institution. Salaries and working conditions vary, of course, but they compare favorably with those of other institutional work.

Community Health Nursing

The public health, visiting, and home health care nurse goes *out* to nurse patients and participates in local or state public and private health programs. The public health nurse usually works for an official health agency, whereas the visiting nurse represents various voluntary community health care agencies. Included in the public health programs are school and preschool health programs, communicable disease control clinics with immunization and treatment programs, health supervision of expectant and delivered mothers and newborn infants, home visits for health education, specific treatments or bedside care for patients, as well as other curative and preventive programs. The home health care or visiting nurse provides skilled nursing care and supportive services to a sick or disabled person at the place of residence. These services are both therapeutic and preventive.

Usually, the practical nurse employed by the public or private health agency must be able to drive and be one of the experienced practitioners of home nursing. Perhaps the most important qualifications for a community health nurse include an interest in people, the ability to get along with them and to accept them for what they are, without any racial or religious prejudices, and the ability to help others to help themselves. An RN is usually responsible for the practical nurse, and your "case load," clinic assignments, school nurse responsibilities, and other duties will be assigned to you by your supervisor once your personality and nursing ability have been evaluated. Working conditions and salaries are equivalent to those in institutions. Since these agencies are usually closed after 5 PM, as well as on weekends and holidays (with nurses on call for emergencies), many nurses have found that this type of position permits more convenient working hours than any other.

EVALUATING POSITIONS

Every job has advantages and disadvantages; there is never a perfect one. However, by knowing personnel policies, regulations, job responsibilities and duties, salary scales, travel and transportation factors, work environment, relationships with employer and other employees, reputation of employer-to-be, and other factors, you will be able to compare preferred positions and thereby make an intelligent choice.

Salary

Very often you may read an advertisement stating that the salary for a certain position is $900 monthly. Do you know how this will be paid per day if you are ill? Are you entitled to sick leave, holidays, and vacation time? It is also important to know whether you work five days (40 hours) or more per week, and whether or not your benefits are calculated on a five-day week. Let us compare two positions and see which choice should be yours, provided that all other conditions are equal.

One position offers $920 monthly for a 40-hour week, 12 days annual sick leave cumulative to 36 days, eight legal or religious holidays, plus two weeks vacation with pay upon completion of 12 months of consecutive employment. The other position pays $225 a week for a 40-hour week, offers 10 work days sick leave per year cumulative to 30 work days, eight legal or religious holidays per year, and two weeks vacation with pay upon completion of 12 months of consecutive employment. At first glance you might select the position paying $920 a month, but let us examine these positions more closely. What are the annual salaries? Twelve times $920 equals $11,040, whereas $225 times 52 weeks equals $11,700; therefore, if you chose the $225-a-week position, you would be earning $660 more annually, or about $55 more per month. Those 12 sick days cumulative to 36 would mean five weeks plus one day sick time with pay, if you had a serious illness. The other position would mean six weeks of pay, since 30 days calculated on a five-day week would entitle you to four more days with pay. If you average around $45 per day, this would mean an additional $180. Your eight holidays would mean one week plus one day in the first position, whereas in the other it would mean one week plus three days; therefore, an additional $90 would be yours. It is plain to see that it is important to calculate your earnings realistically and understand the value of comparing the weekly scale versus the monthly scale, as well as the five-day benefit and the weekly one. This illustration should prove to you that you must find out as much as possible about financial arrangements; no position should ever be accepted on the salary alone.

Increment scales, tour differentials, merit increases based on additional educational or on-the-job experience and inservice training, as well as the job responsibilities involved, will all determine your present and future earnings and your satisfaction.

Usually, your employer will make the following paycheck deductions: Social Security, Federal withholding tax, and your insurance payments (depending on what policies you carry). These deductions are actually to your advantage, since you will be able to have accurate reports for your income tax filing given to you at the required time.

Vacations and Sick Leave

These benefits are usually granted to permanent employees in institutions and agencies upon completion of one to 12 months of consecutive employment. During the first year of employment, vacation and sick days may be prorated or accumulated on a monthly basis. Usually, this means that you will earn one day of sick leave and/or vacation time for every month worked. Sometimes vacations are not accumulated from year to year unless special arrangements are made. Also, in some places of employment you must take your vacation at an assigned time with no choice in the matter. Sick leave with pay is usually granted to those employees who are ill and not able to work. It is not meant to be additional time off with pay, although some institutions calculate these days and add them to a "pool" to be used by you as extra vacation days or leaves of absence. Upon your return from a sick leave, your employer may ask that you report to the personnel physician, or that you bring a note from your private physician, stating that you are able to return to work.

Leaves of Absence and Holiday Time

It is customary to use holiday time to make up for those days when you actually cannot work. Some institutions may grant a leave of absence with pay for a few days when there is a death in the employee's immediate family. If you are on jury duty, you may be paid the difference between jury pay and your actual salary. On Election Day you should be allowed time to vote. Each employer has a set standard for religious and legal holidays, which usually are not cumulative from year to year and may not always be granted on the actual day of the holiday. In each instance these days with pay must be arranged for you through your superior. If you are absent without reason or explanation, your employer may terminate (fire) you. Therefore, as soon as you know that you will be unable to report on duty, you should notify your supervisor immediately, so that this absence may be accounted for properly, and a replacement found.

Transportation

Although not many nurses consider their transportation expenses an important aspect in choosing employment, you should give this matter some serious thought. The location of your job in relation to your home should be considered, since both time and the mode of transportation to be used are expensive and add up. If you live in the nurses' residence or on the premises, there are many savings involved, since you will usually have lower rent and are withing walking distance of your work. If you have your own car or share transportation expenses with someone else, it might be interesting for you to figure out what this would amount to on an annual basis. Carfare and distance of travel, type of connections in case you might be delayed, and other points should be considered carefully before accepting a position. However, do not let this govern your choice entirely. I know of a nurse who spends $1 a day for carfare in preference to working in an institution just across the street from where she lives. She feels that the $5 a week more she would be making in that institution would not compensate for her "peace of mind" and the satisfaction of doing the work for which she is suited. This is something that only you can decide, but do remember that money is not everything, even though it is important.

Reputation of Employer

Just as you are expected to give references to the employer so that your credentials, character, and ability may be checked, it is also important for you to know whether your employer is an honest, capable, understanding, and otherwise desirable person or institution to work for. Health and welfare agencies, hospitals, nursing homes, physicians, and others employing nurses can be checked for reputation standards at the County Medical Society, the Welfare Board, the Health

Department, or other controlling boards. The larger the institution, the more rigid its standards may be. Research and teaching hospitals are usually accredited by the Joint Commission on Accreditation of Hospitals, the American Medical Association, the American College of Surgeons, and State Boards of Nursing. Nursing homes fall under the inspection of health and welfare departments. Physicians and dentists must be licensed in the state in which they are practicing and are usually listed with the County Medical or Dental Societies. It is important for the office-nurse-to-be to check on the licensure and the reputation of the physician hiring you so as not to endanger your license by malpractice or assisting in illegal medical or nursing practices.

Insurance Benefits

For the welfare of employees, many employers have made various insurance policies and types of coverage available. Some of this coverage may be optional, and in other situations it may be mandatory. It is necessary that you realize the importance of insurance and perhaps compare the available plans with others of a similar nature to evaluate the saving you may realize. Blue Cross and Blue Shield insurance plans are usually required, often as a part of your employment conditions. Since you would be a member of group insurance, your payments probably would be much smaller than if you carried this protection on your own. Group life insurance policies may be available at nominal cost, with perhaps part of the payment met by your employer. In addition, there may be pensions, retirement programs, and other plans available to you. Worker's Compensation is usually provided to employees in institutional settings, which will entitle you to receive certain benefits while recovering form any disabling accident connected with your work. This cost is met entirely by the employer, and you should be acquainted with the accident policy. Malpractice insurance is carried by some physicians, who may decide to protect their nursing personnel as well, and since lawsuits for malpractice are becoming more and more prevalent, you should decide to carry this type of insurance for yourself. State LPN associations and NAPNES should have information as to the savings and the advantages of group policies.

Promotional Opportunities

Even though the practical nurse's duties are subject to certain legal restrictions, in deciding on a position you might like to know whether there are regular salary increments and perhaps a merit system by which you would have annual, monthly, or weekly financial increases as you grow in responsibility and the performance of your duties. Some institutions also may have a classification system by which your salary is determined. In one hospital, for instance, the Class 3 practical nurse is one with or without a license (but eligible for licensure) who is able to perform all nursing duties with the exception of dispensing medications; the Class 2 nurse can give medications and does total patient care; and the Class 1 practical nurse is able to assume total patient care and, in addition, may have had some specialized or postgraduate education or experience. The salary differential from Class 3 to Class 1 may be as high as $40 a week, or $2,080 annually.

Laundry and Uniforms

One of the fringe benefits that most nurses welcome is the availability of free laundry services for their uniforms. When you consider the expense and the time involved in doing your own uniforms, you will appreciate an employer who may furnish this service to you free of charge. However, new synthetic fabrics have simplified laundering problems; therefore, you will find that more and more employers are no longer assuming the responsibility for laundering of uniforms.

Inservice Education

One of the most important educational programs in today's hospital or agency is that of Inservice and Orientation, whereby you will be able to keep yourself up to date on the current trends in patient care as well as specific nursing procedures. In some institutions special inservice classes may be conducted in medications, leadership, and in specific types of nursing, such as nursery, recovery room, emergency room, or labor and delivery, thereby offering you additional training without the necessity of a postgraduate course. You earn your regular salary while attending these classes in many institutions and meet the continuing education requirements for relicensure in some states.

Other Points to Consider

Only the most important aspects of selecting a position have been discussed, and although appearances may be deceiving, the physical environment in which you work will influence your morale and therefore your work performance as well. The availability and the condition of equipment, the hours of work, rotation policies, uniform regulations, and the prevailing morale should be considered. Is the employer progressive, or hard to convince that times have changed, and that there are more modern methods which can make work more pleasant and enable you to give more efficient and safer care to your patients? Keep such questions in mind as you make up a list of preferred positions. Inquire about the employer's policies, so that you may obtain full understanding of the responsibilities and the benefits involved.

FINDING A POSITION

Since nurses are in constant demand, you should have no difficulty in finding a position. Positions may be found through word of mouth, advertisements, placement agencies, your school, and by directly contacting hospitals and other health care agencies. Let us examine the advantages and the disadvantages of all of these methods of obtaining employment.

Word of Mouth

You hear about an opening in a doctor's office, your friend tells you that a neighbor needs a nurse, a patient asks you if you know someone who could take care of him while he convalesces at home, or perhaps your head nurse asks you to work on after graduation. What's wrong here? Nothing, certainly, but be sure that you approach your employer-to-be with some knowledge of duties involved, salary scale, working conditions, and so on, before you accept a position on someone else's word. A personal interview in which you can exchange your ideas with the employer is most certainly indicated.

Advertisements

A look at the classified section of the daily newspapers, professional magazines, journals, and other media will indicate that nurses are needed and wanted. Read the advertisement through and understand what it tells you. Do not presume that the position has a 40-hour week or excellent personnel policies until you have had a chance to see some of this in writing, and if you are writing to the advertiser, ask for an application blank as well as a copy of the salary scale and the personnel policies. If a visit can give you the answers, ask for an interview to discuss the position offered. An advertisement is only a lead; it cannot tell you the whole story.

Placement Agencies

There are many employment agencies in every community that, for a fee, will be very happy to find a position for you. The commercial registry or employment office is in many instances interested only in the fee you pay them and will not investigate the position for you, or they may give you only the information that they have obtained from the person who contacted them. The Official Registry of LP/VNs sometimes combined with that of RNs and operated under the auspices of the state Nurses Association, will usually be more seriously concerned with the standards of the nurse as well as those of the employer. The care of the patient, the reputation of the nurse, and the dignity and the conduct of all involved are the Registry's concern. The Official Registry usually maintains a 24-hour service, seven days a week, and caters primarily to private duty nurses. Members of the Official Registry pay registry dues that are far less than the percentage (sometimes the weekly salary fee) charged by the commerical registries. Members must be in good standing with the local Licensed Practical Nurse Association, which sets the employment standards and the salary scale and also disciplines its members when indicated. Although the Official Registry does not guarantee employment to all its registrants, it distributes the calls for private duty, hospital staff relief, and other nursing positions according to the duties required as well as the nurse "on call." Official Registries are preferred by employers; therefore, you should look for one in your community before applying to a commercial registry. Registries usually advertise in newspapers and journals, and are listed also in the "yellow pages" of the telephone book.

Schools

Around graduation time most directors of schools of practical nursing receive calls and letters regarding opportunities for the graduates. Look on your bulletin board and discuss your hopes for employment with your director or representative. Your school faculty members are interested in placing their graduates in the best-suited positions, hoping thereby to build a sound reputation for their program. Some alumnae associations may decide to run their own registries and contact hospitals, physicians, nursing homes, or public health agencies asking for lists, each fall or spring, of the positions they need filled, thereby giving alumnae members a free placement service.

Hospitals and Other Health Care Facilities

Openings in institutional settings for the practical nurse are usually obtained by contacting the personnel or nursing office of the agency concerned. You may save yourself a registry fee by writing or calling the hospital or the agency of your choice to ascertain if there are any vacancies. If there are none at that time, you may ask for and submit an application, so that it will be on file if an opening should occur, and you can call for an interview.

The Interview

A personal interview is advantageous both to the employer and the prospective employee. It will give you a first-hand opportunity to obtain answers to your questions regarding the position, you will see the place where you hope to work, and perhaps you will have the opportunity to observe some of the activities and the people. The employer will be able to ask you questions regarding your education and experience and to observe your general appearance and your personality. Prepare for an interview carefully. First impressions, although not always accurate, are most important in selling yourself. Be neat and well-groomed and arrive on time. Ask questions concerning the position, your responsibilities, the work conditions, personnel regulations, and any other matter important to you. Remember, the interviewer will judge you by the questions that you ask or do not ask. If you are required to fill out an application form, be sure that you do so in ink—neatly, accurately, and completely. Know your license and Social Security numbers, your school graduation dates, the names and the addresses (with correct spelling) of your references, and any other vital information usually asked for on applications. When listing or using names as references on an application form or during the interview, be sure that you have permission to do so. It is customary for an employer to check references as well as former places of employment. In order to select the best qualified applicant, some employers may administer pre-employment examinations to test your nursing knowledge and skills.

You should call or write the employer for a definite interview appointment to discuss the position for which you are applying. If you have an appointment, it usually means that you do not have to wait. Larger institutions may have someone in the personnel department available five days a week to screen applicants and refer the best candidates to the nursing department for final decisions. If you are waiting to see an employer, be sure that you know his or her name. During your interview, relax, be natural and friendly, and think your sentences through. If you have some questions written down that you wish to discuss, refer to your list unobtrusively and ask them in an intelligent manner. Do not boast of your abilities or exaggerate your potentials; discuss your former duties in a simple, matter-of-fact fashion. Your employer will be able to judge your capabilities in a very short time; if you have oversold yourself, you may not meet the qualifications as you continue in the position. Be sure that you know exactly what position you are being interviewed for or are accepting, and that you know the duties, the salary, and the personnel policies before you accept. If there are several applicants for a position that you are seriously interested in, make your interest known before you leave. Thank the interviewer, and ask to be notified whether or not you are acceptable, so that you may look elsewhere for employment if need be. Conversely, if the position is not what you want, say so frankly thanking the interviewer for the granted time.

The Written Application and Resume

If you are moving into another community and would like to find out what positions are available to you, you can write to the hospitals and registries in that area to ascertain possible openings. Another method might be to send for the local newspapers, check the advertisements, and correspond with the persons placing the ads. Letters of application should always be neatly written in ink or typewritten. Prospective employers will judge you by your application; its appearance and content are all that they have to go on. If it is well written, it may pave the way for further consideration. Write your letter carefully, observing the principles of correct letter writing; be brief and accurate and do not enclose any photographs, references, diplomas, or other materials unless the advertisement specifies this. Be careful of legibility, spelling, and punctuation, and be courteous. State the position for which you are applying, the source of your information, your experience and qualifications, and the dates when you are available for an interview and for starting employment, if you are accepted. If you are writing to a large institution, you may merely request an application form.

When applying to smaller institutions, you may wish to include a personal resume. Your resume should include your education, work experience, organizational membership, continuing education, publications, and honors. The information should be listed in chronological order and be brief.

Sample letters and resume follow.

190 Maple Street
Lake George, N.Y. 12845
January 5, 19-

Ms. Elizabeth Van Metre, R.N.
Director of Nursing
Jackson Hospital
Jackson, New Jersey 08527

Dear Ms. Van Metre:

Through Dr. Hubert Kennedy I learned that you might be in need of licensed practical nurses. I am a graduate licensed practical nurse and will apply for endorsement in New Jersey in the near future.

My husband and I are moving to Jackson after March 1, since he has accepted a position with General Aircraft Corporation. Would you please send me an application form, as well as a salary scale, a statement of personnel policies, and a listing of the positions that you have available? If you do have a position available, I would then write again to arrange for a personal interview at a mutually convenient time.

Sincerely yours,
(Mrs.) Josephine Malloy, L.P.N.

Nurses Residence
Mount Sinai Hospital
Miami Beach, Fla. 33141
February 12, 19-

Mr. Roger Wilson, L.P.N.
Division No. 9, Registry Chairman,
Licensed Practical Nurse Association of Florida, Inc.
Security Building
Miami, Fla. 33040

Dear Mr. Wilson:

Through one of your members, Mrs. Hanna Hermle, I learned that you are looking for private duty nurses. Please consider me an applicant as of March 15, when I will be leaving my present position, since I find hospital nursing too strenuous for me.

I have been a member of your organization for the past three years but need a copy of the Registry rules, as well as an application form.

Sincerely yours,
(Miss) Anita Reynolds, L.P.N.

165 N.W. 85th Street
Jamaica Heights, N.Y. 11414
February 8, 19-

Dr. Angela Jacobs
Physicians Building
Jamaica Heights, N.Y. 11433

Dear Doctor Jacobs:

Please consider me as an applicant for the position you advertised in today's copy of <u>The Herald</u>. From the description of the position I feel that this would appeal to me, since I am seriously considering office nursing as a career.

I am a graduate licensed practical nurse and for the past year have been working for a pediatrician; however, I feel that I cannot do my best with children, and would prefer adult patients. I am familiar with billing, office schedules, laboratory work-ups, as well as with injections, treatments and other nursing procedures.

May I have an interview at your earliest convenience? You may reach me at the above address, or by calling 782-3611 between 9 A.M. and 6 P.M., or 866-1636 after 7 P.M. The physician for whom I am currently working realizes that I am anxious to make a change and has given me permission to use his name as a reference. He is Dr. Meyer Weil, located in the Medical Building; I believe that you might know him.

I will be happy to send you any further information that you may desire.

Sincerely yours,
(Ms.) Kitty Galen, L.P.N.

1940 West Street
Homeville, Florida 33148
July 21, 19-

Mrs. Henrietta Walsh, R.N.
Get-Well Home Health Care
23 Recovery Road
Plantation, Florida 33194

Dear Mrs. Walsh:

Enclosed you will find my resume. Please keep it on file in case a vacancy in your L.P.N. staff occurs. I am attending Homeville Community College to become a registered nurse and, since I must rotate tours of duty at Mercy Hospital, I find that I cannot do justice to my classes. When I spoke to your secretary she advised me that you like to have resumes on file. I would be happy to come for an interview and take your pre-employment medication examination.

I look forward to hearing from you.

Sincerely,
Susan L. Smith

Resume of

Mrs. Susan L. Smith, L.P.N.
1940 West Street
Homeville, Fla. 33148
305-126-9345

Education:
1981	Part-time student in L.P.N./A.D.N. Transition Program, Homeville Community College
1980	Diploma – South East Technical Center, Homeville, Fla. 33148
1979	Diploma – Homeville H.S., Homeville, Fla. 33148

Experience:
1980	Graduate Practical Nurse and L.P.N., Mercy Hospital, Medical–Surgical Unit, Homeville, Fla. 33156
1978-80	Nursing Assistant, Homeville Convalescent Center, Homeville, Fla. 33148

Membership and Offices Held:
1981	Board member, Florida Licensed Practical Nurse Assn., Div. #9
1980	Nominating Committee, Florida Licensed Practical Nurse Assn., Div. #9
1979	Secretary, Practical Nursing Student Organization, S.E. Technical Center

Continuing Education:
8/80-12/80	3 CEUs Spanish for Health Care Personnel, Homeville Community College

Honors:
1980	Certificate of Appreciation, American Cancer Society

RESIGNATIONS

If you are unhappy in your position, are offered more money elsewhere, have opportunities for further education and advancement, or perhaps must leave the community in which you are living, you probably will resign from the position that you now hold. However, you should remember that there are no perfect positions; and before you decide to "just quit," it would be well for you to look around and see whether you would be happier if you made a change. It might be helpful to discuss certain problems concerning job dissatisfaction with your supervisors or employer to see if at least some of them could be resolved. If you are planning to leave because of a personality clash, an unsatisfactory work situation, or other differences, you might discuss these difficulties with the person responsible for personnel management. Perhaps a transfer to another tour or area in a large institution might remedy the situation. You would thereby keep your seniority and your employment benefits, which include sick, holiday, and vacation time, as well as perhaps a salary increase that may be due. It is important to realize that it usually takes from six months to a year for an employee to get to know the job's responsibilities and to be able to carry them out competently. During the second year you will probably be a good practitioner of your position, and by the third year you should be a valuable member of the staff. Before resigning from your position you should always discuss your prospects with your immediate supervisor, so that you can be fair to your employer and, at the same time, try to solve your problems. However, even when you are definitely planning to resign, you should continue to do your very best and to remain loyal to your employer.

It is always best to leave with a good feeling toward your coworkers and superiors. You are usually required to give notice of resignation equivalent to the number of vacation days you are entitled to. If possible, an even longer period of time should be given. Consider the importance of your position as well as the responsiblities involved; if you will have to train your replacement, you should consider how long it might take to find a suitable person, and also how much time will be required to have him or her assume your duties competently. If you leave without adequate notice, regardless of the reasons, you will automatically forfeit your accrued benefits; and in most instances your future references from this employer will contain that information. If it is impossible for you to give proper notice, be sure that you express your regrets and explain the situation fully, so that your employer will understand the circumstances.

Some institutions have official resignation forms, and on these you are asked to state your reason or reasons for leaving. In other situations you might wish to write your own letter of resignation. Sometimes you may discuss this with your employer, and this may preclude a written notification. In a brief and courteous manner, state your reasons for leaving and then discuss these matters more fully during your terminal interview. A resignation should not include accusations, resentment, or bitterness, but rather an expression of regret that you are leaving. If you have enjoyed your work and your associations have been pleasant, say so. Remember that gratitude is appreciated, and that once you have left the position, you will not want to have done or said things that you may regret, or that might be held against your record at a later date.

The date you expect to leave should be stated clearly in your resignation. If you expect to have your days off, holidays, or vacation benefits included in your terminal paycheck, or if you expect to take this time before you leave, such information should be included. The resignation, in a sealed envelope, should be addressed to your immediate supervisor or to your employer. If you were hired by the director of nursing, or, in some instances, the director of personnel, your resignation should be sent to that person. In your work relationships you must remember that your resignation usually becomes part of your permanent record; therefore, you should conduct yourself in an ethical manner. To be able to use your last employer as a reference is most essential in obtaining a new position. Below are samples of resignations.

271 Avenue C
New York City, N.Y. 10009
December 12, 19-

Mrs. Florence Jennings, R.N.
Director of Nursing
New York General Hospital
900 Fifth Avenue
New York City, N.Y. 10021

Dear Mrs. Jennings:
  After our discussion yesterday, and after much serious thought, I have come to the conclusion that I must resign from my position as Staff L.P.N. on 4th Floor North. I would like to be able to devote more time to my family and perhaps do staff relief nursing for you when you need me.
  I would like to leave as of January 15, and would appreciate it if I could have my accrued benefits added to my terminal check. I have enjoyed my association with the staff members at General Hospital, and I feel that your in-service programs have assisted me considerably in rendering better nursing care.

                    Sincerely yours,
                    (Mrs.) Norma Stacey, L.P.N.

---

                              45 West 23rd Street
                              New York City, N.Y. 10010
                              December 30, 19-

Dr. Harold Brown
239 Central Park South
New York City, N.Y. 10019

Dear Dr. Brown:
  My husband has been transferred to Homestead Air Force Base in Florida as of January 15; therefore, it is with regret that I must resign from my position as office nurse with you.

I have enjoyed my employment with you during the past two years and have benefited from your guidance and understanding. I hope that I shall be able to train someone to accept my duties before I leave. However, I cannot remain on duty after January 12, since we are leaving for Homestead that evening. I would appreciate being released from duty before that date, if at all possible.

Sincerely yours,
(Mrs.) Helen Jones, L.P.N.

---

475 Riverdale Avenue
Brooklyn, N.Y. 11207
January 18, 19-

Ms. Trudy White, R.N.
Executive Director of
  Visiting Nurse Service of New York
10 West 58th Street
New York City, N.Y. 10019

Dear Ms. White:
  Due to unforeseen circumstances I must resign immediately from my position as staff nurse. My sister died of a heart attack yesterday afternoon, and there is no one to care for her two children.
  I am sorry that I could not give sufficient notice and therefore am forfeiting my benefits; however, I would appreciate anything that you could do for me in that regard, considering the situation. It has been a pleasure working for your agency, and I hope to be able to return someday.

Sincerely yours,
(Mrs.) Abbe Foster, L.P.N.

DISMISSALS

There may be circumstances in which you would be asked to resign from your position, if this were not agreeable to you, you would be dismissed. There are two types of dismissals:

1. An employee may be given notice of termination equivalent to the number of vacation days allowed (usually two weeks). In some instances an employer may decide to give compensation instead of notice. An employee who is dismissed during the probationary period or who was hired for a temporary position, may be discharged without notice and without being entitled to any accrued benefits. This type of dismissal will vary with the policies of the employer, and sometimes the director of personnel may be requested to review any grievances that you may have.

2. An employee may be discharged without notice and paid in full up to the time of dismissal if dishonesty, disobedience, insubordination, or malfeasance (any unlawful or wrong action) is cited as the cause. If terminated under these circumstances, the employee will forfeit all accrued benefits, which usually include holidays and vacation time. In these situations, as in the other type of dismissal discussed, the employee does have the right to discuss the termination further with the supervisor. If the matter is not settled to the employee's satisfaction, it may go to the director of personnel. In situations in which there is no personnel department, the director of the agency or the institution will make the final decision.

LABOR LAWS

There are both state and federal laws that affect all workers, including children. The purpose of these laws is to improve the conditions under which you will work and to give you some protection from hazards such as accidents, unemployment, exploitation, and discrimination. Your state employment and labor service offices will have the most current information available at your request.

The Federal Wage and Hour Law sets wage and hour standards for various workers and requires equal pay for both men and women who have the same work assignment. The law also requires payment of at least a state minimum wage per hour and overtime pay at the rate of one and a half times the regular rate for every hour worked over the 40-hour week. Hospitals and nursing homes are now affected by this law, and your state labor department would be in the best position to advise you regarding the minimum scale in your state. Worker's compensation laws set up a speedy and simple procedure for medical care and for the payment of benefits when an employee is injured in the course of employment. If you should be injured while at work, you may be entitled to medical care and cash benefits for the time you are not able to work, as provided under the state worker's compensation law. All states have these laws but the degree of coverage varies from state to state. Wage payment and collection laws are also in effect, and the state Department of Labor offers help in collecting your salary, which you are entitled to receive promptly and regularly.

Collective Bargaining

Collective bargaining is the process that involves employers and representatives of employees who try to reach agreements covering the employment conditions under which employees should contribute to the organization and how they should be compensated for their contributions. Although the original National Labor Relations Act (NLRA) (or the Wagner Act) became law in 1935, it was not until 1974 that hospitals and other health care institutions were identified as being able to have bargaining units. Licensed practical nurses are usually considered technical employees.

Before the collective bargaining process can begin, it is necessary that a union be recognized as the exclusive bargaining representative for that particular group.

This means that usually 30% of the employees must file a petition and this petition must be filed with the National Labor Relations Board. The union, or representative group. then negotiates a contract with the health care agency and this negotiated contract then becomes a legal means of holding employees and employers accountable. The contract includes negotiated clauses relating to wages, hours, and conditions of work, which are usually called personnel policies. Equity is usually the issue with wage and salary negotiations. Position descriptions will assist in defining the responsibilities.

Whenever there is a deviation from the contract, a grievance may occur and an established grievance procedure may then be followed. You should be familiar with the grievance procedure in any employment setting so that you may follow it. Usually grievances may be resolved by discussion with the immediate supervisor. However, if this is not possible the process continues through management, and may be resolved only at the arbitration level. The arbitration is conducted by an independent outsider or third party who has been given the authority to make final decisions on the issue. This decision is binding to both the employee and the employer. If this decision is not followed, it constitutes a violation of the contract and can be enforced through the judicial system or courts.

State laws take precedence over federal law when certain state laws meet specific standards. It is imperative that you become acquainted with your state law on this topic. Additionally, you should be familiar with the employee organization that would represent you when you select a health care institution as an employer.

YOUR INCOME AND YOU

Money is of basic importance to everyone. Most people waste much of their earnings learning by experience (usually the hard way) how to make the most of their incomes. When you shop, you can stretch your dollars and get more for your money if you plan what to buy, make wise decisions, and know where to shop. Have you ever figured out how much money will pass through your hands during your working years? If you are like most people, you will work between 30 to 45 years. If your average income is about $10,000 and you will be working 30 years, the impressive total is $300,000. This should help you develop an appreciation for your earning and spending capacity. If you are having difficulty in making ends meet, the reason may be a poorly organized budget.

The Budget

There is no ready-made spending or saving plan that will fit everyone. An economic security plan that will work for you personally must be based on your income and the expenses that you must, or want to, incur. You might ask, "What should it cost me to go to school, to support my family, or, exactly how much should it cost me to live?" Some of your friends may manage on less than what you have available, whereas others may have trouble getting along on much more. A good money management plan must be tailored to fit your living requirements

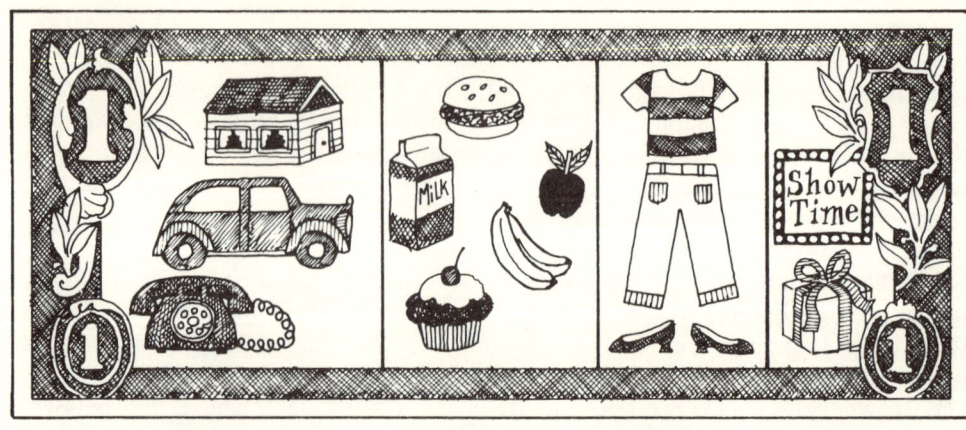

| 30–45% | 30–35% | 25–30% | 10–15% |
| Housing, utilities, transportation | Food | Career expenses, personal items | Recreation, savings |

FIGURE 9-1.   *The budget dollar.*

and your wishes. It cannot be based on the standards of an average or imaginary nurse, since the size of your family, your income, where you live, and other aspects of family life will determine when the necessities end and the luxuries begin.

Once you know what your goals are, you will find a way of fitting them into your spending plan or budget. In addition, you must be able to set up reserves for future fixed expenses, like taxes, or special expenses, such as emergency repairs.

There are several reasons why there can be no simple formulas for budget percentages that automatically supply a satisfactory basis for a spending plan. People are different and even individuals needs differ from time to time. It has been suggested that the budget dollar be allocated as follows: (1) housing, utilities, and transportation 35 to 45%, (2) food, 30 to 35%, (3) clothing, professional expenses and beauty aids, 25 to 30%, and (4) gifts, recreation and savings, 10 to 15% (Figure 9-1). However, with inflation, personal spending has been increasing and savings have been dropping to an all-time low. The cost of housing has risen faster than inflation and mortgage rates are increasing. Wise money management is a must. It is most important to ask yourself before you buy anything: ''Can I afford it? Do I really need it? Could I live without it?''

Your Earnings

Table 9-2 presents a sampling of hourly earnings for licensed practical nurses. The median hourly rate of all practical nurses in 1978 was about $4.76. In the Pacific Coast region practical nurses usually earn higher salaries than those working in the Southeast or the Southwest. Practical nurses employed in doctors' offices, community health agencies, industrial health organizations, and other fields earned higher salaries than those in hospitals. It has been generally accepted that the practical nurse earns approximately three fourths of what the RN earns; however, supply and demand, as well as the salary scales of other employees in the hospital or in the community, will determine the basic nursing salaries.

In estimating your income, consider your take-home pay rather than gross salary. Deductions made from your salary for federal and state taxes, insurance, and Social Security, are not part of your take-home pay. Actual income is figured on your take-home salary plus miscellany, such as stipends, investment returns (dividends from stocks and bonds, and so forth), interest on savings, bonuses, gifts, allowances, and any profit from exchange of property. In budgeting you should consider whether you are paid monthly, twice monthly, or weekly. If you have an irregular income, it is especially important that you manage to keep your expenses at a minimum when your income is at its lowest. Adjustment may also be indicated when your earnings fall below the amount originally estimated. It might be easiest to list the sources of your income, your budget periods, and the total for each period on a chart. Use 12 or 13 lines, depending on when you are paid. If you are paid monthly or twice monthly, use 12 lines and work out your budget on a monthly basis. If you are paid weekly, or every two or four weeks, use 13 lines, working out your budget on a four-week basis.

TABLE 9-2.　AVERAGE HOURLY EARNINGS OF LICENSED PRACTICAL NURSES IN NONGOVERNMENT HOSPITALS AND NURSING HOMES

	Straight time in nursing homes Hourly rate—1978	Full-time in nongovernment hospitals Hourly rate—1978
Atlanta, Ga.	[1]	[1]
Baltimore, Md.	4.80	5.59
Boston, Mass.	4.76	[1]
Buffalo, N.Y.	4.00	4.69
Chicago, Ill.	4.75	5.61
Cleveland, OH.	4.44	5.18
Dallas-Ft. Worth, Tex.	4.52	4.19
Denver-Boulder, Colo.	4.33	4.63
Detroit, Mich.	4.97	5.94
Houston, Tex.	[1]	4.57
Kansas City, Mo.-Kans.	4.30	4.62
Los Angeles-Long Beach, Calif.	5.78	[1]
Miami, Fla.	[1]	[1]
Memphis, Tenn.-Ark.-Miss.	[2]	[1]
Milwaukee, Wisc.	5.40	4.98
Minneapolis-St. Paul	4.91	4.91
New York, N.Y.-N.J.	7.16	6.31
Philadelphia, Pa.	4.78	5.26
Portland, Oreg.	[2]	5.27
St. Louis, Mo.-Ill.	[1]	4.79
San Francisco-Oakland, Calif.	5.30	6.45
Seattle-Everett, Wash.	4.74	4.98
Washington, D.C.-Md.-Va.	4.70	[1]

Source: U. S. Department of Labor, Bureau of Labor Statistics, *Individual Releases*, 1978.
[1] From individual releases. Data for some areas have not yet become available. Releases will be available from the Atlanta, Ga. Regional Office of the Bureau.
[2] This area was not surveyed for Nursing and Personal Care Facilities.

Your Expenses

Your fixed expenses include taxes (federal, property, and sometimes state); monthly rent or mortgage payments, including utilities (electricity, gas, water, and telephone); insurance payments for life, health, accident, fire, theft, liability, personal property, and other types of insurance; interest on loans, as well as regular payments on furniture, car, tuition, and other loans; and miscellaneous expenses, such as licenses, textbooks, and dues.

Expenses that occur daily include food (eaten at home or out); household supplies; transportation; laundry; clothing and clothing repairs; personal needs, such as cosmetics, toiletries, newspapers, postage, entertainment and recreation; gifts; and many more. To find out how much you actually spend, keep a small notebook or other record and write down the actual expenses for a month or two and total them. In planning for them, use the same budget periods as for income and divide them accordingly.

For example, if you are planning to start your budget in January, and your membership dues for the year as well as a quarterly insurance premium totaling $96 are due by April 1 (if you have not as yet saved for these two items in advance), you must set aside $32 monthly in January, February, and March. From then on, however, if you are on a 12-month budget plan, you must set aside one twelfth of the amount of your annual dues and one fourth of the sum of your insurance premium, so that the next time they are due you will have this money in a reserve fund for that purpose.

The first step in successful money management or budgeting is a genuine *desire* to plan and to keep track of your finances. An incentive is to find out what you want and what you need, and once you determine these, you can have fun trying to fit these items into your spending plan. If you can manage your money wisely, you will have many advantages over those who do not. Considerable self-control is needed to maintain a financially secure life. By selecting your purchases with care and not jumping at the first attractive item, you will be able to get the greatest value for your money. You can stretch your dollars further if you become an expert shopper and spend according to a carefully planned budget. A bargain is a bargain only when you really need it.

Credit

If used wisely, credit enables you to get the things you really need, to cover unexpected expenses, and to take care of emergencies. Credit is a means of having now and paying later. Your credit rating usually depends on how promptly you pay your bills, your current salary, how much you owe, and how long you have been employed at and have lived in the same place. Evaluate the need for credit and think carefully before using it; you must be able to afford the extra monthly payments. To figure the cost of credit and credit charges it is simplest to add up all the payments (including the down payment, if there was one) and, from this total, subtract the cash price. The amount left is the cost of the credit. This may vary substantially for different accounts. Be sure you read and understand what you sign. A credit contract can be enforced by law and may include a garnishment clause requiring that a part of the borrower's wages be paid to the creditor. Most employers forbid their employees to involve them in their credit contracts and do not wish to become involved in wage assignments.

FEDERAL INCOME TAX

Like everyone else in the United States, you must file a yearly income tax return. If you are employed by a hospital or in a doctor's office, by industry, or in any other permanent position, you should make sure that you secure the W-2 form, which is a statement of your annual earnings and federal income tax withheld by your employer, if any. This form also includes the total of your Social Security payments. (See Social Security Administration and Account Number Cards, Chapter 8.) If you have been employed in more than one position during the calendar year (January 1 through December 31), you must make certain that you receive these statements from all your employers. If you have been self-employed, either through a registry or through your own efforts, you must keep a record of your income from the various patients you cared for. You may not receive statements from patients and other persons who employed you; the Department of Internal Revenue expects you to have correct and detailed records.

In declaring your income, include not only total regular salary but also other income such as gifts, stipends, investment returns, bank interest, bonuses, and allowances.

Here is a list of items you should keep accurate records of, since they are some of the deductions to which you are legally entitled:

Professional Expenses

Uniforms (including shoes and hose) and maintenance

Nursing Association dues, liability insurance

Books, journals, and educational expenses for advancement

Registry and licensure fees

Advertisements for employment

Convention and meeting expenses (when not reimbursed)

Telephone, if used for professional reasons

Automobile, if used for and in the care of patients (not transportation to and from work)

Equipment and supplies (thermometer, scissors, watch, and so forth)

Personal Expenses

Contributions to charities, churches, and qualified tax-exempt (nonprofit) institutions

Taxes (state purchase taxes, state income tax, and taxes on cigarettes and other items)

Interest on loans and mortgages

Medical and dental expenses

Miscellaneous

Be sure you check this list against the tax form, since these allowed deductions may vary from year to year. You are entitled to exemptions for your dependents, provided that you pay for the bulk of their support. If you are married, it is usually advantageous to file a joint return, in which the incomes are merged, and a lower tax rate applies.

Many states have a state income tax in addition to the federal income tax. This is an added responsibility and should, if possible, be deducted from salary by your employer. Conversely, a city wage tax, when one exists, is usually deducted.

SAVINGS AND INVESTMENTS

Saving is accomplished by reserving some of your present income for use sometime in the future. The greatest incentive is having a specific purpose, such as an emergency, home, wedding, or educational fund. Of the many different ways of saving money, your choice depends on *when* you will need *how much*. The sooner you start, the greater the amount will be.

Bank accounts include the checking account, the regular savings account (pays you interest), and the *certificate of deposit* (also pays interest). A *savings account* can be opened in a bank with a deposit of $1 or more, and any amount may be deposited thereafter. Withdrawals can be made at will as long as the amount withdrawn does not surpass the deposit, but this is done infrequently as the purpose here is to save. The passbook is a duplicate of your account, and records the deposits, the withdrawals, and the interest earnings on your money. Interest is credited daily, quarterly, or semiannually on the balance you have in your account at that time; therefore, it may be to your advantage to avoid making withdrawals just before an interest-crediting date. A bank note offers higher interest rates than a regular savings account. However, it has a requirement that you deposit a fixed amount for six months, or one, two, or six years with a promise that you will not withdraw money during that time. Should you withdraw your money, you would forfeit some interest. The checking account makes it possible to put money in the bank that is readily available for the payment of bills, and your canceled check when returned to you by the bank serves both as a record and as proof of payment. Some banks may have a monthly charge for the account or may charge a definite amount for each check used.

In 1962 Congress passed the Keogh Act or the Self-Employed Individuals Tax Retirement Act. Since that date the law has been amended to broaden the tax benefits; now self-employed individuals can contribute up to 15% of earned income into a special savings account. If you are not self-employed and not under a pension plan, you may open an individual retirement account (IRA), which allows you to contribute up to $1500 annually. Under these plans, you pay income tax only after you retire, at which time you would probably be in a lower tax bracket. Most banks have a pension plan counselor who would be very happy to assist you in compiling a contribution formula and also work out a tax shelter pension plan.

Miscellaneous savings methods include the purchase of United States Savings Bonds. This method is characterized by a high degree of safety. The bonds may be redeemed without charge and will always have a fixed rate of return, which is not usually the case with some other bonds and most stocks. Almost everybody needs advice before putting savings into the stock market. Perhaps the best advice that can be given on the subject of investments is to investigate before you invest and know your source of information well. Beware of get-rich-quick schemes. If in doubt, it may be better to invest in durable, tangible goods—a car or an air conditioner for the sake of your personal comfort and convenience or, better yet, a house or antique furniture, which may very well increase rather then depreciate in value.

Life Insurance

A method of saving money that will provide an income to the survivors when someone dies is known as life insurance. There are various types, and some are linked with retirement rather than death, so that payments will supplement Social Security and a pension. Among the most popular types are term, straight life, limited payment and endowment insurance.

Today, pension and retirement plans are becoming more and more popular. They provide extra income for you in addition to the Social Security benefits that you may have when you retire. Whether you are single or married has very little bearing on your need for life insurance, but is does affect the amount and the type needed. If you are responsible wholly or partially for others; if you wish to have a guaranteed retirement income; or if you do not want those "last expenses," such as funeral expenses and medical bills, to bring financial responsibilities to others, you should discuss your needs with a competent insurance agent representing a reliable agency.

Liability Insurance

In addition to health and life insurance, the average nurse should think also in terms of liability insurance. This covers the claims as well as the cost of legal counsel that may arise from negligence and damage resulting from services rendered. The constant increase in lawsuits involving alleged malpractice makes this type of insurance a necessity. With it you are covered whether the claim is false, groundless, or fraudulent. Most state LPN associations and NAPNES have this insurance available at group premium rates. These premiums are deductible for federal income taxes.

CONTINUING YOUR EDUCATION

Once you have graduated, your responsibilities to keep current in your chosen career begin. No program in practical nursing could possibly encompass all you will need to know for skilled nursing practice in the future. Additionally, some states may require a periodic review of your qualifications for practicing as an LP/VN as a condition for licensure renewal. Regardless, education for nursing practice must be continuous, to counterbalance the rapid obsolescence of practice and skills. Although inservice education is a form of continuing education, other forms include academic study, workshops, seminars, conferences, and other types of instruction available through institutions, schools, and official and voluntary organizations. The nursing organizations encourage their members to participate in various programs by offering continuing education certification.

Present-day nursing education programs are continually developing. "Transition programs" from LP/VN to an associate degree and to the baccalaureate level are being explored and tried. You may want to consider going on to become an RN, in which case the newer concept of the open curriculum in nursing education may take into account some of your past achievements.

One way that you may receive academic credit for the general knowledge that you have gained through reading and correspondence, television, and other courses is by taking the College Level Examination Program (CLEP). The examinations offered by the College Entrance Examination Board enable colleges to evaluate your personal achievements and give you credit. A wide range of college level examinations are offered and include subjects such as American history, government, literature, biology, English, psychology, human growth and development, and sociology. Each college or university determines what examination will be accepted for credit and the amount of credit to be granted.

Another way that you may receive academic credit for the nursing knowledge that you have gained from reading, clinical practice, workshops, seminars, conferences, inservice education, and other programs is through the proficiency and/or equivalency examinations offered by some schools of nursing. These examinations are teacher-constructed tests, and some include patient-care experiences to demonstrate your clinical proficiency. The amount of credit and what examinations are offered will vary with each school. Therefore, it is advisable that you contact the school(s) of your choice for further information.

SELF-PROTECTION RULES

Unfortunately, many nurses, because of their irregular working hours, the location of their employer, and their transportation needs, are victims of criminal attacks. Every nurse should take sensible precautions when traveling alone, particularly at night. The self-protection rules listed below are meant primarily for women, although everyone should exercise common sense and good judgment while traveling at night. Many courses in self-defense are now available to men and women. I strongly encourage the participation of all nurses in such courses.

1. If you must walk alone at night, avoid shortcuts through deserted parks, vacant lots, and poorly lighted streets and passageways. Stay away from building lines to avoid dark doorways, and walk near the

curb. If the sidewalk offers no safe margin, walk down the middle of the street. A friend, a working colleague, or a relative should know your planned traveling route and the time it should take to reach your destination, so that an unusual delay in your arrival can be investigated.

2. If you are being followed, run toward a lighted store or a bright intersection and yell as loud as you can. Even louder than your voice is a police whistle. Carry one in your pocket, not in a purse which may be pulled away from you.

3. If you are attacked and cannot break away, yell as loud and angrily as you can and strike back aiming at any part of the attacker's body that presents itself. If you are attacked from the front aim a blow or kick to your attacker's groin. If attacked from behind aim for the solar plexis with your elbow. There are no ethical standards for a mugging. Be prepared to use any possible weapon that presents itself, including shoes, pocketbook, pens, or umbrella. *Try not to panic.* Fear can be your worst enemy.

4. While waiting on a street corner for a trolley or bus, never accept a ride from anyone you do not know. If an auto should stop near you and the driver asks for directions, furnish the information if you wish, but do not approach the car too closely.

5. If you use your own car for transportation, look inside before you enter to see if anyone is crouching between the seats. (This should be done even though you routinely lock your car when it is parked.) Once inside the car, keep the doors locked and the windows up as high as possible. Remember that corners with stop signs and red traffic signals are the favorite hangouts for car-invading muggers. Should a suspicious-looking person approach you, use your horn to attract attention.

6. Never pick up a stranger or a hitchhiker, even one who looks like an honest person who needs transportation.

7. Keep your garage, porch, and home well lighted. Do not enter if you feel that someone has broken into your home. Leave as quietly as possible and go to the nearest telephone to call the police. If you live in an apartment building, make an effort to avoid entering an elevator with a lone man. Should one enter at another floor, stand facing the alarm bell.

8. Do not wear enticing clothing when traveling alone at night. You want to avoid attention, not attract it, and the tight, low-cut dress may provoke a criminal attack. In addition, self-defense is easier when you're wearing pants (not too tight) and shoes that will remain on your feet if it is necessary to kick or run.

9. Finally, if you display large sums of money—as in counting your salary, for instance—or talk indiscriminately about the fact that you live alone, do not be surprised if you are attacked and robbed en route or when you arrive at home! Your personal conduct and common sense may well protect you from becoming a victim.

Rape-Sexual Assault

Rape has been defined as the act of sexual intercourse committed by one person against another person without her or his consent. Rape occurs between strangers, acquaintances, and friends. Victims have ranged in age from four months to 89 years. The national frequency indicates that rape is reported every two minutes; even more frightening is the fact that 80 to 90% of all rapes go unreported. Criminologists have estimated that as many as 500,000 rapes occur each year. Four fifths of all rapes occur in the victim's own home, school, or office building. The average age of the rape victim is between 15 and 20 years and most rapists are young men between the ages of 17 and 25 years. The victims and the rapist may be of any race, ethnic group, or socioeconomic group. Contrary to common belief, the rapist is not a sex-starved individual, but rather a person who has difficulty relating to people, and to women in particular.

Police departments, women's centers, and rape crisis centers help rape victims and assist with the prosecution of rapists. Rapes are considered a crime of violence. As women have become emancipated it seems their vulnerability to street crimes and especially rape has increased. Perhaps the best advice is for every woman to become more conscious of potential danger from a rape assault. Every woman can take certain precautions until she gets to know someone. Double date with friends and never allow a man whom you have just met drive you home alone. If confronted by a rapist, try to remain calm and emotionally stable. Treat the rapist as a human being, trying to gain his confidence by using your imagination and good judgment. There is no typical rapist and there is no way of recognizing a rapist before he strikes. Become involved in groups that work to educate the public about the misconceptions of rape and those that work for treating rape victims with compassion and understanding. Help prevent rape by reporting any rape and assisting the victim and the police in every way possible. Encourage women to become involved in rape prevention programs and support the rape crisis centers.

Questions

A. Select the correct answer and circle the number that answers the question best.

1. When resigning, it is best (A) to give as much notice as possible, (B) to work at your best until leaving, (C) to state your honest reasons, (D) to discuss your dissatisfactions with your employer.
   1. All of these
   2. All except B
   3. All except C
   4. All except D

2. An LPN (A) knows all limitations, (B) stays within boundaries of the law, (C) follows employers' policies, (D) performs RN duties if no RN is available.
   1. All of these
   2. All except B
   3. All except C
   4. All except D

3. When doing private duty nursing in the home, the nurse (A) leaves unused drugs with patient, (B) leaves unused drugs with the physician, (C) is responsible to the physician, (D) is responsible to the patient.
   1. A, D
   2. A, C
   3. B, C
   4. B, D

4. In institutional nursing the LPN is directly responsible to (A) the patient, (B) the physician, (C) the RN, (D) the Director of Nursing.
   1. A
   2. B
   3. C
   4. D

5. In home private duty nursing, the nurse (A) charts as in a hospital, (B) keeps an informal chart, (C) gives chart to patient when discharged from the case, (D) gives chart to the physician.
   1. A, C
   2. A, D
   3. B, C
   4. B, D

6. As a practical nurse, you should (A) admit what you do not know, (B) assume duties you know how to do but have not been "cleared in," (C) ask for clarification on orders, (D) fulfill duties ethically.
   1. All of these
   2. All except B
   3. All except C
   4. All except D

7. Fixed expenses in a budget include (A) taxes, (B) rent, (C) insurance, (D) loan payments.
   1. All of these
   2. All except B
   3. All except C
   4. All except D

8. In evaluating a position you should consider (A) base pay, (B) vacation time, (C) transportation, (D) reputation of employer.
   1. All of these
   2. All except B
   3. All except C
   4. All except D

9. When writing a letter to a prospective employer, it is best (A) to type or to write legibly, (B) to send diplomas and State Board certificates, (C) to be brief and concise, (D) to state your qualifications.
   1. All of these
   2. All except B
   3. All except C
   4. All except D

10. You may be terminated without notice if you were (A) dishonest, (B) insubordinate, (C) disobedient, (D) malfeasant.
    1. All of these
    2. All except B
    3. All except C
    4. All except D

B. Complete the following statements.
   1. The salary for private duty nurses is suggested by the _____
   2. Private duty nurses are paid by the patient and are directly responsible to the _____
   3. The W-2 form is a statement of your earnings and _____
   4. If you are paid weekly and would like to calculate your monthly salary, you would multiply by _____
   5. Social Security payments are made by the _____ only if self-employed.
   6. Claims for legal counsel and malpractice would be covered by _____ insurance.
   7. When resigning, it is best to give _____ notice.
   8. The role of the practical nurse, as published by NFLPN, is defined in the _____

   9. The LP/VN earns approximately _____% of what the RN may earn.
   10. The hospitals that meet minimum standards are accredited by the _____

C. True or False. Write *T* or *F* in answer space.

_____ 1. Leadership skills are inherited.
_____ 2. As soon as postmortem care is performed, the private duty nurse may leave her case.
_____ 3. Only RNs may be charge nurses in extended care facilities.
_____ 4. "Transition programs" are uniform in nature.
_____ 5. Eight hundred dollars a month is equal to $200 a week.
_____ 6. An employer does not have to pay Social Security for you.
_____ 7. County medical societies can be checked for the reputation of physicians.
_____ 8. Commercial and official registries usually charge the same fees.
_____ 9. CLEP examinations are used for testing nursing skills.
_____ 10. Insubordination may be cause for immediate termination.

Answers (3⅓ points each)

A. Multiple Choice

1. 1
2. 4
3. 3
4. 3
5. 2
6. 2
7. 1
8. 1
9. 2
10. 1

C. True of False

1. F
2. F
3. F
4. F
5. F
6. F
7. T
8. F
9. F
10. T

B. Completion

1. LPN association's Registry
2. physician
3. Social Security and federal income taxes withheld
4. 4⅓
5. employee
6. liability or malpractice
7. two weeks
8. Nursing Practice Standards
9. 75%
10. Joint Commission on Accreditation of Hospitals

Appendices

A. Directory of State Boards of Nursing or Nurse Examiners
B. National Association for Practical Nurse Education and Service, Inc. Declaration of Functions
C. Self-Evaluation
D. LPN Charge Nurse—A Job Description
E. Review Test
F. Answer Section

APPENDIX A
DIRECTORY OF STATE BOARDS OF NURSING OR NURSE EXAMINERS

Alabama
State Administration Bldg.
Montgomery, AL 36104

Alaska
142 E. Third Ave.
Anchorage, AK 99501

Arizona
1645 West Jefferson St.
Phoenix, AZ 85007

Arkansas
4120 W. Markham St.
Little Rock, AR 22205

California
1020 N St.
Sacramento, CA 95814

Colorado
1525 Sherman St.
Denver, CO 80203

Connecticut
79 Elm St.
Hartford, CT 06115

Delaware
Federal and Court Sts.
Dover, DE 19901

District of Columbia
614 11 St., N.W.
Washington, DC 20001

Florida
111 E. Coastline Dr.
Jacksonville, FL 32202

Georgia
166 Pryor St., S.W.
Atlanta, GA 30303

Guam
P.O. Box 2816
Agana, GU 96910

Hawaii
P.O. Box 3469
Honolulu, HI 96801

Idaho
413 W. Idaho #203
Boise, ID 83702

Illinois
320 W. Washington
Springfield, IL 62786

Indiana
700 N. High School Rd.
Indianapolis, IN 46224

Iowa
  300 Fourth St.
  Des Moines, IA 50319
Kansas
  503 Kansas Ave.
  Topeka, KS 66601
Kentucky
  4010 Dupont Cr. #430
  Louisville, KY 40407
Louisiana
  150 Baronne St.
  New Orleans, LA 70112
Maine
  295 Water St.
  Augusta, ME 04330
Maryland
  201 W. Preston St.
  Baltimore, MD 21201
Massachusetts
  100 Cambridge St.
  Boston, MA 02202
Michigan
  905 Southerland Ave.
  Lansing, MI 48909
Minnesota
  717 Delaware St., S.W.
  Minneapolis, MN 55141
Mississippi
  135 Bounds St.
  Jackson, MS 39206
Missouri
  Box 656
  Jefferson City, MO 65101
Montana
  Wheat Bldg. (201)
  Helena, MT 59601
Nebraska
  P.O. Box 95065
  State House Station
  Lincoln, NB 68509
Nevada
  1135 Terminal Way #209
  Reno, NV 89502
New Hampshire
  105 Loudon Rd.
  Concord, NH 03301

New Jersey
  1100 Raymond Blvd.
  Newark, NJ 07102
New Mexico
  2340 Menuel, N.E.
  Albuquerque, NM 87107
New York
  Cultural Education Center #3031
  Albany, NY 12230
North Carolina
  Box 2129
  Raleigh, NC 27602
North Dakota
  418 E. Rosser
  Bismarck, ND 58505
Ohio
  65 S. Front St. #509
  Columbus, OH 43215
Oklahoma
  4001 N. Lincoln Blvd.
  Oklahoma City, OK 75105
Oregon
  1400 S.W. Fifth Ave.
  Portland, OR 97201
Pennsylvania
  279 Boas St.
  Harrisburg, PA 17120
Puerto Rico
  Box 759
  Hato Rey, PR 00919
Rhode Island
  75 Davis St. #104
  Providence, RI 02908
South Carolina
  1777 St. Julian Place
  Columbia, SC 29204
South Dakota
  304 Phillips Ave. #205
  Sioux Falls, SD 57102
Tennessee
  301 7th Ave., N.
  Nashville, TN 37219
Texas
  5555 N. Lamar Blvd.
  Austin, TX 78751

Utah
330 E. 4th St., S.
Salt Lake City, UT 84111

Vermont
10 Baldwin St.
Montpelier, VT 05602

Virginia
3600 W. Broad St.
Richmond, VA 23230

Virgin Islands
Charlotte Amalie
St. Thomas, VI 00801

Washington
Business and Professional Division
P.O. Box 9649
Olympia, WA 98504

West Virginia
922 Quarrier St.
Charleston, WV 25301

Wisconsin
1400 E. Washington Ave.
Madison, WI 53702

Wyoming
2300 Capitol Ave.
Cheyenne, WY 82002

APPENDIX B
NATIONAL ASSOCIATION FOR PRACTICAL NURSE EDUCATION AND SERVICE, INC. DECLARATION OF FUNCTIONS OF THE LICENSED PRACTICAL/VOCATIONAL NURSE

This statement was originally approved in 1969 and was revised by the Education Committee and approved by the Board of Directors in June 1976.*

PURPOSE

This statement is intended to guide administrators of nursing services to develop sound and consistent written policies for assignment of functions to the licensed practical/vocational nurse.

The LP/VN recognizes and is able to meet the basic needs of the patient. The LP/VN is taught the underlying principles of nursing care and is prepared to execute therapeutic and technical skills. The LP/VN may assist in teaching and demonstrating nursing procedures to other personnel.

DEFINITION OF THE ROLE OF THE LP/VN

An LP/VN through education and clinical experience has acquired the necessary knowledge, skill, and judgment to provide nursing care at the direction of a registered nurse, a licensed physician, or a licensed dentist. Through continuing education, the LP/VN prepares to assume progressively more complex nursing responsibilities.

FUNCTIONS

1. Participates in the planning, implementation, and evaluation of nursing care, and teaches the maintenance of health and prevention of disease.
2. Observes and reports to the appropriate person significant symptoms, reactions, and changes in the condition of the patient, and records pertinent information.

* Education Committee: *Declaration of Functions of the Licensed Practical Nurse* (New York: National Association for Practical Nurse Education and Service, Inc., 1976).

3. Performs and/or assists in nursing functions such as:
   a. the administration of medications as prescribed.
   b. therapeutic and diagnostic procedures.
   c. procedures requiring the use of medical/surgical aseptic technique.
4. Assists with the rehabilitation of the patient and family according to the patient care plan:
   a. provides support for emotional needs.
   b. teaches appropriate self-care.
   c. advocates use of community resources.
5. Assists in performing nursing services in specialized units, with appropriate preparation.
6. Assumes responsibilities as a charge nurse under direction, with appropriate preparation.

VOCATIONAL RESPONSIBILITIES
The LP/VN:
1. practices nursing according to state law.
2. performs those nursing functions for which he/she has been prepared.
3. seeks further growth through educational opportunities.
4. participates in nursing organizations.

CLOSING STATEMENT
The LP/VN should by example of dignity and grace maintain a spiritual approach to all nursing care.

APPENDIX C
SELF-EVALUATION

Perhaps one of the hardest tasks a person faces is to be honest with oneself. This unit deals with you. Are you the kind of nurse that will be an asset to nursing? Self-appraisal takes insight. It is not based on "Mirror, mirror on the wall, who is the fairest of them all?" Rather, the question to ask is, "Now that I know what my shortcomings are, what will I do to correct them and improve myself?"

Throughout this book it has been stressed that the personality of the nurse and the relationships established with patients and coworkers are of vital importance to a successful career. Try these evaluations.

1. Check the column that applies to you, and after you have done so, fold it under or cover it and then get someone else, a classmate, a friend, a supervisor, an instructor or even a member of your family, to judge you, too. This might prove to be interesting, especially if you do not know the identity of the judge.

	Never to Seldom	Usually to Always
Do you take the responsibility for your own mistakes?		
Do you "cheat" on tests, assignments, or in patient care?		
Do you know your limitations?		
Do you tell the truth, the whole truth?		
Do you make excuses frequently?		

	Never to Seldom	Usually to Always
Do you judge before you know all the facts?		
Do you feel resentful about regulations?		
Do you refrain from spreading rumors and gossip?		
Do you criticize the people you work for or with?		
Do you hold grudges?		
Do you assist others?		
Do you listen to what others have to say?		
Do you do things without having to be told?		
Would you work overtime or an extra day?		
Do you save time and effort?		
Do you know the right way, and do it that way?		
Are you economical in your use of supplies?		
Do you use equipment safely?		
Do you think of new ideas for better working methods?		
Do you make adjustments easily?		
Are you impatient?		
Can you control your emotions?		
Can you substitute supplies and equipment if necessary?		
Do you accept changes?		
Do you face your problems?		
Do you welcome criticisms?		
Do you thank people?		
Do you follow through on requests?		
Do you keep promises?		
Do you show humility and consideration?		
Do you give others credit for what they do?		
Can you laugh at yourself rather than at others?		
Do you greet people in a friendly manner?		
Do you engage in continuous shop talk?		
Do you treat people as individuals rather than as types?		
Do you express yourself clearly?		
Are you tactful?		
Do you keep things in their proper place?		
Do you keep a current inventory of supplies and report the need for replacements?		
Do you systematize your work?		
Is your handwriting legible?		
Do you clean up after yourself?		
Are you accurate in your charting?		
Do you use the proper forms and supplies?		
Do you give good nursing care regardless of patient's age, sex, color, or creed?		
Do you have a sense of humor?		

	Never to Seldom	Usually to Always
Do you derive personal satisfaction from nursing? _____	_____	_____
Do you know where to find the answers to problems in both your private and professional lives? _____	_____	_____
Are you dressed for the occasion? _____	_____	_____
Are you neat and clean? _____	_____	_____
Are you more than 10 pounds overweight? _____	_____	_____
Are the heels of your shoes run down? _____	_____	_____
Have you had annual physical examinations? _____	_____	_____
Is the six-month visit to your dentist a "must"? _____	_____	_____
Do you smoke? _____	_____	_____
Do you sleep about eight hours a day? _____	_____	_____
Have your eyes and ears been checked lately? _____	_____	_____
Do you abuse drugs and/or alcohol? _____	_____	_____

2. Evaluate your general relationships with others, and check the proper space:

	All the Time	Usually	Seldom
I am able to inspire confidence _____	_____	_____	_____
I am cooperative _____	_____	_____	_____
I am tolerant _____	_____	_____	_____
I am ethical _____	_____	_____	_____
I am respectful and courteous _____	_____	_____	_____
I am tactful _____	_____	_____	_____
I am loyal _____	_____	_____	_____
I have insight _____	_____	_____	_____
I follow directions _____	_____	_____	_____
I follow the proper channels _____	_____	_____	_____
I strive for teamwork _____	_____	_____	_____
I am responsible for my acts _____	_____	_____	_____
I understand human behavior _____	_____	_____	_____
I recognize my own feelings and can control them ___	_____	_____	_____
I appreciate individual differences _____	_____	_____	_____

3. In respect to the qualities listed above, how do you get along with the following people? Grade yourself on your work relationships by checking the proper space:

	Above	Average	Below
Patients _____	_____	_____	_____
Their family _____	_____	_____	_____
Their friends or visitors _____	_____	_____	_____
Physicians _____	_____	_____	_____

	Above	Average	Below
Registered nurses	———	———	———
Supervisors	———	———	———
Charge nurses	———	———	———
Private duty nurses	———	———	———
Licensed practical nurses	———	———	———
Student nurses	———	———	———
Nursing aides	———	———	———
Orderlies	———	———	———
Clerks/receptionists/unit managers	———	———	———
Dietary personnel	———	———	———
Housekeeping personnel	———	———	———

Now that you have completed the evaluation, write down and outline the steps that you might take to improve those traits that you should develop and to correct those that are a liability to you. (Seek assistance from those who can help you.)

Establishing Standards

In establishing standards for LPNs at a hospital, the following list was developed. Although this evaluation was intended for graduate practical nurses, those of you in the last phase or your program may find it very beneficial. Ask your instructor or supervisor to evaluate you by using *U* for usually or within average range, *A* for always or in the excellent to outstanding group, and *S* for seldom, which would indicate an unsatisfactory rating. This is a useful guide for establishing your own work objectives.

I. *Technical skills*
_____ 1. Is able to perform "LPN Skills," with minimal supervision and reteaching
_____ 2. Has been cleared to give medications
_____ 3. Does total patient care with ease
_____ 4. Checks all orders and patient's identity before carrying out assignments
_____ 5. If not cleared to give medications, is making every effort to attend a medication course for the purpose of being cleared

II. *Organizes work*
_____ 1. Gets assignment promptly
_____ 2. Sees all patients, takes inventory of patients' needs, extra procedures to be done, and so forth, and plans work for the tour
_____ 3. Completes work in good order, with units having a finished appearance
_____ 4. Reports back to charge nurse whenever necessary, and at completion of assignment
_____ 5. Is aware of factors that may interfere with the completion of the assignment, and reports them so that cooperative planning may be instituted
_____ 6. Offers patients extra services without being asked
_____ 7. Knows the importance of making an organized plan of work for the next day

III. *Use of equipment/supplies*
_____ 1. Knows and properly uses equipment to perform patient care procedures
_____ 2. Is economical and careful with equipment, supplies, and linen

_____ 3. Cares properly (cleans, stores, disposes of) equipment and supplies

_____ 4. Uses linen safely, economically (only when needed) and correctly (for instance, using washcloths only to wash patients, not to clean equipment), and disposes of same immediately after use

_____ 5. Does not hide or store equipment or linen. Makes self responsible for picking up linen and equipment hidden away, or no longer in use, and returning these to their correct place

_____ 6. Makes sure that equipment and supplies are immediately returned when no longer needed. Properly identified, so that patients will not be charged needlessly

_____ 7. Reports equipment that is in need of repair

_____ 8. Checks instructions and follows these when using unfamiliar equipment

_____ 9. Treats hospital property economically and with respect

IV. *Observes, reports, records*

_____ 1. Has a good understanding of the assignment, diagnosis, and what to watch for in patient care

_____ 2. Knows and recognizes symptoms of emergency situations and improper reactions to medications and treatments

_____ 3. Knows how to take and evaluate vital signs

_____ 4. Knows when to call for help and seeks assistance as needed

_____ 5. Reports results of treatments, changes in condition, untoward reaction to drugs, and other data when necessary, and not at the end of the tour

_____ 6. Does correct, accurate, meaningful charting without unnecessary details

_____ 7. Checks chart forms for patient's name, proper dating, page number, important information

V. *Follows instructions*

_____ 1. Gets and completes assignment

_____ 2. Checks orders for patients with the Doctor's Order Sheet, not the Kardex

_____ 3. Follows procedures and policies as written in a procedure manual

_____ 4. Carries out any additional instructions as given

_____ 5. Makes every effort, insofar as possible, to understand the reasons for instructions given. "When in doubt, find out!"

VI. *Communication skills*

_____ 1. Communicates with patient, visitors and hospital personnel by maintaining an "air of competency," creating confidence in nursing skill

_____ 2. Converses pleasantly

_____ 3. Knows how to direct conversation with patients so that they are able to communicate fear, anxiety, symptoms, or anything else that may be important in giving them care

_____ 4. Reports accurately and completely on patient's condition and nursing care to charge nurse

_____ 5. Charts accurately

VII. *Judgment*

_____ 1. Knows and recognizes untoward reactions and symptoms of treatments and medications

_____ 2. Knows when and what to report

_____ 3. Understands how to assign auxiliary personnel and volunteers, maintaining responsibility for them and for the care given to the patients

VIII. *Teaching ability*

_____ 1. Uses positive approach with patients and visitors, recognizing and using opportunities for teaching good basic hygiene—covering cough, using tissues, observing trays for good dietary regimen daily instead of just before discharge

_____ 2. Knows procedures in order to determine when others are doing them incorrectly, and can give proper direction, especially to nursing aides and orderlies

_____ 3. Is familiar with procedures to teach patients how to cough safely, how to take insulin, how to get out of bed, and so forth

IX. *Contributes to good relationships*

_____ 1. Understands that the bedside nurse is the hospital representative most frequently seen by patient and visitors, and that the public's opinion of the hospital depends on bedside care of the patient

_____ 2. Is courteous to patients, visitors, and other personnel

_____ 3. Is proud to be an LPN and understands that role

_____ 4. Respects privacy and knocks before entering a room

X. *Tact and courtesy*

_____ 1. Speaks in a well-modulated voice, using proper English

_____ 2. Takes time to answer questions, no matter how rushed

_____ 3. Keeps promises to patients, no matter how inconvenient

_____ 4. Remembers that the LPN should always be polite

_____ 5. Keeps patient information in confidence and does not gossip

XI. *Appearance and grooming*

_____ 1. Wears a neat, clean, well-fitting, pressed uniform

_____ 2. Wears shoes that are polished and not down at the heels

_____ 3. If required, wears a cap that is clean and in good condition

_____ 4. Wears all necessary emblems and name pin

_____ 5. Uses a plain white sweater for cool weather

_____ 6. Adheres to common sense in standards of cleanliness and grooming

XII. *Adaptability*

_____ 1. Handles heavy assignments without complaining, knowing they are necessary (because of illness of personnel, vacation schedules, and so forth)

_____ 2. Understands the necessity for occasional reassignment to another area or tour

_____ 3. Does day-off work or double tour when asked, understanding the necessity for this

_____ 4. Changes the assignment organization when patient's condition or needs warrant same

_____ 5. Accepts new or revised procedures, even if the reasons are not clear, and carries them out as required

XIII. *Cooperation*

_____ 1. Understands the Table of Organization and follows established protocols

_____ 2. Takes care of patients and performs duties even if they are assigned to someone else

_____ 3. Helps other individuals without being asked

_____ 4. Helps students as indicated, instead of disappearing when the students come on duty

XIV. *Punctuality*

_____ 1. Reports on duty in full uniform before tour starts

_____ 2. Signs the time sheet without being reminded

_____ 3. Is ready to take the report on time

_____ 4. Goes on breaks when assigned, if this is not possible, reports to charge nurse in sufficient time, so that proper planning can be done

_____ 5. If unable to report for work on time, telephones early enough for proper planning

_____ 6. Completes patient care and other assignments; charts and reports to team leader on time

XV. *Contributes to improvement*

_____ 1. Reports to charge nurse or supervisor ideas or suggestions for improving procedures, forms, the unit, and so forth

_____ 2. Uses equipment and supplies economically

XVI. *Attendance*

_____ 1. Makes every effort to be on duty when scheduled

_____ 2. Plans for transportation, baby sitters, and so forth, to accomplish this

_____ 3. If ill, reports this early enough to allow for proper planning

_____ 4. Communicates with nursing office if several days off are needed

XVII. *Inservice attendance*

_____ 1. Attends inservice, understanding the responsibility for continued self-improvement in the job

_____ 2. Plans ahead in order to attend inservice

_____ 3. Plans assignment to attend patient-care and other conferences

XVIII. *Follows regulations*

_____ 1. Knows the regulations taught in orientation, and follows them carefully

_____ 2. Gets answers to questions about regulations, policies, and procedures, from charge nurse, supervisor, or administration and procedure manuals

_____ 3. Knows how to report on duty following illness

_____ 4. Does not leave the unit at the completion of the tour without the team leader's permission

_____ 5. Knows all routines and regulations—treatment, medication, admission, transfer, discharge, expiration, equipment, operation and anesthesia, incident, fire, disaster, and safety

_____ 6. Reads log, bulletin, administrative and procedure manuals to be completely informed, and whenever in doubt, refers to these for clarification

XIX. *Interest in self-improvement*

_____ 1. Understands own evaluation by the supervisor, and makes plans to improve weak areas

_____ 2. Takes advantage of inservice, patient-care, and unit conferences, and courses in medications and other subjects, both professional and of general interest

_____ 3. Maintains *active* membership in alumnae organization, local division of the LPN Association, other nursing organizations, and civic and religious organizations

_____ 4. Reads the newest books in nursing and periodicals such as *The Journal of Practical Nursing* and *Journal of Nursing Care*

_____ 5. Refers to the floor library frequently

_____ 6. Participates in continuing education programs

XX. *Meets patient's needs*

_____ 1. Understands the physical, emotional, social, and spiritual needs of people, especially when they become patients (knows patients as individuals)

_____ 2. Reassures patient, when need is indicated, by manner, as well as by word and deed

——— 3. Organizes work to conform with the condition of patients or their special needs and changes plans for nursing care whenever necessary, instead of working in a routine way in order to get finished

——— 4. Knows and accepts the philosophy underlying patient care and conforms to it

——— 5. Shares the guiding principles of the hospital's nursing department and abides by them

XXI. *Sets a good example*

——— 1. Is a model of what we mean when we say, "This is a *good nurse!*"

——— 2. Is the sum total of all the factors mentioned in this evaluation

APPENDIX D
THE LPN CHARGE NURSE—
A JOB DESCRIPTION

Although the charge nurse's duties may vary from employer to employer, generally they will involve the following responsibilities.

1. Receiving reports from and giving reports to:
   a. off-going charge nurse (on-coming charge nurse)
   b. patient care personnel
   c. personnel from other departments
   d. community agencies
   e. physicians
   f. patients, families, visitors
   g. headnurse, supervisor, director of nursing

2. Making rounds to:
   a. assess condition and needs of patients
   b. evaluate patient care being given
   c. observe personnel giving care
   d. check on fire-fighting and other emergency care equipment
   e. accompany visitors, physicians, other personnel, as necessary
   f. evaluate physical condition of unit

3. Making a nursing care plan that:
   a. individualizes patient care
   b. recognizes patient's needs (long- and short-term)
   c. is accurate, concise, current, and comprehensible
   d. is used by all patient-care personnel

4. Making assignments based on:
   a. needs of patients
   b. capabilities of patient care personnel
   c. experience and potentials of personnel
   d. job satisfaction of personnel
   e. continuity of patient care
   f. learning needs of patients and personnel
   g. time necessary to complete care
   h. location of patients

     i. number of personnel available

     j. policies and regulations regarding the assignment of certain pro-cedures, special duties, and so forth to the right employee

5. Holding conferences for:

     a. assignment-making and clarification

     b. planning patient care with patient-care personnel

     c. teaching and orientation of patient-care personnel

     d. evaluation and guidance of patient-care personnel

     e. counseling patients and patient-care personnel

     f. communication with doctors, other personnel, or head nurse, as indicated or made necessary

6. Giving direct patient care to:

     a. determine patient's needs and condition

     b. demonstrate and teach correct nursing skills to patient care personnel

     c. evaluate care given

     d. communicate with patient

     e. teach patient and family

     f. act as a model for patient-care personnel

7. Using leadership skills, so that:

     a. medications, linens, supplies, and equipment are readily available

     b. patient care is coordinated with other departments

     c. patients are available for treatments, medications, laboratory tests, and so forth

     d. records and patient charts are kept according to policies

     e. regulations and employer's policies are enforced and followed

     f. job satisfaction is produced

     g. grievances reported and acted upon

     h. patient-care personnel is informed of changes and "happenings"

     i. good morale is produced

In summary, as a charge nurse, you have the full responsibility for a specific area during a given time period. Your main duty and primary objective is always the same—to provide the best possible nursing care to all patients under your supervision. You are given personnel, supplies, equipment, and supervisory help (as needed) to accomplish this goal. If for one reason or another you cannot accept your employer's patient-care philosophy and you have tried your best to advocate changes but nothing constructive has been done, feel free to leave and find another position in which job satisfaction can be yours. Being a charge nurse is not an easy task. It takes a lot of skill, judgment, personal involvement, and commitment. (See also The LPN Charge Nurse, Chapter 9.)

A Final Word

Gibran in *The Prophet* wrote: "Work is love made visible. And if you cannot work with love but only with distaste, it is better you should leave your work and sit at the gate of the Temple and take alms of those who work with *joy.*"

This important message should have meaning to you as a nurse and suggest to you that it is indeed better to leave nursing than to contribute nothing. These standards should be your goal, toward which you constantly work.

Good luck to you in your chosen career!

APPENDIX E
REVIEW TEST

This final examination may help you in testing your general knowledge of material in this book. (Highest possible score—100%.)

A. Select the correct answer and circle the number that answers the question best.

1. Licensure laws are (A) uniform throughout the United States, (B) controlled by the State Board of Education, (C) enforced by the State Board of Nursing, (D) protection for the patient.
   1. All of these
   2. All except B
   3. C, D
   4. C

2. Licensure for *practical nurses* in the United States (A) is required in all states, (B) may be mandatory or permissive in nature, (C) may have been by waiver, (D) is by examination usually, (E) may be by endorsement.
   1. All except E
   2. All except B
   3. A, D, E
   4. All of these

3. Licensure for *graduate practical nurses* is usually by (A) passing State Board, (B) reciprocity, (C) waiver, (D) 18 months of professional nurse education.
   1. A
   2. A, B
   3. All except C
   4. All of these

4. Licensure renewal is (A) uniform throughout the United States, (B) done routinely by State Boards of Nursing, (C) the responsibility of the individual nurse, (D) on the anniversary of State Board examination.
   1. C
   2. A, C
   3. All except D
   4. All except A

5. The state sets the title that the practical nurse may use in its licensing laws. Some of the titles are: (A) LPN, (B) RN, (C) PN, (D) LPA, (E) LVN.
   1. All except B
   2. All except D
   3. A, B, D
   4. A, C, E

6. Nurse Practice Acts are (A) administered by the State Board of Nursing, (B) enforced by the American Nurses Association, (C) protection for the nurse, (D) uniform throughout the United States, (E) mandatory or permissive in nature.
   1. A, C
   2. All of these
   3. A, B, D
   4. A, C, E

7. *Registered Nurses* may have graduated from the following nursing programs: (A) vocational, (B) diploma, (C) junior college, (D) correspondence, (E) university.
   1. A, B, C
   2. B, C, E
   3. All except D
   4. All of these

8. Accredited practical nurse programs are conducted in (A) junior colleges, (B) hospitals, (C) correspondence schools, (D) vocational schools.
   1. A, C, D
   2. All except C
   3. All except B
   4. All of these

9. Maslow's hierarchy of needs is grouped into five categories. Which is the proper order of importance? (A) security and
   1. B, D, A, C, E
   2. D, A, B, E, C

safety, (B) basic (physiological) survival, (C) self-esteem and respect, (D) affection, love, or belonging, (E) self-actualization.

3. A, B, C, D, E
4. B, A, D, C, E
5. D, B, A, C, E

10. Hospitals may be supported financially by (A) taxes, (B) endowments, (C) Community Chest-United Fund, (D) patient charges, (E) state grants.

1. All of these
2. B, D, E
3. A, B, C
4. All except E
5. All except D

11. Hospitals are usually classified as (A) voluntary, (B) official, (C) clinical, (D) nonprofit, (E) specific, (F) general, (G) vocational, (H) investor-owned.

1. All except C, G
2. A, B, D, F
3. All except C
4. All except G
5. All of these

12. The modern hospital has the following functions: (A) treatment and prevention of disease, (B) research, (C) rehabilitation, (D) custodial care of the aged, (E) education of personnel and patients.

1. All of these
2. A, C, D
3. All except D
4. A, C, E
5. All except E

13. Official hospitals may be supported financially through (A) taxes, (B) the United Fund, (C) the Public Health Service, (D) patient charges, (E) state and federal grants.

1. All except B
2. All except C
3. A, D, E
4. A, C, E
5. All of these

14. The Department of Health and Human Services includes the (A) Social Security Administration, (B) Food and Drug Administration, (C) World Health Organization, (D) National Health Council, (E) Welfare Council.

1. All except E
2. All except C, E
3. A, B, C
4. A, B

15. NAPNES (A) publishes *The Journal of Practical Nursing,* (B) accredits schools, (C) sponsors summer schools, (D) prepares a list of approved schools, (E) was founded in 1941.

1. All except E
2. All except C
3. All except D
4. All of these

16. NFLPN (A) prepares a list of approved schools, (B) was founded in 1949, (C) has LPN and LVN members, (D) has state and local divisions, (E) was at one time directed by Hilda Torrop.

1. All except E
2. All except B, E
3. C, D
4. B, C, D

17. The NLN (A) publishes the *American Journal of Nursing,* (B) publishes *Nursing and Health Care,* (C) is interested in registered nurse education only, (D) founded a Practical Nurse Division in 1950, (E) organized the Council of Practical Nursing programs in 1957.

1. All except D, E
2. B, C
3. B, E
4. B, D

18. In problem-oriented records, the nursing notes are written according to the following: (A) PSRO; (B) SOAP; (C) HMOS; (D) NFLPN

1. All of these
2. A, B, D
3. B
4. B and D

19. The field of vital statistics includes: (A) birth and death, (B) divorce and marriage, (C) accident and fire prevention, (D) morbidity, (E) census, (F) mental health.

   1. All of these
   2. A, B, D, E
   3. A, B, C, F
   4. A, C, E

20. In meeting the needs of the patient, the nurse must be familiar with his (A) religion, (B) illness, (C) visitors, (D) fears, (E) ambitions.

   1. B only
   2. All except C
   3. All except E
   4. All of these

21. A patient observing the kosher diet could drink milk and eat (A) steak, (B) peas, (C) potato, (D) eggs, (E) lobster, (F) cucumbers, (G) chicken, (H) halibut.

   1. C, D, F, G, H
   2. A, B, D, F
   3. B, D, F, G
   4. B, C, D, F, H

22. Progressive patient care usually includes the following units: (A) intensive care, (B) functional care, (C) intermediate care, (D) self-care, (E) group care.

   1. A, C, D
   2. A, C, E
   3. All except B
   4. All of these

23. The Drug Abuse Prevention and Control Act regulates the use of (A) pentothal sodium, (B) empirin no. 3, (C) codeine, (D) morphine sulphate, (E) alcohol, (F) meperidine, (G) cyclopropane, (H) hydromorphone hydrochloride (Dilaudid).

   1. C, D, F, G, H
   2. A, B, C, F
   3. B, D, F, G
   4. B, C, D, F, H
   5. B, D, G, H

24. Narcotics are safeguarded by (A) being counted three times a day, (B) being kept in a single-locked cabinet, (C) being kept in a double-locked cabinet, (D) recording their use on special records, (E) reporting all discrepancies, wastes, errors and breakages.

   1. All of these
   2. All except B
   3. All except C
   4. C, D, E

25. Nursing team members giving direct patient care include: (A) registered nurses, (B) practical nurses, (C) aides, (D) clerks, (E) floor managers, (F) orderlies.

   1. All except D
   2. All except E, F
   3. All except C, E
   4. All except D, E

26. Nursing care plans should take into account (A) special circumstances in the dispensing of medical care, (B) factors that affect the method of performing any nursing technique, (C) decisions about whether certain information should or should not be given to the patient's family, (D) aspects of the interpersonal relationship between patient and employee.

   1. All of these
   2. A and C
   3. A, B, C
   4. B

27. A written application for employment should include: (A) salary you desire, (B) date you are available, (C) preference of tour and type of nursing, (D) friends as references, (E) relatives as references.

   1. All of these
   2. All except D
   3. All except E
   4. A, B, C

28. When resigning it is best to (A) give two weeks notice or longer, (B) discuss your dissatisfactions with your employer, (C) state your regret for leaving, (D) work at your best until you leave, (E) give your honest reasons for leaving.

   1. All of these
   2. All except A
   3. All except B
   4. All except C

29. In selecting a position you should (A) evaluate working conditions, (B) know the reputation of employer, (C) know the job responsibilities, (D) accept the highest paying one, (E) consider transportation, vacation and holidays, sick time allowance, and so on as part of your total salary.

    1. All of these
    2. All except B
    3. All except D
    4. All except E

30. An LPN always (A) stays within boundaries of the law, (B) performs RN duties if no RN is available, (C) performs all that has been taught, (D) follows orders exactly, (E) refuses to do something not qualified to do.

    1. All of these
    2. All except B
    3. All except E
    4. A, E

31. A derogatory remark may be considered (A) defamation, (B) negligence, (C) slander, (D) "malice aforethought," (E) libel.

    1. A, C
    2. A, E
    3. A, C, E
    4. A, C

32. Malpractice suits may result from: (A) patient being burned from hot-water bottles, (B) patient falling out of bed when side rail was left down, (C) giving wrong medication, (D) using an oral thermometer on an unconscious patient, (E) improper use of patient's personal belongings.

    1. All of these
    2. All except D
    3. All except E
    4. C only

33. A nurse may refuse to carry out a physician's order if (A) the nurse has not been taught or supervised in this procedure, (B) the patient requests this, (C) the order goes against the nurse's judgment or common sense, (D) the handwriting is unreadable, (E) the order is incomplete.

    1. All of these
    2. All except B
    3. All except C
    4. D, E

34. The Department of Health and Human Resources (A) is supported through taxation, (B) is administered by the United Nations, (C) includes the Public Health Service, (D) has Civil Service employees, (E) has regional offices.

    1. All of these
    2. All except A
    3. All except B
    4. All except C

35. The Public Health Service (A) provides medical and hospital care for American Indians, (B) has research programs, (C) establishes quarantine laws, (D) supervises immigrants' medical and psychiatric examinations, (E) constructs health and medical facilities.

    1. All of these
    2. All except A
    3. D only
    4. C, D

36. Easter seals are used to raise funds for the (A) Red Cross, (B) Crippled Children's Association, (C) Cancer Society, (D) Lung Association.

    1. A
    2. B
    3. C
    4. D

37. The majority of practical nurse education programs are conducted in (A) hospitals, (B) junior or community colleges, (C) vocational technical schools, (D) community agencies.

    1. A
    2. B
    3. C
    4. D

38. Research to eliminate the leading cause of death in the United States would be conducted by the (A) Lung Association, (B) Cancer Society, (C) Heart Association, (D) Mental Health Association.

    1. A
    2. B
    3. C
    4. D

39. The organization that coordinates the efforts of voluntary and

    1. A

official agencies is the (A) National Foundation, (B) Public   2. B
Health Service, (C) State Health Department, (D) Health   3. C
Systems Agency.   4. D

40. Morbidity rate in the field of vital statistics applies to (A)   1. A
deaths, (B) stillborns, (C) disease, (D) epidemiology.   2. B
    3. C
    4. D

B. True or False. Write *T* or *F* in the answer space.
_____ 1. You may practice as an LPN during the time your license has lapsed.
_____ 2. LVN and LPN are legally the same.
_____ 3. A graduate practical nurse is always an LPN.
_____ 4. The nurse's act of negligence may result in a liability suit.
_____ 5. Nurses may permit their names to be used in advertisements.
_____ 6. All State Boards of Nursing have uniform licensure laws.
_____ 7. There are more graduate licensed practical nurses than waiver practical nurses.
_____ 8. Communication involves the five senses.
_____ 9. The WHO is supported through the United Fund.
_____ 10. The American Cancer Society is supported through Easter seals.
_____ 11. All RNs have black bands on their school caps.
_____ 12. The "Patient's Bill of Rights" was published by the ANA.
_____ 13. The Eskimos are considered to be a racial group.
_____ 14. A Catholic must abstain from food for three hours and from liquids for two hours to receive baptism.
_____ 15. Voluntary agencies are usually tax-supported.
_____ 16. Clara Barton founded the Red Cross.
_____ 17. Associate degree programs are four years in duration.
_____ 18. Florence Nightingale wrote *Notes on Nursing*.
_____ 19. During the Dark Ages (400–1000) several great hospitals were founded.
_____ 20. Medicare is part of social security.
_____ 21. When a nurse is negligent, only the hospital is sued, since the hospital takes full legal responsibility for the nurses employed.
_____ 22. The suit-prone patient will not generally sue for malpractice unless there has existed a poor nurse/patient relationship prior to the act of malpractice.
_____ 23. There are more hospital than vocational schools of practical nursing.
_____ 24. A nurse may walk "off duty" if assignment is not appropriate.
_____ 25. Schools of nursing should be accredited by the Joint Commission on Accreditation.
_____ 26. Annie Goodrich founded the National League for Nursing.
_____ 27. Functional nursing is the best method for giving patient care.
_____ 28. In California, practical nurses are called vocational nurses.
_____ 29. You need not visit the dentist regularly if you have dentures.
_____ 30. Only Catholic nurses may baptize Catholics.

C. Complete the following statements.
    1. The killing of a human by another is called _____
    2. The Drug Abuse Prevention and Control Act controls the use of narcotics and _____ (state other classification of drugs).
    3. The "Statement of Functions and Qualifications of the Licensed Practical Nurse"

was approved by the National Federation of Licensed Practical Nurses, Inc., and
updated in _____

4. Lillian Wald founded the _____
5. Interstate licensure is usually done by _____
6. Oral defamation is called _____
7. Unwarranted restriction of the freedom of another is called _____
8. A threat or an attempt to contact the body of another person without consent is

_____

9. Diploma programs are usually _____ years in duration.
10. Associate degree programs are usually _____ years in length.
11. The Jewish New Year is called _____
12. Flammable liquids (gasoline, paint, oil, and so forth) are classified as type _____
13. Blood transfusions are objected to and refused by _____
14. Seventh-Day Adventists usually will not eat _____
15. When resigning, at least _____ weeks' notice should be given.
16. The Day of Atonement is known also as _____
17. LPN and _____ are legally the same.
18. Hospitals are accredited by the _____
19. The legal title for licensed registered nurse is _____
20. In 1893 the first PN school was founded. It was known as the _____
21. The "Father of Medicine" was _____
22. Clara Barton founded the _____
23. The Supreme Head of the Roman Catholic Church is called _____
24. Official agencies are supported through _____
25. The *National Formulary* is approved by the _____
26. Medicare programs are administered by the _____
27. Vaccines are tested and spot checked by the _____
28. Florence Nightingale died in (year) _____
29. Hilda Torrop was a founder of the _____
30. The competencies of graduates of educational programs in practical nursing was
published by _____

APPENDIX F
ANSWERS, REVIEW TEST
(1 POINT EACH)

A. Multiple Choice

1. 3	11. 1	21. 4	31. 1
2. 1	12. 3	22. 1	32. 1
3. 1	13. 1 or 5	23. 4	33. 1
4. 1	14. 4	24. 2	34. 3
5. 4	15. 4	25. 4	35. 1
6. 4	16. 4	26. 1	36. 2
7. 2	17. 3	27. 4	37. 3
8. 2	18. 3	28. 1	38. 3
9. 4	19. 2	29. 3	39. 4
10. 1	20. 4	30. 4	40. 3

B. True or False

1. F	11. F	21. F
2. T	12. F	22. T
3. F	13. F	23. F
4. T	14. F	24. F
5. F	15. F	25. F
6. F	16. T	26. F
7. F	17. F	27. F
8. T	18. T	28. T
9. F	19. T	29. F
10. F	20. T	30. F

C. Completion
1. homicide, manslaughter, murder
2. barbiturates
3. 1970
4. Henry Street Settlement House
5. endorsement
6. slander
7. false imprisonment
8. assault
9. two to three
10. two
11. Rosh Hashanah
12. B fire
13. Jehovah's Witnesses
14. pork (and some other meats)
15. two
16. Yom Kippur
17. LVN (Licensed Vocational Nurse)
18. Joint Commission on Accreditation of Hospitals
19. Registered Nurse (RN)
20. Ballard School
21. Hippocrates
22. American Red Cross
23. Pope
24. taxes
25. Food and Drug Administration
26. Social Security Administration (SSA)
27. Food and Drug Administration
28. 1910
29. NAPNES
30. National League for Nursing, Division of Practical Nursing Programs.

Index